AF556773

Intracranial Atherosclerosis: Pathophysiology, Diagnosis and Treatment

Frontiers of Neurology and Neuroscience

Vol. 40

Series Editor

J. Bogousslavsky Montreux

Intracranial Atherosclerosis: Pathophysiology, Diagnosis and Treatment

Volume Editors

Jong S. Kim Seoul
Louis R. Caplan Boston, Mass.
Ka Sing Wong Hong Kong

60 figures, 3 in color, and 9 tables, 2016

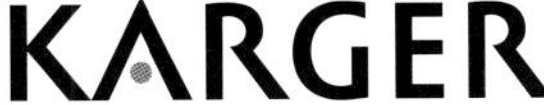

Basel · Freiburg · Paris · London · New York · Chennai · New Delhi · Bangkok · Beijing · Shanghai · Tokyo · Kuala Lumpur · Singapore · Sydney

Frontiers of Neurology and Neuroscience
Vols. 1–18 were published as Monographs in Clinical Neuroscience

Jong Sung Kim
Department of Neurology
Asan Medical Center, University of Ulsan
138-600 Seoul (South Korea)

Louis R. Caplan
Department of Neurology
Beth Israel Deaconess Medical Center
Boston, MA 02115 (USA)

Ka Sing Wong
Division of Neurology
Department of Medicine and Therapeutics
Chinese University of Hong Kong
Prince of Wales Hospital
Shatin, New Territory, HKSAR (China)

Library of Congress Cataloging-in-Publication Data

Names: Wong, Ka Sing, editor. | Kim, Jong S., editor. | Caplan, Louis R., editor.
Title: Intracranial atherosclerosis : pathophysiology, diagnosis, and treatment / volume editors, Jong S. Kim, Louis R. Caplan, Ka Sing Wong.
Other titles: Intracranial atherosclerosis (2016) | Frontiers of neurology and neuroscience ; v. 40. 1660-4431
Description: Basel ; New York : Karger, 2016. | Series: Frontiers of neurology and neuroscience, ISSN 1660-4431 ; vol. 40 | Includes bibliographical references and indexes.
Identifiers: LCCN 2016037224| ISBN 9783318027587 (hard cover : alk. paper) | ISBN 9783318027594 (e-ISBN)
Subjects: | MESH: Intracranial Arteriosclerosis--physiopathology | Intracranial Arteriosclerosis--diagnosis | Intracranial Arteriosclerosis--therapy
Classification: LCC RC388.5 | NLM WL 355 | DDC 616.8/1--dc23 LC record available at
https://lccn.loc.gov/2016037224

Bibliographic Indices. This publication is listed in bibliographic services, including Current Contents® and Index Medicus.

Drug Dosage. The authors and the publisher have exerted every effort to ensure that drug selection and dosage set forth in this text are in accord with current recommendations and practice at the time of publication. However, in view of ongoing research, changes in government regulations, and the constant flow of information relating to drug therapy and drug reactions, the reader is urged to check the package insert for each drug for any change in indications and dosage and for added warnings and precautions. This is particularly important when the recommended agent is a new and/or infrequently employed drug.

www.karger.com
Printed on acid-free and non-aging paper (ISO 9706)
ISSN 1660–4431
e-ISSN 1662–2804
ISBN 978–3–318–02758–7
e-ISBN 978–3–318–02759–4

Contents

Preface

Intracranial atherosclerosis is a leading cause of stroke in Asians and Africans. Considering that these ethnic groups account for more than 70% of the world's population, it could be said that intracranial atherosclerosis is the major cause of ischemic stroke worldwide. Nevertheless, as compared with extracranial atherosclerosis, intracranial atherosclerosis has been largely neglected in the literature. Nowadays, partly due to the development of imaging technologies, such as magnetic resonance, computed tomography angiography and Transcranial Doppler, that can easily assess the intracranial arterial diseases and partly because of the active research happening in Asia, the importance of intracranial atherosclerosis is being more appreciated. Moreover, recent development of technologies pertaining to stenting/angioplasty has sparkled both interest and controversy.

The aim of this book is to provide our readers with up-to-date knowledge of intracranial atherosclerosis, ranging from vascular anatomy, pathology, epidemiology, stroke mechanisms and syndromes and diagnostic methods to treatment strategies, including antithrombotics, angioplasty/stenting and surgical operations. In addition, nonatherosclerotic intracranial arterial diseases such as Moyamoya disease, dissection, vasculitis and other miscellaneous disorders are extensively discussed.

The chapters are written by experts from various parts of the world, both East and West. We believe that readers will find interesting results from cutting edge research, such as the application of high-resolution magnetic resonance imaging or the development of interventional procedures. In controversial areas, such as angioplasty/stenting, readers will be exposed to different yet balanced points of view, so that they may form an unbiased opinion on these issues. Finally, readers will also notice that despite extensive research, vague areas, yet to be investigated, still remain, such as the answers to the following questions: Why are there East–West differences in the location of atherosclerosis? What is the best medical therapy? What are the factors that best predict outcome of the patients? Who are the patients who may benefit from angioplasty/stenting or bypass surgery? Thus, we hope that this book is informative, interesting and stimulating for readers, and serves as a useful guide in their clinical and research activities.

Finally, we sincerely thank all the contributors, who dedicated their valuable time to write excellent manuscripts, and also Karger for allowing us to formulate a vehicle to communicate with our readers.

Jong S. Kim, Seoul, Korea

Kim JS, Caplan LR, Wong KS (eds): Intracranial Atherosclerosis: Pathophysiology, Diagnosis and Treatment.
Front Neurol Neurosci. Basel, Karger, 2016, vol 40, pp 1–20 (DOI: 10.1159/000448264)

Intracranial Arteries – Anatomy and Collaterals

David S. Liebeskind[a] · Louis R. Caplan[b]

[a]UCLA Stroke Center University of California, Los Angeles, Calif., and [b]Department of Neurology, Beth Israel Deaconess Medical Center, Harvard Medical School, Boston, Mass., USA

Abstract

Anatomy, physiology, and pathophysiology are inextricably linked in patients with intracranial atherosclerosis. Knowledge of abnormal or pathological conditions such as intracranial atherosclerosis stems from detailed recognition of the normal pattern of vascular anatomy. The vascular anatomy of the intracranial arteries, both at the level of the vessel wall and as a larger structure or conduit, is a reflection of physiology over time, from *in utero* stages through adult life. The unique characteristics of arteries at the base of the brain may help our understanding of atherosclerotic lesions that tend to afflict specific arterial segments. Although much of the knowledge regarding intracranial arteries originates from pathology and angiography series over several centuries, evolving non-invasive techniques have rapidly expanded our perspective. As each imaging modality provides a depiction that combines anatomy and flow physiology, it is important to interpret each image with a solid understanding of typical arterial anatomy and corresponding collateral routes. Compensatory collateral perfusion and downstream flow status have recently emerged as pivotal variables in the clinical management of patients with atherosclerosis. Ongoing studies that illustrate the anatomy and pathophysiology of these proximal arterial segments across modalities will help refine our knowledge of the interplay between vascular anatomy and cerebral blood flow. Future studies may help elucidate pivotal arterial factors far beyond the degree of stenosis, examining downstream influences on cerebral perfusion, artery-to-artery thromboembolic potential, amenability to endovascular therapies and stent conformation, and the propensity for restenosis due to biophysical factors.

Introduction

Comprehensive knowledge of intracranial arterial anatomy and their corresponding collateral circulation forms the basis for consideration of intracranial atherosclerosis. Anatomy defines the location of such neurovascular lesions, delineates the extent and involvement of branching perforators [1], and consequently determines the effects on downstream perfusion that be balanced by corresponding collaterals. Anatomy is intimately intertwined with pathophysiology, as vessel morphology influences hemodynamic variables that promote plaque growth and vessel wall constituents predispose to atherosclerotic involvement. Once an atherosclerotic plaque has formed, the arterial territories within the brain shift, reflecting diminished perfusion beyond a stenosis and compensatory collateral flow via anastomoses from adjacent arterial sources [2–4]. The anatomical features of these arteries or pipes and their perforators determine perfusion, penumbra and the parenchymal consequences of brain ischemia. These intracranial vessels differ in anatomy from other circulatory beds in the heart or periphery, with only limited correlates noted in comparative anatomy of intracranial arteries across species. Arterial anatomy adds to the complexity of neurological localization, providing a unique classification of neurovascular disorders. Consideration of intracranial arterial anatomy is most germane to clinical management; recognition of particular stroke syndromes influences treatment decisions. Identification of a culprit atherosclerotic lesion also hinges on anatomical details of the case and consideration of collateral perfusion.

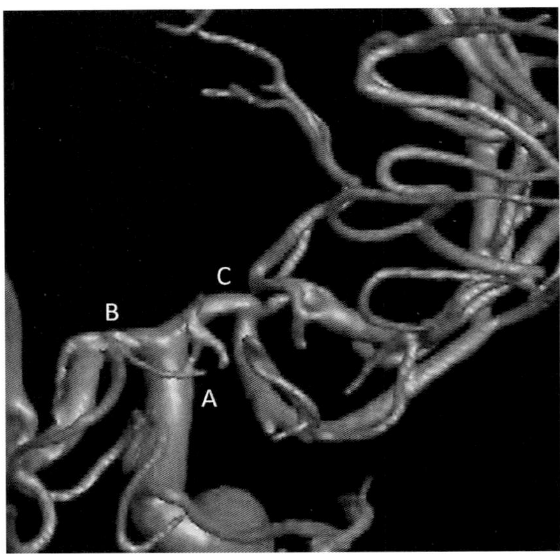

Fig. 1. Three-dimensional rotational angiography illustrating the proximal segments of the anterior circulation, including bifurcation of the ICA (**A**) into the ACA (**B**) and MCA (**C**).

The historical perspective on characterizing anatomy of the intracranial arteries includes an ironic twist where only marginal advances regarding pathology of these arterial segments have been made since autopsy series performed hundreds of years ago. Angiography reigns as the definitive modality for defining these structures almost a century after its introduction. Pathology related to atherosclerotic involvement of the major intracranial arteries has largely eluded modern imaging techniques due to the small size of these vessels and the orientation of these segments that defy conventional imaging planes. Numerous noninvasive methods have been developed to image intracranial arterial anatomy [5, 6], yet these modern vascular imaging techniques including transcranial Doppler ultrasound (TCD), computed tomographic angiography (CTA), high-resolution MRI (HR-MRI) and magnetic resonance angiography (MRA) do not reliably reflect the reference standard of conventional or digital subtraction angiography (DSA) [7, 8]. Recently, the advent of angioplasty and stenting for intracranial atherosclerotic disease has reinforced the importance of DSA, as arterial access is needed for such interventional strategies [9]. Noninvasive imaging modalities including TCD, CTA, and MRA each provide differing information regarding a balance of anatomical information such as measures of the arterial lumen versus physiological data reflecting flow through a specific arterial segment and distal perfusion. HR-MRI delineates the architecture of vessel wall derangements in isolation from luminal details and impact on cerebral blood flow. DSA remains the prevailing method for evaluating vascular anatomy and collaterals in the brain, although modifications such as three-dimensional rotational angiography (fig. 1) have allowed for expansion across numerous frames of reference.

This introductory chapter considers vascular anatomy of the major intracranial arterial segments supplying blood flow to the brain, emphasizing proximal segments where atherosclerotic lesions or stenoses are often noted and the sources of collateral perfusion that offsets ischemia. The extracranial segments of these vessels are not discussed and only marginal attention has been devoted to distal branches beyond the primary or secondary intracranial arterial divisions. For each artery, the discussion reviews embryologic development, basic morphology such as orientation and luminal dimensions, functional aspects such as perforators, territories, or collateral anastomoses, and common variants encountered in standard anatomy [10].

Embryology

The arteries of the central nervous system originate from mesenchymal elements that coalesce to form channels that cover the surface of the neural tube [11]. Over time, certain channels persist and enlarge to become principal conduits whereas others involute. A single ventral median artery forms with paired or symmetrical branches that spread out in a circumferential pattern over the surface. A segmental pattern of blood flow predominates from the 4 to 12 mm human embryo stage, arising from the branchial arches. Intracranial blood flow at this stage is distributed by the primitive trigeminal, otic or acoustic, and hypoglossal arteries. Early arterial blood flow is centripetal, extending from the periphery to center. Beyond the 12 mm stage, longitudinal connections develop, including the vertebral arteries that form with involution of the cervical intersegmental arteries. The embryologic development of the circle of Willis is also important to consider when these segments are recruited to later shunt blood flow due to stenosis or occlusions in the anterior or posterior circulations. Previously hypoplastic segments may be recruited and progressively enlarge over time, whereas others involute due to disuse. The specific events that characterize the embryologic development of particular intracranial arteries are detailed in the discussion below.

Arterial Wall

The majority of anatomical descriptions consider the cerebral vasculature as a mere conduit to supply and return blood through the brain, yet these vascular channels play an active role in the regulation of brain blood flow. The proximal segments of the intracranial arteries distribute flow to specific areas of the brain to match metabolic demand during development and thereafter. Cerebral perfusion depends on intraluminal pressure and downstream resistance. Because arterial blood pressure is so readily measured and commonly used as a principal vital sign, the presumption is that cerebral blood flow is principally mediated by blood pressure. Most of the pressure head or arterial pressure gradient is lost before blood flow reaches terminal branches feeding the cortical surface and deep regions of the brain. These proximal arterial circuits and their vessel wall constituents, in addition to other biophysical factors and metabolic orchestration within the intracranial compartment, directly modulate resistance. Unlike the peripheral vasculature, where precapillary sphincters mediate pressure gradients, the cerebral circulation lacks such structures and pressure gradients are modified in the arteries and arterioles of the brain. Flow is also readily shunted or equilibrated via unique anastomotic structures such as the circle of Willis. These features underscore the importance of recognizing the unique role of the proximal arterial circulation in the brain, not just as pipes for flow distribution, but as active physiological elements in metabolic homeostasis. Recent development of MRI sequences can now measure elasticity of vessel segments [12]. The structural characteristics in the vessel wall that enable such functional capacity are an important anatomical aspect to consider.

Several features distinguish intracranial arteries from arteries of similar caliber elsewhere in the body. Arteries in the brain have a well-developed internal elastic lamina with only a minimal degree of elastic fibers scattered in the media [13]. Unlike arteries elsewhere throughout the body, the intracranial arteries do not have an external elastic lamina. Other distinctive features of the intracranial arteries include the presence of tight endothelial junctions with a relative paucity of pinocytic vesicles, and differing distribution of enzymes within the vessel wall. The adventitial layer is typically thin compared to systemic arteries. In general, the cerebral arteries have a smaller wall-to-lumen ratio than arteries elsewhere in the body [14]. Overall, the intimal layer accounts for about 17% of total vessel wall thickness, with the media comprising 52% and adventitia only 31% [15, 16].

The arterial lumen is defined by the adjacent architecture of the vessel wall. Cerebral endothelial cells with tight junctions form a critical element of the blood-brain barrier [17]. These endothelial cells are not fenestrated and the tight junctions bestow only selective permeability to this boundary, preventing exchange of numerous substances. This boundary is often referred to as the 'blood-brain barrier'. Under pathophysiologic conditions, this selective permeability boundary is deranged [18]. The number of endocytotic vesicles is also limited compared to the endothelial lining of other vascular beds. Cerebral endothelial cells have a high concentration of mitochondria, denoting their active metabolic role and possibly, their vulnerability to ischemia [19]. Endothelial cells in cerebral arteries and arterioles play an active role in regulation of hemodynamics. This capacity is partially related to the expression of a wide array of vasoactive substances, including endothelin and nitric oxide [20]. The internal elastic lamina of intracranial arteries is fenestrated, with holes that vary in size according to the arterial segment [21]. Beyond the endothelial layer, the cerebral arteries have protuberances at distal branching sites that also modulate flow. These structures have been variably defined as intimal cushions, bifurcation pads or subendothelial protuberances. Underneath the luminal surface, these structures contain groups of smooth muscle cells arranged in irregular fashion, with intertwined collagenous fibrils and are encompassed by the split internal elastic membrane [22]. Although the exact role of these structures in titration of arterial pressure has not been fully elucidated, it appears that these structures help alter flow via fluid shear stress mechanisms. Fluid shear stress is a critical physiological variable both in the development of atherosclerosis and in compensatory arteriogenesis [23–26]. A circumferential orientation of the smooth muscle cells at branching sites is be related to titration of arterial inflow resistance by acting via a sphincter-like mechanism.

In normal intracranial arteries, smooth muscle cells compose 72% of the media whereas this composition is radically altered under pathophysiologic conditions such as intracranial atherosclerosis or chronic hypertension [13]. Age-related changes are found in the composition of the media. Autonomic nerves located in the tunica adventitia have connections with these subendothelial structures via intercellular smooth muscle cell contacts. Within the media, smooth muscle cells are oriented in a pattern circumferential to the lumen except at bifurcations [15]. Adjacent collagen and elastin fibers run perpendicular to the smooth muscle layer or in parallel with the long axis of the vessel. The thin medial layer of intracranial arteries compared to systemic vessels is related to compliance differences associated with surrounding cerebrospinal fluid. The number of smooth muscle cell layers within the media diminishes distally. A basement membrane associated with the adjacent smooth muscle cells forms the framework for adjoining layers of the intima and adventitia. Nerve fibers approach the media from the adventitial layer. Within the adventitia, loose connective tissue surrounds autonomic nerve fibers. All vessel wall structures are enclosed by spindle-shaped fibrocytes. Once beyond the dura mater, the intracranial arteries have no vasa vasorum. The external surface of the intracranial arteries in these regions is in direct contact with surrounding cerebrospinal fluid. A rete vasorum in the adventitia is permeable to large proteins, allowing ingress or exchange with cerebrospinal fluid in the subarachnoid space [27].

Characteristics of the intracranial arterial wall in humans typically consider the proximal intracranial arteries such as the middle cerebral artery (MCA) separately from much smaller intracerebral or pial arterioles. As the ICA courses distally, there is progressive disappearance of the external elastic lamina. The MCA is a terminal continuation of the ICA with a gradual change in blood vessel wall characteristics and histopathology. The relative amounts of intima, media and adventitia in the MCA are less than the equivalent amount per vessel size in the more proximal ICA. The MCA internal elastic lamina is thicker and partially fenestrated. Compared with similar sized extracranial arteries, the MCAs have less adventitia with less elastic tissue and few perivascular supporting structures, including an absence of vasa vasorum [28].

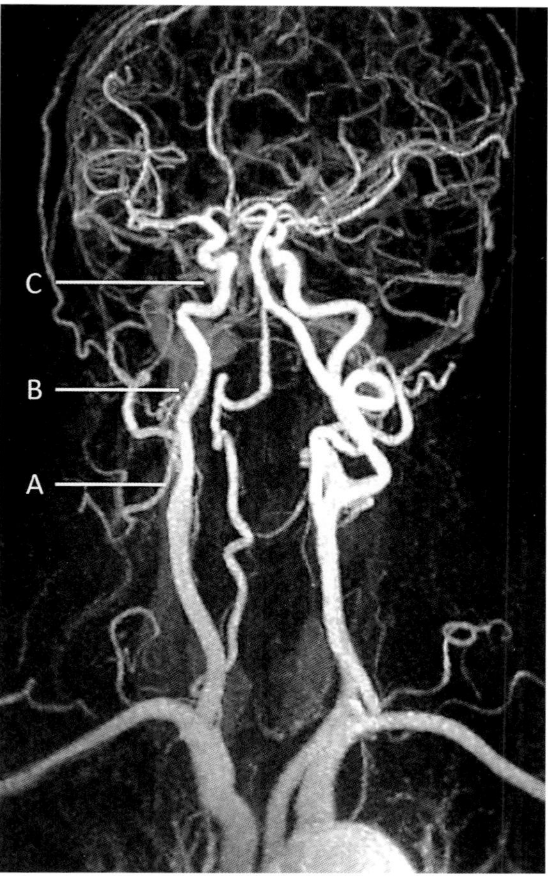

Fig. 2. Gadolinium-enhanced MRA depicting the course of the right ICA, from its extracranial origin at the carotid bifurcation (**A**), through the carotid canal at the skull base (**B**), to become the intracranial ICA (**C**).

Internal Carotid Artery

Each ICA supplies approximately 40% of total perfusion to the brain. The internal carotid artery (ICA) develops from the third primitive aortic arch. The distal cervical segment of the ICA arises from the junction of the distal aspect of this third primitive aortic arch with the dorsal aorta. The ICA arises from the common carotid artery in the neck, extending into the head at the skull base via the carotid canal (fig. 2). There are three named segments of the intracranial ICA, including petrous, cavernous, and supraclinoid segments (fig. 3). The petrous ICA extends for about 25–35 mm anteromedially from the skull base to the cavernous sinus [29]. The shape of the petrous ICA varies depending on the development of the surrounding bony structures skull. Along this course, it bends anterior to the tympanic cavity near the apex of the petrous bone and traverses the posterior aspect of the foramen lacerum. The ICA crosses the membranes of the cavernous sinus, winding anteriorly and superomedially, then ascending vertically in a groove along the sphenoid bone and then passing along the medial aspect of the anterior clinoid process [30]. On exiting the cavernous sinus, the ICA extends through the meninges to become the supraclinoid segment. The cavernous ICA typically averages 39 mm in length. The supraclinoid or cerebral

ICA bends posteriorly and laterally between the oculomotor (III) and optic (II) nerves. Because of this sinuous course of the ICA, the cavernous and supraclinoid segments are often collectively referred to as the carotid siphon. Beyond the supraclinoid segment, the ICA terminates at the bifurcation into the anterior (ACA) and MCA. This bifurcation is often referred to as the 'carotid T' because of its shape or the 'top-of-the carotid' because of its location.

Along the course of the intracranial ICA, branching progressively increases with more distal locations [31]. The petrous segment gives rise to the caroticotympanic artery, supplying the tympanic cavity, and the pterygoid or vidian branch passing through the pterygoid canal [29]. This vidian artery anastomoses with the internal maxillary artery. On occasion, the persistent stapedial branch of the petrous segment traverses a bony canal and continues as the middle meningeal artery [29]. The cavernous portion, however, has far more tributaries including the meningohypophyseal trunk, the anterior meningeal artery, the artery to the inferior portion of the cavernous sinus and the ophthalmic artery. The meningohypophyseal trunk further subdivides into diminutive branches that include the basal and marginal (artery of Bernasconi and Cassinari [32]) tentorial arteries, the inferior hypophyseal artery, and the dorsal meningeal artery. The inferolateral trunk arises from the inferolateral aspect of the cavernous ICA, supplying many small branches to the tentorium and trigeminal (V) nerve divisions. Collateral anastomoses between the ICA and ECA are formed by the inferolateral trunk extending to the internal maxillary artery. The supraclinoid ICA also has numerous branches including the superior hypophyseal perforators to the anterior pituitary and stalk, posterior communicating artery (PCoA), and anterior choroidal artery (AChA) before bifurcating into the ACA and MCA [33].

The two ACAs connect through the anterior communicating artery (ACoA) thus joining the left and right carotid circulations. The PCoA extends posteriorly to connect with the primary segment of the posterior cerebral artery, allowing collateral flow to pass between the anterior and posterior circulations [4, 34]. This vascular network, referred to as the circle of Willis (fig. 4),

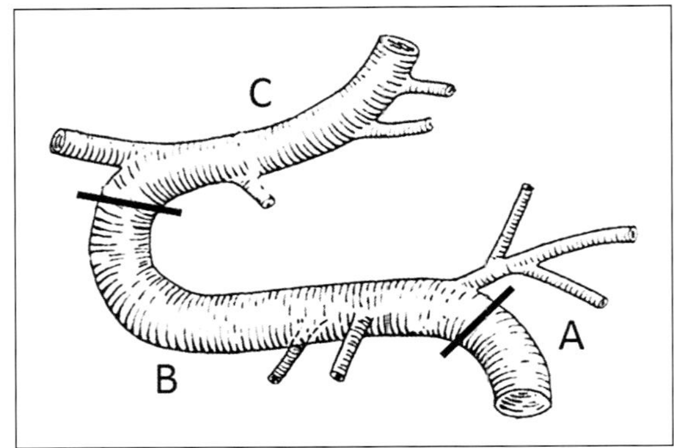

Fig. 3. Line drawing of the intracranial ICA, depicting the petrous (**A**), cavernous (**B**), and supraclinoid (**C**) segments.

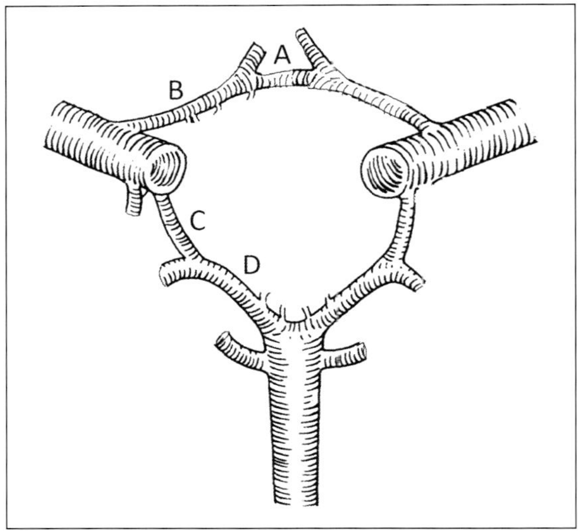

Fig. 4. Line drawing of anastomotic connections at the circle of Willis, including the ACoA (**A**), the proximal or A1 segment of the ACA (**B**), the PCoA (**C**), and the proximal or P1 segment of the PCA (**D**).

plays a critical role in shunting blood flow between adjacent territories in the brain. At its origin, the PCoA often has a widened segment referred to as the infundibulum. The PCoA passes ventral to the optic tract, with perforators that supply the optic tract, posterior aspect of the chiasm, posterior hypothalamus, and anterior and ventral nuclei of the thalamus. In 15% of individuals, this vessel continues distally as the posterior cerebral artery [35, 36]. Great variability is noted in the caliber of PCoA, ranging from less than 1 mm to greater than 2 mm. The anatomy of the PCoA differs in various populations and in clinical conditions associated with ischemia [36, 37]. Hypoplasia or absence of the PCoA is found in a minority of cases at autopsy, with bilateral hypoplasia in only 0.25% of individuals [35]. The configuration and size of the PCoA also differs between rates gleaned from autopsy studies and angiography series.

There are numerous variant configurations of the ICA, including its rare absence or hypoplasia. The amount of blood volume supplied to distal structures can vary depending on the caliber of the terminal ICA. The course of the ICA sometimes varies, coursing through the middle ear or bending towards the midline in a configuration termed 'kissing ICAs' at the cavernous segments. Anomalous origins of the posterior fossa arteries from the ICA, including the SCA, AICA, or PICA, may also occur. Persistent fetal connections to the posterior circulation involve the PCoA, trigeminal, otic or acoustic, hypoglossal, and proatlantal intersegmental arteries [38]. The persistent trigeminal artery is the most common persistent embryonic connection (85%), arising from the cavernous ICA and joining the upper basilar artery [39]. The persistent otic artery is very rare, connecting the petrous ICA with the basilar artery inferior to AICA. The persistent hypoglossal connects the distal cervical ICA with the distal vertebral artery. Intercavernous ICA collaterals also allows for blood to flow laterally to either hemisphere.

Anterior Choroidal Artery

The AChA arises from the posterior aspect of the ICA, about 2–4 mm distal to the origin of the PCoA and about 5 mm proximal to the carotid terminus [40]. The AChA is relatively small, yet serves as an important landmark in delineating important structures at angiography [41]. There are two segments of the AChA, including the cisternal and plexal segments. The AChA may have a single origin or consist of several smaller vessels (4% of individuals) [40, 42]. The AChA arises from the MCA or PCoA in 2–11% of individuals [42]. Complete absence of the AChA has also been reported [41]. The external diameter of this vessel is often only 0.5–1 mm, although a reciprocal relationship has been noted in the caliber of this vessel with the ipsilateral PCoA. The cisternal segment passes posteriorly from the lateral to medial aspect of the optic tract in close proximity to the PCA, extending for about 12 mm, extending to a total length of about 26 mm. The AChA gives off penetrating branches to the optic tract in this segment. As the AChA courses posteriorly it gives off penetrating branches to the globus pallidus and the genu and posterior limb of the internal capsule. Subsequent branches extend laterally to supply the medial temporal lobe cortex, hippocampal and dentate gyri, caudate, and amygdala. Medial branches supply the cerebral peduncle, substantia nigra, red nucleus, subthalamus and ventral anterior and lateral nuclei of the thalamus. The AChA is the only branch of the ICA that supplies a portion of both the anterior and posterior circulation although the midbrain and thalamic supply is very variable. More distally, the AChA extends through the choroidal fissure to become the plexal segment. The juncture of the AChA at the choroidal fissure is often referred to as the plexal point. The plexal segment then enters the choroid plexus near the posterior aspect of the temporal horn. Arterial supply of this segment includes the lateral geniculate body, optic radiations, and posterior limb of the internal capsule. The AChA anastomoses with lateral branches of the posterior choroidal artery, PCoA, PCA, and MCA [41, 43]. Variants include AChA origin from the PCoA or MCA. Although atherosclerotic disease rarely directly involves the AChA, the potential of collateral flow between the AChA and the posterior choroidal artery is an important anastomotic route to offset hypoperfusion, balancing flow between the posterior and anterior cerebral circulations. Proliferation of collaterals at this juncture is common in other disorders with stenotic lesions at the terminal ICA such as moyamoya.

Middle Cerebral Artery

The MCA provides arterial blood flow to the largest extent of the intracranial circulation. The MCA is typically 75% of the caliber of the parent ICA [33]. After diverging from the terminal ICA below the anterior perforated substance, it course horizontally and slightly anteriorly to reach the Sylvian fissure where branches perfuse the frontal, parietal, and some extent of the temporal and occipital cortices (fig. 5). The proximal or horizontal segment of the MCA averages around 15 mm in length yet may be as long as 30 mm [33]. At younger ages, the M1 segment rises obliquely but this segment tends to course more inferiorly or anteriorly with increasing age later in life [44]. Between the 7 and 12 mm (7 weeks) embryonic stage, small perforators that are precursors of the MCA arise from the ICA. The MCA is smaller than the AChA at these early stages and then grows larger. During the second month of fetal life, the Sylvian fissure develops as a groove over the cerebral hemisphere and the MCA grows within this depression. The MCA becomes enveloped in the sulcation of the cerebral cortex, following the growth of each specific brain region.

The proximal or M1 division of the MCA provides lenticulostriate arteries that feed the globus pallidus, putamen, internal capsule, corona radiata, and caudate nucleus. This segment is typically around 2.5 mm in internal diameter [33]. These end arteries originate from the M1 segment in almost perpendicular fashion to penetrate the brain parenchyma. The lateral lenticulostriates ascend for 2–5 mm posteromedially from the M1 and then course laterally and superiorly for an additional 9–30 mm to penetrate the internal capsule. The medial lenticulostriates generally arise from more proximal segments of the MCA or from distal reaches of the terminal ICA and proximal ACA [45–48].

There is considerable variation in the relative distribution and origins of medial versus lateral lenticulostriate perforators. The arterial diameter of lateral lenticulostriates is typically greater than the medial lenticulostriate perforators. Overall, there are typically 5 to 17 lenticulostriate arteries, although all are barely identifiable at angiography [33]. There are three principal patterns that have been described for the anatomy of the lenticulostriates. Grand et al. described a pattern where either one or more of the larger lenticulostriates arise just beyond the MCA bifurcation (49%), all arise proximal to the major bifurcation (39%), and a minority of cases where some of the larger perforators arise from the medial portion of the stem [46]. According to Jain, 54.1% originate from the MCA trunk, 25.6% from the division point, and 20.3% from one of the branches of the MCA [47]. The lateral lenticulostriates supply the lateral portion of the anterior commissure, the putamen, lateral segment of the globus pallidus, superior half of the internal capsule, adjacent corona radiate, and body and head of the caudate nucleus. The medial lenticulostriates arise perpendicular to the parent MCA or ACA, yet bend medially. The areas supplied by the medial lenticulostriates, including the prominent recurrent artery of Heubner, and the AChA are adjacent to the territories of the lateral lenticulostriates. The relative territorial extents are reciprocal in size and depend on the development of each of these arterial groups.

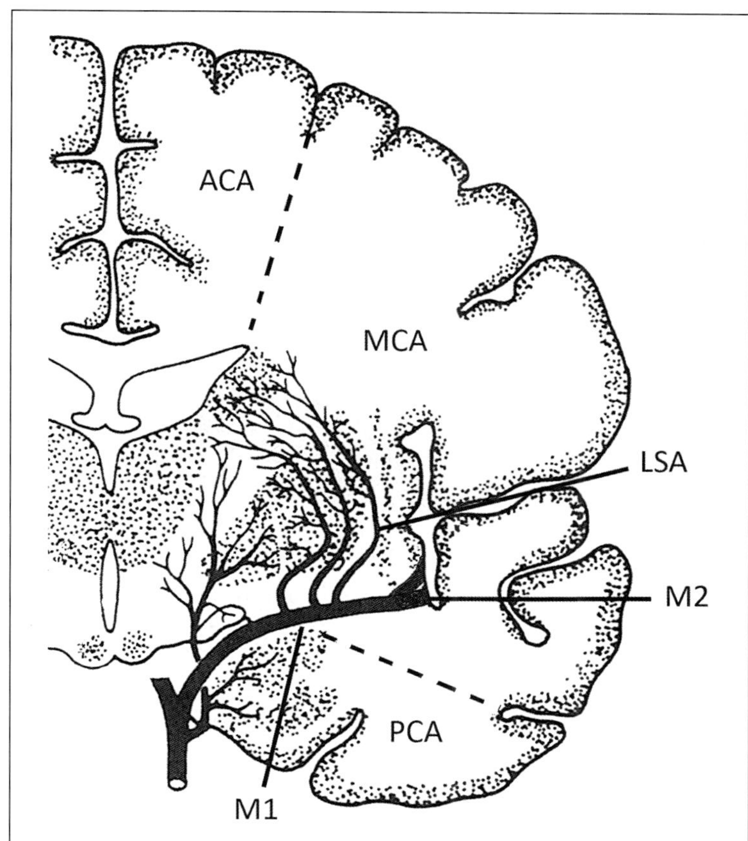

Fig. 5. Schematic of MCA, illustrating proximal segment or M1, lenticulostriate arteries (LSA), and bifurcation into M2, with downstream territories delineated between adjacent ACA and PCA regions.

The largest branch of the proximal MCA is the anterior temporal artery, extending from the middle of the proximal MCA and winding anteriorly and inferiorly. Although the configuration of the proximal MCA often varies, the vessel most often splits into two or more main divisions near the Sylvian fissure. Although prior studies have suggested symmetry in the morphology of bilateral MCAs, no clear correlations exist. The anterior and posterior divisions of the MCA extend into the Sylvian fissure and spread out over the hemisphere. These cortical branches include the temporopolar, frontobasal, operculofrontal, precentral, postcentral, posterior parietal, angular, anterior temporal, middle temporal, and posterior temporal arteries. As the MCA branches loop over the insula in the Sylvian fissure, they form the Sylvian triangle, a landmark classically used to identify mass lesions on angiography. Terminal branches of the MCA form collateral anastomoses with the ACA and PCA [4]. These leptomeningeal and pial collaterals have been studied extensively in the setting of acute ischemic stroke, yet collateral flow from these adjacent territories also influences the outcome of patients with M1 stenoses.

Variation in MCA anatomy is less common than variants in other intracranial arteries. Fenestration of the M1 segment occurs and duplicated M1 segments may also arise from the ICA [49]. Angiographic demonstration of MCA fenestration is evident in approximately 0.26% of

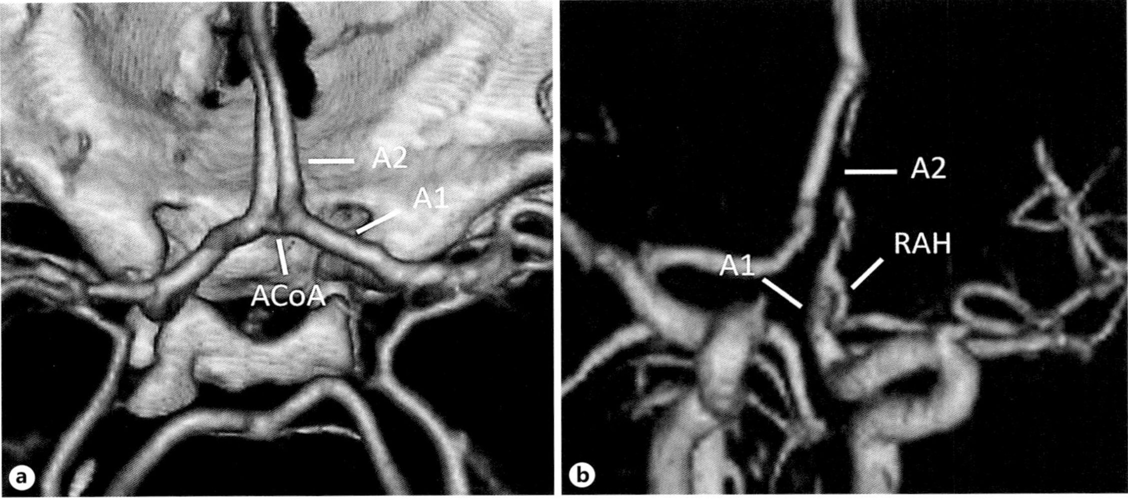

Fig. 6. CT angiography illustration of two different configurations in the ACA complex and ACoA anastomosis. **a** A patent ACoA provides interhemispheric flow between left and right ACAs. **b** ACoA is absent, yet a prominent recurrent artery of Heubner (RAH) is demonstrated.

individuals [50, 51]. Yamamoto et al. described 14 accessory MCAs and 7 duplicated MCAs in a series of 455 bilateral carotid angiographies [52]. The M1-M2 junction is characterized by a bifurcation in 64–90% of individuals, trifurcation in 12–29%, and complex branching in isolated individuals [33]. Some controversy has surrounded specific landmarks and associated classification of the MCA segments. Whereas many identify the segments of the MCA based on each successive branch point, others use a nomenclature that relates each of these MCA segments with a specific adjacent anatomical structure. For instance, some refer to the M2 origin at the initial bifurcation of the proximal or M1 MCA, whereas others identify the M2 segment as the arterial segment that overlies the insula.

Anterior Cerebral Artery

The ACA develops from residual elements of the primitive olfactory artery at the terminus of the ICA. The paired primitive olfactory arteries from each side form a plexus in the midline that gives rise to the ACoA. During development, the ACA extends superiorly and then posteriorly over the hemispheres in the midline whereas the remainder of the primitive olfactory artery regresses to become a small perforating vessel. The ACA is typically 50% of the caliber of the parent ICA [53]. The internal diameter of the A1 is usually 0.9–4 mm, with hypoplasia defined as a diameter less than 1 mm. The A1 segment measures 7–18 mm, with an average span of 12.7 mm [53]. The ACA extends anteromedially between the optic chiasm (70% of individuals) or optic nerve (30% of individuals) and the anterior perforated substance to join the contralateral ACA through an anastomosis via the ACoA.

The ACoA forms the anterior aspect of the circle of Willis, a critical route for collateral flow between the cerebral hemispheres. The ACoA is the shortest cerebral artery, measuring only 0.1–3 mm in length [53]. The anatomy of the ACAs-ACoA is variable (fig. 6) with hypoplasia of different segments, including absence of the ACoA. Accessory routes, fenestrations, and other complex azygous connections between the proximal ACAs are also described.

The proximal ACA or A1 segment gives off numerous perforating arteries that supply the adjacent optic nerves and chiasm inferiorly, and the hypothalamus, septum pellucidum, anterior commissure, fornix, and corpus striatum. These mesial lenticulostriate vessels often include a prominent recurrent artery of Heubner that supplies the caudate head, putamen, and anterior limb of the internal capsule [54]. The A2 segment begins at the juncture of the ACA with the ACoA and extends to the genu of the corpus callosum. The recurrent artery of Heubner arises from the A2 segment in 49–78% of individuals [53]. The recurrent artery of Heubner may be a single vessel or can be represented by a number of parallel arteries. Beyond the proximal segment of the ACA, azygous connections allow for shunting of flow between the cerebral hemispheres. The ACAs course over the cerebral hemispheres in the interhemispheric fissure as paired vessels, with their distal extent typically determined by the corresponding anatomy of the PCAs. Subsequent divisions including the pericallosal and callosomarginal arteries divide to provide arterial supply to the corpus callosum and anteromesial cortices. Several variations in distal ACA anatomy have been described, including the observation that the left pericallosal artery is located more posteriorly than the corresponding right-sided vessel in 72% [55]. Similarly, absence of the callosomarginal artery has been noted in 18–60% of cases studied [55].

Cortical branches of the ACA include the orbitofrontal, frontopolar, callosomarginal, and pericallosal arteries. As the terminal portion of the ACA travels along the corpus callosum, its anterior pericallosal branches form anastomoses with the posterior pericallosal branches of the PCA [55].

Variant anatomy of the ACA most commonly includes hypoplasia or absence of the A1 segment (10% of individuals) [53]. Other variations include anomalous origin of the ACA from the ICA, agenesis or accessory branches, direct connection of bilateral A1 segments, or other combinations that involve azygous orientation of distal ACA segments.

Vertebral Artery

The vertebral artery enters the skull at the level of C1 through the foramen magnum. The intracranial or intradural (V4) segment of the vertebral artery ascends anteriorly to the medulla, approaching midline at the pontomedullary junction where it meets the contralateral vertebral artery to form the basilar artery. The paired longitudinal arteries that form the arterial supply to the posterior circulation during early fetal development retain their proximal course as the vertebral arteries. The left vertebral artery is larger than the right in 42% of the time, whereas the right is larger than the left in 32%. In the remainder of individuals, the vertebral arteries are equivalent in caliber.

Vertebral artery hypoplasia is fairly common, often involving the right side. The frequency of this finding depends largely on the modality used to image the vessel, the size threshold used to define hypoplasia, and the study population, including healthy subjects or patients with ischemic stroke. Defining hypoplasia as ≤2 mm by ultrasonography, one group reported a frequency of 1.9% in 451 subjects [56]. Amongst healthy subjects with a threshold of <3 mm, another group noted a frequency of 6% in 50 healthy subjects [57]. Others have recently noted a frequency as high as 35.2% in 529 patients with ischemic stroke [58]. Utilizing a luminal diameter threshold of 2.2 mm, prominent asymmetry in vertebral artery hypoplasia has also been described (7.8% on the right and 3.8% on the left) in 447 subjects [59]. Differentiation of hypoplasia from a diseased arterial segment is difficult to define based on luminal dimensions alone. The configuration or compensatory enlargement of neighboring segments provide clues to this distinction. Definitions vary considerably based on the imaging technique used. The vertebral artery may also terminate in the PICA rather than extend to the junction with the basilar artery. In such cases, the vertebral artery is generally smaller than the contralateral vertebral artery. When a vertebral artery is hypoplastic the foramena transversara on that side are also smaller than the contralateral foramina.

The terminal vertebral artery yields several branches that supply the rostral end of the spinal cord and posterior inferior aspect of the cerebellum. Anterior and posterior spinal arteries extend from this segment. Each anterior spinal artery fuses with its counterpart, supplying the ventral medulla and rostral spinal cord. The posterior spinal arteries do not pair in the midline, but descend the spinal cord at the level of the dorsal roots. The posterior inferior cerebellar artery branches from the vertebral to supply the inferior aspect of the cerebellum.

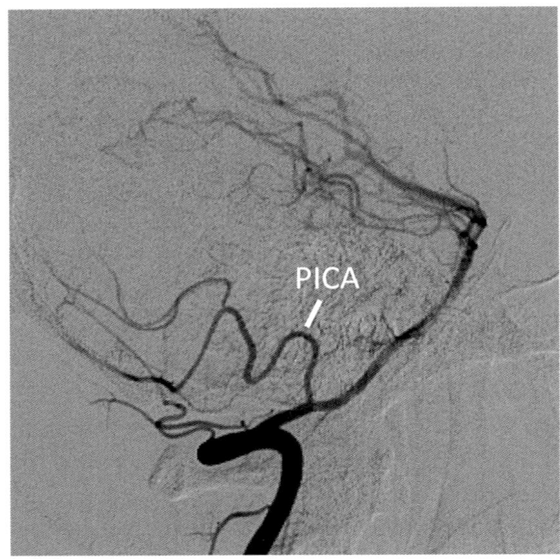

Fig. 7. DSA of the PICA, showing proximal medullary segments and hemispheric tributaries.

Posterior Inferior Cerebellar Artery

The largest tributary of the vertebral artery is the PICA, arising 10–20 mm before the vertebrobasilar junction (fig. 7) [60]. In 20% of individuals, the PICA arises from below the foramen magnum [61]. During embryogenesis, the PICA is be evident as a larger branch of numerous arteries that extend posteriorly from the hindbrain in the 20–24 mm embryo stage. At later stages, this vessel continues to predominate growing into the largest arterial offshoot. There are four segments of this vessel, including the anterior, lateral, posterior medullary, and supratonsillar PICA. The anterior medullary segment travels laterally near the inferior aspect of the olive of the medulla oblangata, continuing in a loop that courses between the cerebellum and medulla. Numerous perforating arteries extend from the first three segments of the PICA to supply anterior, lateral, and posterior aspects of the medulla. The PICA then extends posteriorly in the tonsillomedullary fissure adjacent to the glossopharyngeal (IX) and vagus (X) nerves. Beyond this point, the PICA curves over the cerebellar tonsil to become the supratonsillar segment extending further across the cerebellum as the medial and lateral terminal PICA branches. At the juncture of the posterior medullary and supratonsillar segments of the PICA, perforating vessels arise to feed the choroid plexus of the fourth ventricle. This choroidal point is used as a landmark to identify masses within the posterior fossa.

Variations in PICA anatomy include hypoplasia or absence of this branch (10–20% of individuals), typically accompanied by a prominent ipsilateral anterior inferior cerebellar artery. Absence of PICA is also accompanied by numerous medullary perforators that arise directly from the vertebral artery. Duplication of PICA and double origin with distal arterial convergence of PICA may occur [62]. PICA-AICA connections and other anomalies are seen; the frequencies of such

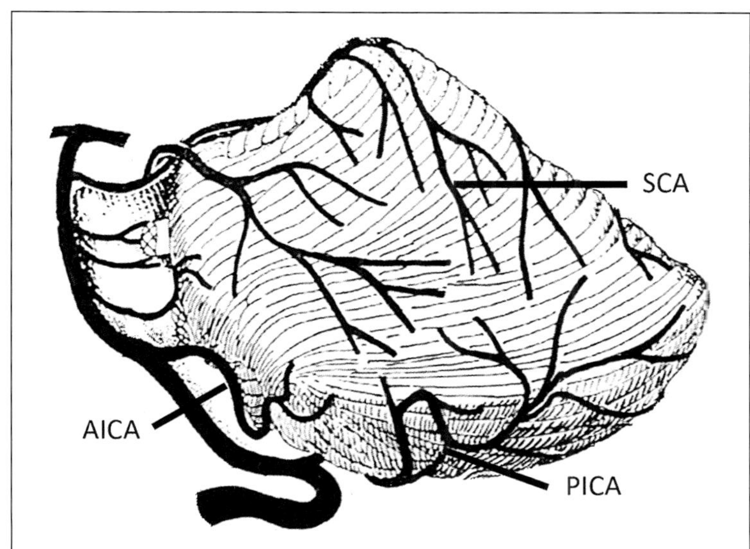

Fig. 8. Schematic of posterior circulation, demonstrating cerebellar arteries including SCA, AICA, and PICA.

anatomic configurations remain unclear. On occasion, both inferior cerebellar territories are supplied by a bihemispheric PICA originating from one vertebral artery [63].

Basilar Artery

The basilar artery extends from the confluence of the vertebral arteries near the pontomedullary junction to the terminal bifurcation as the PCAs at the level of the midbrain. During embryologic development, paired vessels on the ventral surface of the hindbrain fuse to form the basilar artery. Distal segments of these paired basilar arteries have connections with the ipsilateral ICA. Over time, the plexus formed by the paired basilar arteries fuses with progressive disappearance of fenestrations. The basilar artery is often tortuous or serpentine, with a straight course noted in about 25% of the time. Curvature of the basilar artery as it ascends has been associated with the presence of a wider contralateral vertebral artery, suggesting hemodynamic modeling. The length of the basilar artery is consistently 25–35 mm, irrespective of body size [64]. The diameter is about 2.7–4.3 mm at the proximal portion. The luminal diameter of the basilar artery tapers towards the distal end.

The largest branches of the basilar artery include the anterior inferior cerebellar artery (AICA) and superior cerebellar artery (SCA) (fig. 8). Numerous smaller perforators embrace the brainstem, coursing from the midline ventral aspect around the surface to the lateral dorsal surface, and diving deep into the substance of the brainstem between fiber tracts [65]. These pontine perforators are grouped into medial and lateral subdivisions, often referred to as paramedian and circumferential arteries. Lateral pontine perforators extend to also supply the ventrolateral surface of the cerebellum, whereas the medial perforators perfuse midline structures of the midbrain. There is a somewhat downward trajectory of brainstem perforating arteries so that the most rostral portion of the basilar artery supplies penetrators to the pontine tegmentum. The internal auditory or labyrinthine artery arises from the basilar to provide arterial blood flow to the cochlea, labyrinth, and facial (VII) nerve [66].

Alternatively, this artery may arise as a branch of the AICA. Due to the paired structure of posterior circulation arteries, asymmetries or relative dominance of one artery such as the PICA, AICA, or SCA occur. Contralateral cerebellar infarction can result from occlusion or disease of one cerebellar artery. The frequencies of such patterns vary and are difficult to estimate, although the advent of MRI and MRA allows for systematic evaluation of such features. Terminal branches of the PICA, AICA, and SCA form anastomoses that allow for collateral flow to easily shift between their arterial territories [4, 67].

Anterior Inferior Cerebellar Artery

The AICA extends off of the basilar artery approximately one-third to halfway through its course [67]. The AICA arises from the caudal third of the basilar 74% of the time. This artery is the smallest of the principal cerebellar arteries. During development, the AICA appears as one of the larger perforatoring vessels extending to the posterior aspect of the hindbrain. The AICA extends laterally and inferiorly, in close proximity to the abducens (VI) nerve. Similar to the lateral pontine perforators, it courses around the brainstem and then enters the cerebellopontine angle cistern along with the facial (VII) and vestibulocochlear (VIII) nerves. The AICA crosses the anteroinferior aspect of the cerebellum to supply the middle cerebellar peduncle, flocculus, and adjacent cerebellum. The AICAs supply a rather small variable portion of the anterior inferior cerebellum [68]. The supply to the brachium pontis and flocculus is consistent. Numerous pontine perforators arise from its proximal segment. The lateral branch runs across the cerebellum in the horizontal fissure. The medial branch of AICA courses inferiorly to supply the biventral lobule. Similar to absence of the PICA, AICA may be absent or hypoplastic and is typically accompanied by a prominent PICA. Variable infarct patterns are noted in these regions of the posterior circulation, likely reflecting arterial configurations of the principal cerebellar arteries that involve hypoplastic segments or anomalous anastomoses [68, 69]. Combined or multiple territorial infarcts such as PICA and AICA or AICA and SCA reflect dominant patterns of arterial supply originating from the vertebral and basilar arteries. Collateral anastomoses between these territories can provide sufficient arterial inflow to spare distal segments of a particular arterial territory. As individual anatomy is often studied only after stroke onset, the original arterial configuration and mechanistic events may only be surmised. Similarly, the frequency of specific arterial supply patterns are difficult to ascertain in the healthy population as individuals are most often studied after presentation with potential neurovascular disorders.

Superior Cerebellar Artery

The SCA also extends from the basilar artery in a symmetric fashion, just proximal to the terminal bifurcation of the basilar into the proximal PCAs. SCA morphology is most consistent across individuals compared with other cerebellar branches [70]. The SCA courses laterally below the oculomotor (III) nerve, passing around the cerebral peduncles and below the trochlear (IV) nerve [42]. Numerous perforators extend from the proximal or ambient SCA to supply the adjacent pons and midbrain, whereas distal segments split into the lateral marginal and superior vermian branches. These divisions can also arise independently from the basilar artery or even the PCA. Duplication of the SCA is noted in 28% of individuals, with bilateral duplication in 10% [71]. The SCA variably divides into medial SCA and lateral SCA branches. The lateral marginal SCA supplies the anterosuperior cerebellum, superior cerebellar peduncle, middle cerebral peduncle, and dentate nuclei. The superior vermian SCA supplies the superior cerebellar peduncle, tentorium, inferior colliculi, cerebellar hemispheres and dentate nuclei. Anastomoses between this branch and the inferior vermian branch of the PICA allow for robust collateral perfusion across the cerebellar hemispheres [72].

Posterior Cerebral Artery

The posterior cerebral artery (PCA) develops from fusion of several vessels that supply the mesencephalon, diencephalon, and choroid plexus in the fetus [73]. These vessels stem from the terminal aspect of the PCoA at the distal end of the carotid circulation. The PCA most often then extends posteriorly to spread over the ipsilateral cortex, whereas the proximal connection with the PCoA regresses [74]. In this common scenario, the primary arterial supply shifts to a source from the terminal basilar artery. In the remainder of individuals, the PCA supply continues from what has been termed a fetal PCoA. Variants of PCoA anatomy include a diverse range of caliber in this segment, complete agenesis, and anomalous origins of other vessels from this arterial segment [75].

The PCA extends from the terminal portion of the basilar artery in the interpeduncular cistern, passing above the oculomotor (III) nerve to circle the midbrain above the tentorium (fig. 9). As it passes through the peduncular, ambient, and quadrigeminal cisterns, numerous perforators supply adjacent structures [76]. This pattern of arterial limbs includes paramedian perforators, short circumferential and long circumferential branches that typify the general structure of the major arterial territories in the posterior circulation. The perforating arteries from these segments range from 200 to 800 μm in diameter [76]. The artery of Davidoff and Schechter extends from the P1 segment to supply part of the inferior surface of the tentorium. The midbrain receives arterial blood from the peduncular or P1 segment

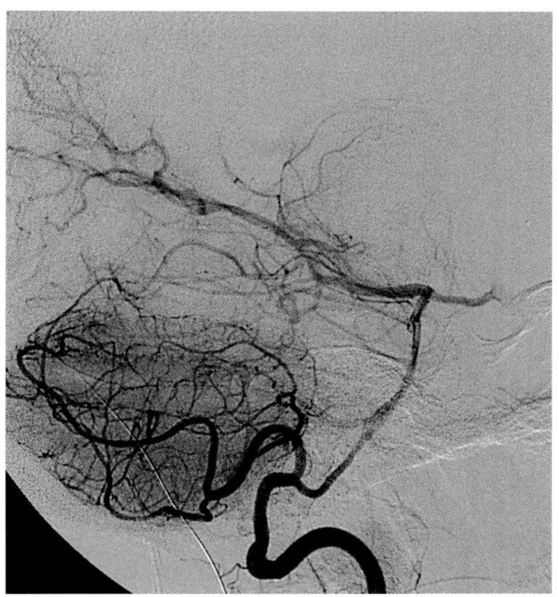

Fig. 9. DSA illustrating PCA anastomosis with PCoA, thalamoperforators, and distal cortical branches.

before posterior thalamoperforators arise. In the successive ambient segment, the thalamogeniculate arteries diverge to supply the lateral geniculate and pulvinar nuclei. Medial and lateral branches of the posterior choroidal arteries extend from this portion of the PCA to supply the pineal gland, third ventricle, dorsomedial thalamus, pulvinar, lateral geniculate body and choroid plexus [77]. These distal posterior choroidal arteries form anastomoses with the AChA.

These deep arterial territories comprised of perforatoring arterioles that encompass the thalamus are often difficult to comprehend due to their complex configuration (fig. 10) [78]. The P1 or proximal PCA serves as an important arterial segment in this configuration, with variable contributions from the basilar, PCoA and AChA [79]. These vessels have perforators that supply these critical structures at the juncture between the anterior and posterior circulations. The anterior thalamoperforating arteries consist of about 7–10 branches that arise from the superior and lateral

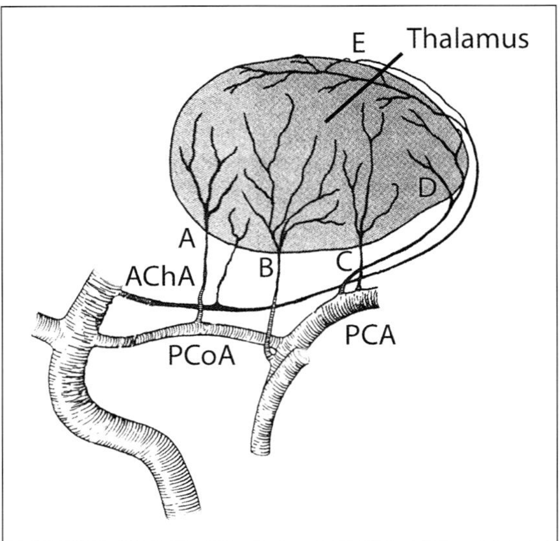

Fig. 10. Schematic of the arterial supply to the thalamus, illustrating premamillary arteries (**A**), interpeduncular perforators (**B**), thalamogeniculate arteries (**C**), posterior choroidal arteries (**D**), and AChA (**E**).

surfaces of the PCoA [79]. A larger branch, the premamillary artery, is often noted [80]. This vessel courses from the posterior aspect of the PCoA, penetrates the hypothalamus and subsequently terminates in branches that supply the anterior and ventroanterior nuclei of the thalamus. Further posteriorly, the thalamus is supplied by a combination of vessels arising from the posterior circulation. Interpeduncular branches from the basilar artery and P1 segment ascend superiorly to perfuse mesial aspects of the thalamus. More lateral aspects of the thalamus, including the ventroposteromedial and ventroposterolateral nuclei are supplied by the thalamogeniculate arteries [81]. These typically consist of 3 to 5 small branches that penetrate the inferior aspect of the thalamus and also supply blood to the geniculate bodies [76]. The most posterior reaches of the thalamus are supplied via the posterior choroidal arteries, arising from more distal aspects of the subcortical PCA. These posterior choroidal branches supply portions of the medial nuclei, habenula, and rostromedial pulvinar, and choroid plexus [82]. The posterior choroidal arteries adjoin and overlap to some extent with distal reaches of the AChA, extending from the ICA to supply lateral and posterior regions of the thalamus.

The PCA passes along the free edge of the tentorium to eventually reach the medial aspect of the occipital lobe. Further branching within the hippocampal fissure produces cortical divisions that course over the inferior and mesial aspects of the hemisphere. The cortical territories of the PCA are supplied via the anterior and posterior divisions, fanning out to follow the architecture of the cortical surface in these regions.

Cortical branches of the PCA include the hippocampal, anterior temporal, middle temporal, posterior temporal, parietooccipital, calcarine, and posterior pericallosal or perisplenial arteries [83]. Anastomoses of the PCA allow for collateral flow into the MCA via the anterior and posterior temporal arteries and into the ACA via pericallosal divisions that arise from the quadrigeminal PCA [4].

Beyond Anatomy – Clinical Implications of Collateral Circulation

The detection or identification of an intracranial stenosis in a proximal cerebral artery is now readily accomplished, yet the implications with respect to downstream ischemia and subsequent stroke remain unclear. As diagnostic techniques have evolved, it has become apparent that the degree of luminal stenosis is solely a marker of disease extent, disjointed from the potential collateral circulation that offset ischemia in the territory downstream of the arterial lesion [84, 85]. Detailed investigations show that collateral perfusion is just as important as the degree of stenosis in characterization of intracranial atherosclerosis [86]. Territorial perfusion downstream of an intracranial stenosis varies due to features of the arterial lesion and the rigor of compensatory collateral perfusion. Noninvasive imaging modalities, such as time-of-flight MRA reveal signal loss that corresponds to the severity of hypoperfusion in the territory downstream of an arterial lesion [87–90]. Local hemodynamic effects such as shear stress induced by the atherosclerotic lesion can be illustrated with computational fluid dynamics on CTA or MRA, that show a variety of flow perturbations in arterial flow [91]. Recent clinical trial results confirmed that imaging of downstream hypoperfusion or low flow beyond an arterial stenosis is an important marker of subsequent stroke [92]. Ongoing work continues to refine HR-MRI characterization of atherosclerotic plaques and relationship with intracranial vascular anatomy [93, 94]. Conventional measures of downstream flow at angiography reveal that functional characterization of an arterial lesion in the brain adds another dimension beyond anatomical delineation of culprit plaques. The striking clinical impact of collateral perfusion in intracranial atherosclerosis demonstrated in recent clinical studies underscores the need to consider functional implications of an arterial stenosis, akin to recent work on fractional flow in the coronary circulation. In the heart, such approaches have revolutionized coronary revascularization, delineating the individual impact of an atherosclerotic lesion based on downstream hemodynamics. Such an individualized approach or precision medicine perspective that incorporates both anatomy and physiology of collaterals will undoubtedly become reality in coming years for intracranial atherosclerosis [95, 96].

References

1 Petrone L, Nannoni S, Del Bene A, Palumbo V, Inzitari D: Branch atheromatous disease: a clinically meaningful, yet unproven concept. Cerebrovasc Dis 2015;41:87–95.

2 Qiao Y, Anwar Z, Intrapiromkul J, Liu L, Zeiler SR, Leigh R, Zhang Y, Guallar E, Wasserman BA: Patterns and implications of intracranial arterial remodeling in stroke patients. Stroke 2016;47:434–440.

3 Hartkamp NS, Petersen ET, De Vis JB, Bokkers RP, Hendrikse J: Mapping of cerebral perfusion territories using territorial arterial spin labeling: techniques and clinical application. NMR Biomed 2013;26:901–912.

4 Liebeskind DS: Collateral circulation. Stroke 2003;34:2279–2284.

5 Parmar H, Sitoh YY, Hui F: Normal variants of the intracranial circulation demonstrated by mr angiography at 3t. Eur J Radiol 2005;56:220–228.

6 van der Kolk AG, Zwanenburg JJ, Brundel M, Biessels GJ, Visser F, Luijten PR, Hendrikse J: Distribution and natural course of intracranial vessel wall lesions in patients with ischemic stroke or tia at 7.0 tesla mri. Eur Radiol 2015;25:1692–1700.

7 Feldmann E, Wilterdink JL, Kosinski A, Lynn M, Chimowitz MI, Sarafin J, Smith HH, Nichols F, Rogg J, Cloft HJ, Wechsler L, Saver J, Levine SR, Tegeler C, Adams R, Sloan M: The stroke outcomes and neuroimaging of intracranial atherosclerosis (sonia) trial. Neurology 2007;68:2099–2106.

8 Dieleman N, van der Kolk AG, Zwanenburg JJ, Harteveld AA, Biessels GJ, Luijten PR, Hendrikse J: Imaging intracranial vessel wall pathology with magnetic resonance imaging: current prospects and future directions. Circulation 2014;130:192–201.

9 Dumont TM, Sonig A, Mokin M, Eller JL, Sorkin GC, Snyder KV, Nelson Hopkins L, Levy EI, Siddiqui AH: Submaximal angioplasty for symptomatic intracranial atherosclerosis: a prospective phase i study. J Neurosurg 2016;8:1–8.

10 Perez-Carrillo GJ, Hogg JP: Intracranial vascular lesions and anatomical variants all residents should know. Curr Probl Diagn Radiol 2010;39:91–109.

11 Raybaud C: Normal and abnormal embryology and development of the intracranial vascular system. Neurosurg Clin N Am 2010;21:399–426.

12 Yan L, Liu CY, Smith RX, Jog M, Langham M, Krasileva K, Chen Y, Ringman JM, Wang DJ: Assessing intracranial vascular compliance using dynamic arterial spin labeling. Neuroimage 2016; 124:433–441.

13 Stehbens WE: Pathology of the cerebral blood vessels. Book, St Louis, CV Mosby 1972.

14 Walmsley JG, Canham PB: Orientation of nuclei as indicators of smooth muscle cell alignment in the cerebral artery. Blood Vessels 1979;16:43–51.

15 Walmsley JG: Vascular smooth muscle orientation in curved branches and bifurcations of human cerebral arteries. J Microsc 1983;131:377–389.

16 Walmsley JG: Vascular smooth muscle orientation in straight portions of human cerebral arteries. J Microsc 1983; 131:361–375.

17 Farrall AJ, Wardlaw JM: Blood-brain barrier: Ageing and microvascular disease – systematic review and meta-analysis. Neurobiol Aging 2009;30:337–352.

18 Bang OY, Buck BH, Saver JL, Alger JR, Yoon SR, Starkman S, Ovbiagele B, Kim D, Ali LK, Sanossian N, Jahan R, Duckwiler GR, Vinuela F, Salamon N, Villablanca JP, Liebeskind DS: Prediction of hemorrhagic transformation after recanalization therapy using t2*-permeability magnetic resonance imaging. Ann Neurol 2007;62:170–176.

19 Oldendorf WH, Cornford ME, Brown WJ: The large apparent work capability of the blood-brain barrier: a study of the mitochondrial content of capillary endothelial cells in brain and other tissues of the rat. Ann Neurol 1977;1:409–417.

20 McCarron RM, Chen Y, Tomori T, Strasser A, Mechoulam R, Shohami E, Spatz M: Endothelial-mediated regulation of cerebral microcirculation. J Physiol Pharmacol 2006;57(suppl 11):133–144.

21 Hassler O: The windows of the internal elastic lamella of the cerebral arteries. Virchows Arch Pathol Anat Physiol Klin Med 1962;335:127–132.

22 Takayanagi T, Rennels ML, Nelson E: An electron microscopic study of intimal cushions in intracranial arteries of the cat. Am J Anat 1972;133:415–429.

23 Heil M, Eitenmuller I, Schmitz-Rixen T, Schaper W: Arteriogenesis versus angiogenesis: similarities and differences. J Cell Mol Med 2006;10:45–55.

24 Schaper W, Scholz D: Factors regulating arteriogenesis. Arterioscler Thromb Vasc Biol 2003;23:1143–1151.

25 Zhao X, Zhao M, Amin-Hanjani S, Du X, Ruland S, Charbel FT: Wall shear stress in major cerebral arteries as a function of age and gender – a study of 301 healthy volunteers. J Neuroimaging 2015;25:403–407.

26 Dolan JM, Kolega J, Meng H: High wall shear stress and spatial gradients in vascular pathology: a review. Ann Biomed Eng 2013;41:1411–1427.

27 Zervas NT, Liszczak TM, Mayberg MR, Black PM: Cerebrospinal fluid may nourish cerebral vessels through pathways in the adventitia that may be analogous to systemic vasa vasorum. J Neurosurg 1982;56:475–481.

28 Clower BR, Sullivan DM, Smith RR: Intracranial vessels lack vasa vasorum. J Neurosurg 1984;61:44–48.

29 Quisling RG, Rhoton AL Jr: Intrapetrous carotid artery branches: radioanatomic analysis. Radiology 1979;131:133–136.

30 Sanders-Taylor C, Kurbanov A, Cebula H, Leach JL, Zuccarello M, Keller JT: The carotid siphon: a historic radiographic sign, not an anatomic classification. World Neurosurg 2014;82:423–427.

31 Allen JW, Alastra AJ, Nelson PK: Proximal intracranial internal carotid artery branches: prevalence and importance for balloon occlusion test. J Neurosurg 2005;102:45–52.

32 Frugoni P, Nori A, Galligioni F, Giammusso V: Further considerations on the bernasconi and cassinari's artery and other meningeal rami of the internal carotid artery. Neurochirurgia (Stuttg) 1964;108:18–23.

33 Gibo H, Carver CC, Rhoton AL Jr, Lenkey C, Mitchell RJ: Microsurgical anatomy of the middle cerebral artery. J Neurosurg 1981;54:151–169.

34 Liebeskind DS, Flint AC, Budzik RF, Xiang B, Smith WS, Duckwiler GR, Nogueira RG, Merci, Multi MI: Carotid i's, l's and t's: collaterals shape the outcome of intracranial carotid occlusion in acute ischemic stroke. J Neurointerv Surg 2015;7:402–407.

35 Alpers BJ, Berry RG, Paddison RM: Anatomical studies of the circle of willis in normal brain. AMA Arch Neurol Psychiatry 1959;81:409–418.

36 Schomer DF, Marks MP, Steinberg GK, Johnstone IM, Boothroyd DB, Ross MR, Pelc NJ, Enzmann DR: The anatomy of the posterior communicating artery as a risk factor for ischemic cerebral infarction. N Engl J Med 1994;330:1565–1570.

37 Eftekhar B, Dadmehr M, Ansari S, Ghodsi M, Nazparvar B, Ketabchi E: Are the distributions of variations of circle of willis different in different populations? – Results of an anatomical study and review of literature. BMC Neurol 2006;6:22.

38 Tubbs RS, Verma K, Riech S, Mortazavi MM, Shoja MM, Loukas M, Cure JK, Zurada A, Cohen-Gadol AA: Persistent fetal intracranial arteries: a comprehensive review of anatomical and clinical significance. J Neurosurg 2011;114:1127–1134.

39 Uchino A, Kato A, Takase Y, Kudo S: Persistent trigeminal artery variants detected by mr angiography. Eur Radiol 2000;10:1801–1804.

40 Rhoton AL Jr, Fujii K, Fradd B: Microsurgical anatomy of the anterior choroidal artery. Surg Neurol 1979;12:171–187.

41 Takahashi S, Suga T, Kawata Y, Sakamoto K: Anterior choroidal artery: angiographic analysis of variations and anomalies. AJNR Am J Neuroradiol 1990;11:719–729.

42 Saeki N, Rhoton AL Jr: Microsurgical anatomy of the upper basilar artery and the posterior circle of willis. J Neurosurg 1977;46:563–578.

43 Morandi X, Brassier G, Darnault P, Mercier P, Scarabin JM, Duval JM: Microsurgical anatomy of the anterior choroidal artery. Surg Radiol Anat 1996;18:275–280.

44 Bouissou H, Emery MC, Sorbara R: Age related changes of the middle cerebral artery and a comparison with the radial and coronary artery. Angiology 1975;26:257–268.

45 Donzelli R, Marinkovic S, Brigante L, de Divitiis O, Nikodijevic I, Schonauer C, Maiuri F: Territories of the perforating (lenticulostriate) branches of the middle cerebral artery. Surg Radiol Anat 1998;20:393–398.

46 Grand W: Microsurgical anatomy of the proximal middle cerebral artery and the internal carotid artery bifurcation. Neurosurgery 1980;7:215–218.

47 Jain KK: Some observations on the anatomy of the middle cerebral artery. Can J Surg 1964;7:134–139.

48 Marinkovic SV, Milisavljevic MM, Kovacevic MS, Stevic ZD: Perforating branches of the middle cerebral artery. Microanatomy and clinical significance of their intracerebral segments. Stroke 1985;16:1022–1029.

49 Komiyama M, Nakajima H, Nishikawa M, Yasui T: Middle cerebral artery variations: duplicated and accessory arteries. AJNR Am J Neuroradiol 1998;19:45–49.

50 Lazar ML, Bland JE, North RR, Bringewald PR: Middle cerebral artery fenestration. Neurosurgery 1980;6:297–300.

51 van Rooij SB, Bechan RS, Peluso JP, Sluzewski M, van Rooij WJ: Fenestrations of intracranial arteries. AJNR Am J Neuroradiol 2015;36:1167–1170.

52 Yamamoto H, Marubayashi T, Soejima T, Matsuoka S, Matsukado Y, Ushio Y: Accessory middle cerebral artery and duplication of middle cerebral artery – terminology, incidence, vascular etiology, and developmental significance. Neurol Med Chir (Tokyo) 1992;32:262–267.

53 Perlmutter D, Rhoton AL Jr: Microsurgical anatomy of the anterior cerebral-anterior communicating-recurrent artery complex. J Neurosurg 1976;45:259–272.
54 Pearce JM: Heubner's artery. Eur Neurol 2005;54:112–114.
55 Perlmutter D, Rhoton AL Jr: Microsurgical anatomy of the distal anterior cerebral artery. J Neurosurg 1978;49:204–228.
56 Delcker A, Diener HC: [various ultrasound methods for studying the vertebral artery–a comparative evaluation]. Ultraschall Med 1992;13:213–220.
57 Touboul PJ, Bousser MG, LaPlane D, Castaigne P: Duplex scanning of normal vertebral arteries. Stroke 1986;17:921–923.
58 Park JH, Kim JM, Roh JK: Hypoplastic vertebral artery: Frequency and associations with ischaemic stroke territory. J Neurol Neurosurg Psychiatry 2007;78:954–958.
59 Jeng JS, Yip PK: Evaluation of vertebral artery hypoplasia and asymmetry by color-coded duplex ultrasonography. Ultrasound Med Biol 2004;30:605–609.
60 Lister JR, Rhoton AL Jr, Matsushima T, Peace DA: Microsurgical anatomy of the posterior inferior cerebellar artery. Neurosurgery 1982;10:170–199.
61 Fine AD, Cardoso A, Rhoton AL Jr: Microsurgical anatomy of the extracranial-extradural origin of the posterior inferior cerebellar artery. J Neurosurg 1999;91:645–652.
62 Lesley WS, Dalsania HJ: Double origin of the posterior inferior cerebellar artery. AJNR Am J Neuroradiol 2004;25:425–427.
63 Cullen SP, Ozanne A, Alvarez H, Lasjaunias P: The bihemispheric posterior inferior cerebellar artery. Neuroradiology 2005;47:809–812.
64 Brassier G, Morandi X, Riffaud L, Mercier P: Basilar artery anatomy. J Neurosurg 2000;93:368–369.
65 Lescher S, Samaan T, Berkefeld J: Evaluation of the pontine perforators of the basilar artery using digital subtraction angiography in high resolution and 3d rotation technique. AJNR Am J Neuroradiol 2014;35:1942–1947.
66 Kim JS, Lopez I, DiPatre PL, Liu F, Ishiyama A, Baloh RW: Internal auditory artery infarction: clinicopathologic correlation. Neurology 1999;52:40–44.
67 Rhoton AL Jr: The cerebellar arteries. Neurosurgery 2000;47:S29–S68.
68 Kumral E, Kisabay A, Atac C: Lesion patterns and etiology of ischemia in the anterior inferior cerebellar artery territory involvement: a clinical – diffusion weighted – mri study. Eur J Neurol 2006;13:395–401.
69 Terao S, Miura N, Osano Y, Takatsu S, Adachi K, Noda A, Sobue G: Multiple cerebellar infarcts: clinical and pathophysiologic features. J Stroke Cerebrovasc Dis 2005;14:193–198.
70 Hardy DG, Peace DA, Rhoton AL Jr: Microsurgical anatomy of the superior cerebellar artery. Neurosurgery 1980;6:10–28.
71 Icardo JM, Ojeda JL, Garcia-Porrero JA, Hurle JM: The cerebellar arteries: cortical patterns and vascularization of the cerebellar nuclei. Acta Anat (Basel) 1982;113:108–116.
72 Brandt T, von Kummer R, Muller-Kuppers M, Hacke W: Thrombolytic therapy of acute basilar artery occlusion. Variables affecting recanalization and outcome. Stroke 1996;27:875–881.
73 Zeal AA, Rhoton AL Jr: Microsurgical anatomy of the posterior cerebral artery. J Neurosurg 1978;48:534–559.
74 Uchino A, Saito N, Takahashi M, Okano N, Tanisaka M: Variations of the posterior cerebral artery diagnosed by mr angiography at 3 tesla. Neuroradiology 2015;58:141–146.
75 Bisaria KK: Anomalies of the posterior communicating artery and their potential clinical significance. J Neurosurg 1984;60:572–576.
76 Milisavljevic MM, Marinkovic SV, Gibo H, Puskas LF: The thalamogeniculate perforators of the posterior cerebral artery: the microsurgical anatomy. Neurosurgery 1991;28:523–529; discussion 529–530.
77 Fujii K, Lenkey C, Rhoton AL Jr: Microsurgical anatomy of the choroidal arteries: Lateral and third ventricles. J Neurosurg 1980;52:165–188.
78 Carrera E, Michel P, Bogousslavsky J: Anteromedian, central, and posterolateral infarcts of the thalamus: Three variant types. Stroke 2004;35:2826–2831.
79 Percheron G: [arteries of the thalamus in man. Choroidal arteries. Iii. Absence of the constituted thalamic territory of the anterior choroidal artery. Iv. Arteries and thalamic territories of the choroidal and postero-median thalamic arterial system. V. Arteries and thalamic territories of the choroidal and postero-lateral thalamic arterial system]. Rev Neurol (Paris) 1977;133:547–558.
80 Gibo H, Marinkovic S, Brigante L: The microsurgical anatomy of the premamillary artery. J Clin Neurosci 2001;8:256–260.
81 Georgiadis AL, Yamamoto Y, Kwan ES, Pessin MS, Caplan LR: Anatomy of sensory findings in patients with posterior cerebral artery territory infarction. Arch Neurol 1999;56:835–838.
82 Liebeskind DS, Hurst RW: Infarction of the choroid plexus. AJNR Am J Neuroradiol 2004;25:289–290.
83 Brandt T, Steinke W, Thie A, Pessin MS, Caplan LR: Posterior cerebral artery territory infarcts: clinical features, infarct topography, causes and outcome. Multicenter results and a review of the literature. Cerebrovasc Dis 2000;10:170–182.
84 Liebeskind DS, Cotsonis GA, Saver JL, Lynn MJ, Turan TN, Cloft HJ, Chimowitz MI, Warfarin-Aspirin Symptomatic Intracranial Disease I: Collaterals dramatically alter stroke risk in intracranial atherosclerosis. Ann Neurol 2011;69:963–974.
85 Liebeskind DS, Cotsonis GA, Saver JL, Lynn MJ, Cloft HJ, Chimowitz MI, Warfarin-Aspirin Symptomatic Intracranial Disease I: Collateral circulation in symptomatic intracranial atherosclerosis. J Cereb Blood Flow Metab 2011;31:1293–1301.
86 Leng X, Wong KS, Liebeskind DS: Evaluating intracranial atherosclerosis rather than intracranial stenosis. Stroke 2014;45:645–651.
87 Leng X, Wong KS, Soo Y, Leung T, Zou X, Wang Y, Feldmann E, Liu L, Liebeskind DS: Magnetic resonance angiography signal intensity as a marker of hemodynamic impairment in intracranial arterial stenosis. PLoS One 2013;8:e80124.
88 Leng X, Ip HL, Soo Y, Leung T, Liu L, Feldmann E, Wong KS, Liebeskind DS: Interobserver reproducibility of signal intensity ratio on magnetic resonance angiography for hemodynamic impact of intracranial atherosclerosis. J Stroke Cerebrovasc Dis 2013;22:e615–e619.

89 Leng X, Wong LK, Soo Y, Leung T, Zou X, Wang Y, Feldmann E, Liu L, Liebeskind D: Signal intensity ratio as a novel measure of hemodynamic significance for intracranial atherosclerosis. Int J Stroke 2013;8:E46.
90 Liebeskind DS, Kosinski AS, Lynn MJ, Scalzo F, Fong AK, Fariborz P, Chimowitz MI, Feldmann E: Noninvasive fractional flow on mra predicts stroke risk of intracranial stenosis. J Neuroimaging 2015;25:87–91.
91 Leng X, Scalzo F, Ip HL, Johnson M, Fong AK, Fan FS, Chen X, Soo YO, Miao Z, Liu L, Feldmann E, Leung TW, Liebeskind DS, Wong KS: Computational fluid dynamics modeling of symptomatic intracranial atherosclerosis may predict risk of stroke recurrence. PLoS One 2014;9:e97531.
92 Amin-Hanjani S, Pandey DK, Rose-Finnell L, Du X, Richardson D, Thulborn KR, Elkind MS, Zipfel GJ, Liebeskind DS, Silver FL, Kasner SE, Aletich VA, Caplan LR, Derdeyn CP, Gorelick PB, Charbel FT, Vertebrobasilar Flow E, Risk of Transient Ischemic A, Stroke Study G: Effect of hemodynamics on stroke risk in symptomatic atherosclerotic vertebrobasilar occlusive disease. JAMA Neurol 2016;73:178–185.
93 Harteveld AA, De Cocker LJ, Dieleman N, van der Kolk AG, Zwanenburg JJ, Robe PA, Luijten PR, Hendrikse J: High-resolution postcontrast time-of-flight mr angiography of intracranial perforators at 7.0 tesla. PLoS One 2015; 10:e0121051.
94 Gounis MJ, van der Marel K, Marosfoi M, Mazzanti ML, Clarencon F, Chueh JY, Puri AS, Bogdanov AA Jr: Imaging inflammation in cerebrovascular disease. Stroke 2015;46:2991–2997.
95 Liebeskind DS, Feldmann E: Imaging of cerebrovascular disorders: precision medicine and the collaterome. Ann N Y Acad Sci 2016;1366:40–48.
96 Feldmann E, Liebeskind DS: Developing precision stroke imaging. Front Neurol 2014;5:29.

David S. Liebeskind, MD
Neuroscience Research Building
635 Charles E Young Drive South, Suite 225
Los Angeles, CA 90095–7334 (USA)
E-Mail davidliebeskind@yahoo.com

Kim JS, Caplan LR, Wong KS (eds): Intracranial Atherosclerosis: Pathophysiology, Diagnosis and Treatment.
Front Neurol Neurosci. Basel, Karger, 2016, vol 40, pp 21–33 (DOI: 10.1159/000448267)

Pathological Characteristics

Xiang-Yan Chen[a] · Mark Fisher[b]

[a]Division of Neurology, Department of Medicine and Therapeutics, Prince of Wales Hospital, Shatin, New Territory, Hong Kong, China; [b]Departments of Neurology and Pathology & Laboratory Medicine, University of California, Irvine, Calif., USA

Abstract

Within the intracranial vasculature, atherosclerosis occurs in two distinctive patterns: (1) in Western populations who have severe extracranial and systemic atherosclerosis, the severity of intracranial involvement is consistently less than that within extracranial arteries; and (2) in Asians, Africans, and Hispanics, who often have isolated intracranial arterial disease that is found to be more often accompanied by brain infarction than comparable extracranial atherosclerotic disease. Compared to coronary and extracranial carotid atherosclerosis, intracranial atherosclerosis has distinct pathological characteristics compared to that of extracranial arteries. Intracranial atherosclerosis (ICAS) had been understudied due to the relative inaccessibility of cerebral artery specimens under current treatment strategies. Acquiring post-mortem cerebral vessel specimens for histology processing is the most direct method to analyze the pathological characteristics of ICAS, in order to analyze both lumen stenosis and plaque components contributing to brain infarctions. The developments in high resolution magnetic resonance imaging (HRMRI) make it feasible to assess human ICAS in vivo. It is nevertheless challenging to understand vessel wall changes within brain vasculature demonstrated on HRMRI, as well as to identify biomarkers for stroke risk stratification and treatment strategy modification. Knowledge about intracranial atherosclerosis remains limited due to lack of human arterial specimens, and the development of proper animal models of human cerebral atherosclerosis is necessary to explore the pathogenesis of intracranial atherosclerosis and to assess various strategies preventing or treating ICAS-related stroke.

Atherosclerosis involves multiple arteries throughout the body, including the aorta, coronary arteries, and the limb arteries. Within the intracranial vasculature, atherosclerosis occurs in two separate patterns: (1) in Western populations who have severe extracranial and systemic atherosclerosis [1–6], the severity of which is consistently less than that of the extracranial arteries; and (2) in Asians, Africans, and Hispanics who often have isolated intracranial arterial disease with little evidence of extracranial, coronary or systemic disease. Similar to coronary or carotid artery atherosclerosis, conventional risk factors [7–12] such as age [13], gender, hypertension, diabetes mellitus, hyperlipidemia and cigarette smoking, may account for the occurrence of intracranial atherosclerosis. It remains unclear, whether race-ethnicity is an independent risk factor of intracranial atherosclerosis (ICAS) or is confounded by differences in stroke risk factors among different ethnic groups.

Atherosclerosis is a lifetime illness evolving slowly over many years [14], beginning with inflammatory reactions and endothelial injury. Platelets gather at sites of endothelial disruption, followed by smooth muscle proliferation and thickening of the arterial wall. Although cholesterol accumulation in the endothelial cells of the arterial wall influences the course and maturation of atherosclerosis [15], the process of atherosclerosis is a complex interaction of cellular events [16] involving intercellular messengers, shear stress, elevated or modified low-density lipoproteins (LDL), free radicals, and vascular risk factors [17]. The cellular contributors to plaque development include monocytes/macrophages, endothelial cells, smooth muscle cells, and, to a lesser degree, lymphocytes and platelets. Circulating monocytes and later macrophages precipitate the formation of early plaque with foam cells, which leads to plaque growth and maturation.

Hemodynamic factors also influence the atherosclerotic process in determining the location of early plaques and subsequently contributing to their eventual destabilization [18]. Within the cerebral vasculature, the origin of the internal carotid artery (ICA) is the most frequent site for severe atherosclerosis in subjects of European ancestry [19], whereas intracranial arteries, especially the first portion (M-1 segment) of middle cerebral artery (MCA), are most commonly affected among persons of African or Asian heritage [8, 20–24]. In the vertebrobasilar system, plaques are most commonly found at the origin of the vertebral artery (VA) and in the proximal portion of the basilar artery (BA).

Compared to extracranial carotid atherosclerosis, ICAS has been understudied due to the relative inaccessibility of specimens. Intracranial vessels have a thinner media, less abundant adventitia, and fewer elastic fibers compared to extracranial arteries of similar size [25] (fig. 1). Vessel wall metabolism of intracranial arteries is distinct from that of extracranial arteries [25], suggesting that ICAS may demonstrate distinct pathological characteristics from coronary or carotid artery atherosclerosis. To delineate the pathology of ICAS, acquiring post-mortem brain vessel specimens for histology processing is crucial [10, 26–28]. A complete examination of the brain vasculature should include the entire ICA, MCA, VA and the circle of Willis (fig. 2). Pathological examination should include gross (macroscopic) examination using the method of Baker et al. [26]. The narrowest parts of the individual arteries should then be taken for histological sectioning (microscopic examination). The presence of thrombotic or embolic occlusion and ulceration should also be recorded. During the process, caution should be taken to ensure perpendicular cutting and embedding. Careful use of correct terminology is a requirement [29].

During the 1960s, several autopsy studies were performed in exploring the distribution and natural history of ICAS [30–33]. A large-scale autopsy study of asymptomatic cohorts extending to patients in their 10th decade of life revealed intracranial atherosclerotic changes occurring from the first to second decade and progressing with age [30–32]. Compared to the relatively linear progression of aortic atherogenesis, ICAS increased more slowly initially and paralleled aortic lesions. Advanced atherosclerotic lesions were almost nonexistent up to the fourth decade [33]. Increased activity of antioxidant enzymes in intracranial arteries may contribute to their greater resistance to atherogenesis; with increasing age intracranial arteries respond with accelerated atherosclerosis probably because their antioxidant protection decreases relatively more than that of extracranial arteries [34]. In Japan, a nation-wide study [35] in 1988 examined atherosclerosis in autopsied patients (from 1 month to 39 years old). This study showed that ICAS occurred later and was less extensive than aortic or

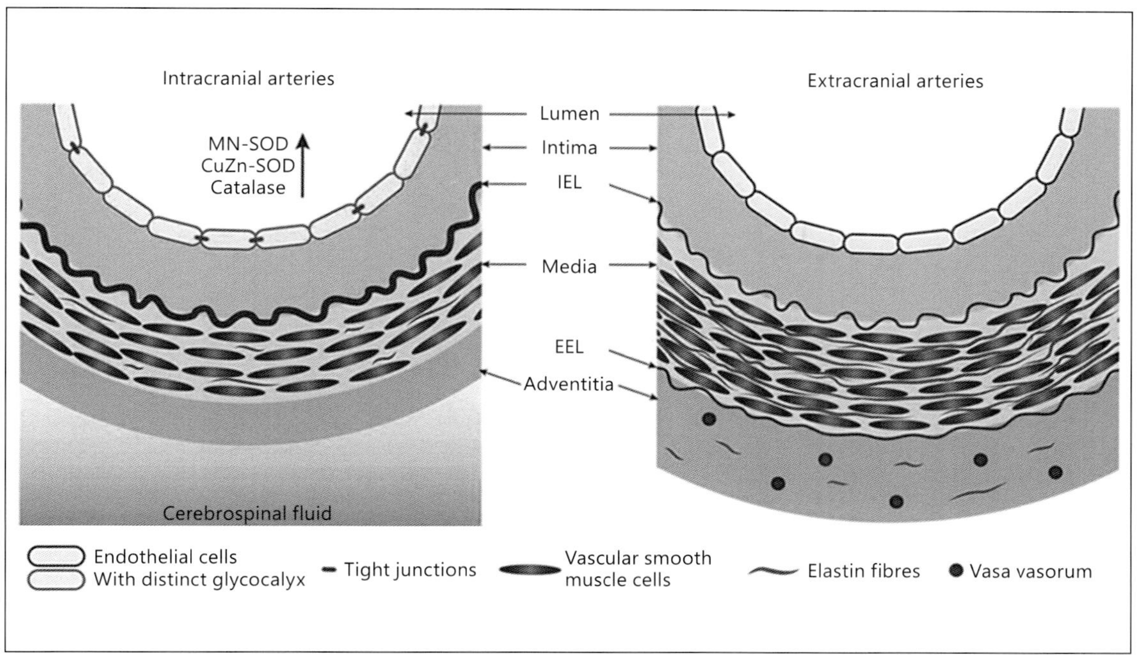

Fig. 1. Major structural characteristics of intracranial and extracranial arteries. Intracranial arteries tend to be muscular arteries with a thin media and adventitia, few elastic medial fibers, thicker and denser internal elastic lamina (IEL), and lacking external elastic lamina (EEL) and vasa vasorum. With permission [91].

coronary artery disease. A later autopsy study among Chinese individuals showed that the extent of ICA was much more severe, while atherosclerotic narrowing of the extracranial ICA was less severe, than that shown in white and Japanese populations [10].

The distribution of atherosclerosis within the brain vasculature shown by early autopsy studies is also consistent with current knowledge from recent epidemiologic and clinical studies [8, 23, 36, 37]. Overall, American and European studies showed a similar pattern: The ICA and intracranial VA were most commonly affected, followed by the BA, MCA, posterior cerebral artery (PCA), and anterior cerebral artery (ACA) [30, 38, 39]. The MCA was most often involved in Asians, followed by the ICA, BA, VA, PCA, and ACA [36, 40]. In all cohorts, cerebellar and communicating arteries were rarely affected. Atherosclerosis of the intracranial ICA was observed mainly in the cavernous and supraclinoid segments [38, 41]. The BA was commonly affected in the upper and lower regions, and less affected in the mid-basilar region [26].

Atherosclerotic plaques consist of cells, connective tissue extracellular matrix, and intra- and extracellular lipid deposits. The proportion of these three components varies in different atherosclerotic plaques, which affects plaque stability (fig. 3) and give rise to a wide spectrum of lesions [42–44]: (1) The so-called fatty streaks are characterized by adhesion of monocytes to the endothelium and migration to the subendothelial potions of the arterial wall [17] in the aorta and the coronary arteries of adolescents and young adults; (2) With increasing age, fatty streaks are

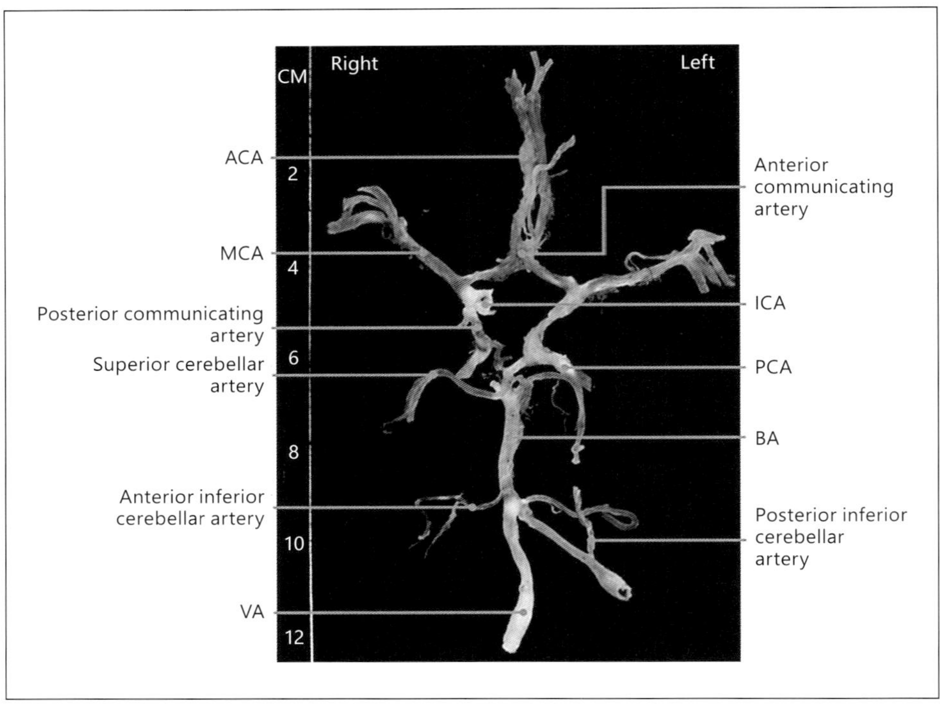

Fig. 2. Circle of Willis from a 90-year-old subject. Atherosclerotic lesions are identified by white vessels, and non-diseased arteries appear transparent. This case shows prominent atherosclerosis in internal carotid, vertebral, basilar, middle cerebral, and posterior cerebral arteries. With permission [91].

transformed into fibrous plaques consisting of a core of cellular debris, free extracellular lipid, and cholesterol crystals under a 'cap' of foam cells, transformed smooth muscle cells, lymphocytes, and connective tissue [17]; (3) The most advanced stage of atherosclerosis is the complicated lesion, which includes calcification, hemosiderin deposition, and lumen surface disruption. Coronary artery atherosclerosis has been well-studied and rupture-prone plaques, the so-called 'vulnerable plaques', are described as having a thin fibrous cap and a large lipid core, which may lead to acute coronary syndromes [44]. For extracranial carotid atherosclerosis, the procedure of carotid endarterectomy provides specimens to examine the pathology and components of carotid atherosclerotic plaques [45]. Conventional pathologic and imaging markers of plaque vulnerability include carotid artery intima/media thickness (IMT), status of fibrous caps, erosion or ulceration, status of the lipid core, intraplaque hemorrhage or neovascularization, thrombus, extent of plaque inflammation, and microembolic signals detected by transcranial Doppler [46–48].

To help define pathological characteristics of intracranial atherosclerosis, we searched the literature for relevant histology information. In Caucasians, Daemen et al. [25] screened 283 circles of Willis segments from 18 asymptomatic elderly individuals (mean age, 70.2 years) to investigate the basic structural features of intracranial arteries (ICA, MCA, VA, and BA) including the smaller arteries (ACA, PCA, and cerebellar and communicating arteries). This study reported an intermediate phenotype sharing structural features of both the larger extracranial and the small-

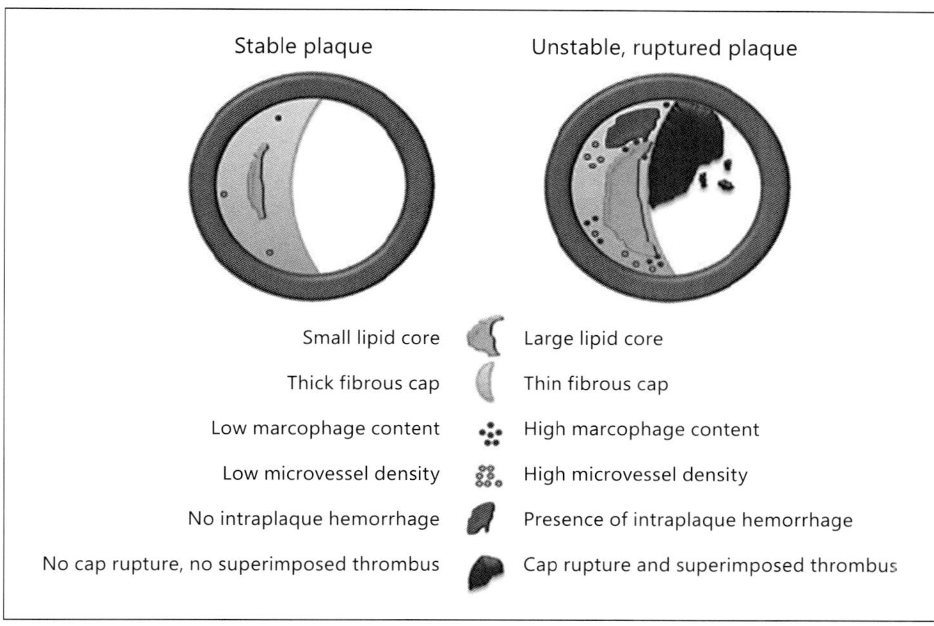

Fig. 3. Schematic overview of a stable atherosclerotic plaque (left) and an unstable atherosclerotic plaque (right). With permission [92].

Table 1. The morphological features of plaques associated and not associated with infarcts in the MCA territory. With permission [93]

	Plaques associated with infarct (n = 46)	Plaques not associated with infarct (n = 65)	p value	95% confidence interval
Degree of area stenosis, %	62.2±16.8	52.4±10.5	0.001	−15.4 to −4.19
Fibrous cap	1.59±0.83	1.46±0.69	0.403	−0.42 to 0.17
Lipid core	2.48±0.91	1.98±0.82	0.004	−0.83 to −0.16
Intraplaque hemorrhage	14/46	10/65	0.066	0.958 to 6.045
Intraplaque neovasculature	13/46	5/65	0.008	1.549 to 14.423
Intraplaque thrombus	7/46	1/65	0.008	1.361 to 96.932
Intraplaque calcification	16/46	15/65	0.202	0.770 to 4.107
CD45RO	2.38±0.78	1.79±0.81	0.007	−0.968 to 0.153
CD68	3.07±0.64	2.58±0.70	0.009	−0.849 to −0.130

er intracranial arteries, such as the lack of vasa vasorum and an external elastic lamina and only a few medial elastic fibers compared with extracranial arteries (table 1). The study also detected mainly early lesions (63%) and only a few advanced atherosclerotic lesions (15%), within which calcifications were rare and macrophage load was relatively low, consistent with a previous study [25]: 0.9 ± 0.7% CD68 positivity per plaque area compared with 1.8 ± 2.4% in coronary arteries [49]. In 1966, Moossy et al. [7] also reported that hemorrhage, ulceration, and calcification in intracranial plaques were much less frequent as compared to extracranial atherosclerotic disease.

Table 2. Data from this review on the basic characteristics of the large intracranial arteries of 18 asymptomatic patients. With permission [91]

	ICA	VA	MCA	BA
Type of lesion, % (n/N)				
Early	57 (17/30)	54 (15/28)	68 (19/28)	75 (24/32)
Advanced	33 (10/30)	25 (7/28)	25 (7/28)	16 (5/32)
High content of elastin fibers, % (n/N)	37 (11/30)	43 (12/28)	29 (8/28)	13 (4/32)
Continuous EEL, % (n/N)	17 (5/30)	79 (22/28)	21 (6/28)	9 (3/32)
Calcification, % (n/N)	20 (6/30)	18 (5/28)	14 (4/28)	9 (3/32)
Vasa vasorum, % (n/N)	53 (16/30)	43 (12/28)	11 (3/28)	16 (5/32)
Macrophages (mean ± SD), %	0.9±0.7	0.4±0.5	0.8±0.7	0.9±0.9

In a recent study, eight subjects with a history of stroke had atherosclerotic lesions present in seven basilar arteries, with a mean estimated stenosis of 34% [50]; lumenal thrombus with disrupted fibrous cap was seen in 1 lesion, neovascularity and calcification were seen in 1 lesion, mild to moderate inflammation was seen in 3 lesions, and necrotic core was present in 4/7 lesions (with one plaque rupture).

Among Asian populations (based on a series of Chinese autopsy adults, mean age, 74.7 years; range, 46–99 years), Chen et al. [51] reported that 69 MCAs out of 152 had more than 40% cross-sectional area luminal narrowing, among which calcification was detected in nearly 30% of atherosclerotic lesions and intraplaque hemorrhage in 20% of lesions. They also found that in addition to lumen stenosis, the percentage of lipid core and intraplaque neovasculature played a key role in leading to clinical ischemic events [52] (table 2); this partly verified the previously hypothesized stroke mechanisms caused by intracranial atherosclerosis [53]. Narrowing of the involved vessel leads to reduced blood flow supplying brain tissue [14], a major mechanism of ischemic stroke related to ICAS [53]. Moreover, vulnerable plaques (those with a large lipid core, intraplaque hemorrhage, or a thin or ruptured fibrous cap) may be prone to rupture, exposing the thrombogenic core to tissue and clotting factors, resulting in thrombus that either occludes the artery locally or embolizes distally; note that artery-to-artery embolism has been verified in stroke patients by multiple clinical studies using TCD monitoring [54–58]. Thirdly, unique to ICAS, plaque extension over small penetrating artery ostia (also known as branch atheromatous disease) [53, 59] results in reduced blood flow in the penetrators, leading to single subcortical infarctions [60].

In clinical practice, current imaging techniques such as CT angiography, digital subtraction angiography, and magnetic resonance angiography (MRA) are of limited utility in the diagnosis of intracranial arterial disease, because they show only the arterial lumen status of intracranial vessels [61]. These methods may underestimate the presence of intracranial arterial pathology because of the presence of non-occlusive atherosclerotic disease (due to arterial remodeling). Detailed visualization of vessel wall changes and the ability to derive information about plaque composition may be clinically important, because rupture of a non-occlusive plaque can potentially cause ischemic stroke [53]. Compared to carotid artery disease, a key factor that complicates detection of intracranial arterial pathology is the smaller diameter of the cerebral arteries, ranging from 2 to 3 mm proximally to 1 mm more distally [25].

The advent of high resolution MRI (3.0T or 7.0T) has been a major advance in image resolution, making it potentially feasible to yield excellent visualization of vessel wall changes by modi-

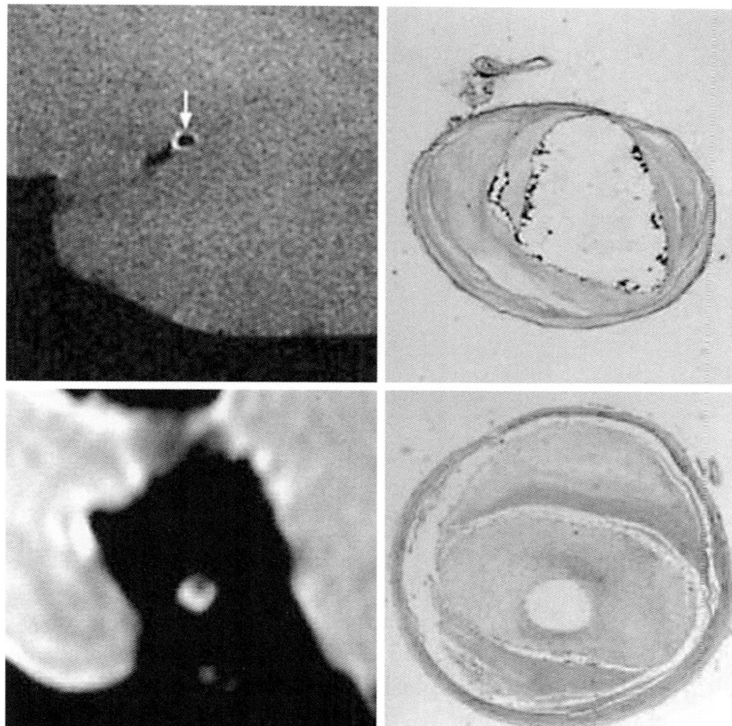

Fig. 4. Examples of the plaques leading to >30% (upper row) and >50% (lower row) stenosis in MCA, corresponding images in MRI T1 sequence (left) and in histopathology (right). With barium distending the artery lumen appears dark and vessel wall appears bright in T1 sequence. With permission [94].

fied scanning techniques [62–64]. Clinical HRMRI studies in recent years have demonstrated the ability of HRMRI vessel wall imaging for quantitative measurement of plaque burden or vessel wall area [65–67]. This technique is more accurate than lumen stenosis in reflecting the degree of intracranial arterial stenosis, especially in the case of non-stenotic atherosclerotic disease. In addition, evaluating thickness of the fibrous cap or identifying intraplaque hemorrhage or lipid component by HRMRI vessel wall imaging has the potential to indicate whether intracranial atherosclerotic plaques are vulnerable [28, 68]. This assumes that intracranial atherosclerosis pathophysiology parallels that in the carotid artery [25, 25]. Histologic validation of HRMRI findings on intracranial vessel walls is needed to confirm the validity of HRMRI as a useful tool for stroke risk stratification and treatment strategy medication.

Pathological data from post-mortem brain artery specimens provide the basis to compare plaque morphology to corresponding vessel wall changes on in-vivo HRMRI. In a histology-MRI comparative study, Chen et al. [27] adopted 1.5T MRI to scan the cross-sections of bilateral MCAs in a series of Chinese autopsy adults and showed agreement between ex vivo MRI and histopathology in identifying MCA stenosis (fig. 4), as well as the relationship between MCA stenosis identified by MRI and radiologically- or histopathologically-evident brain infarcts. For example, a hyperintense signal in T1 sequences was shown to be intraplaque hemorrhage by histology (fig. 5) [28]. Compared to 1.5T MRI, 3.0T or even 7.0T HRMRI is a particularly promising tool for studying intracranial arterial disease in-vivo, with enhanced resolution [64, 69]. In one patient with symptomatic left cavernous carotid stenosis, Turan et al. [70]

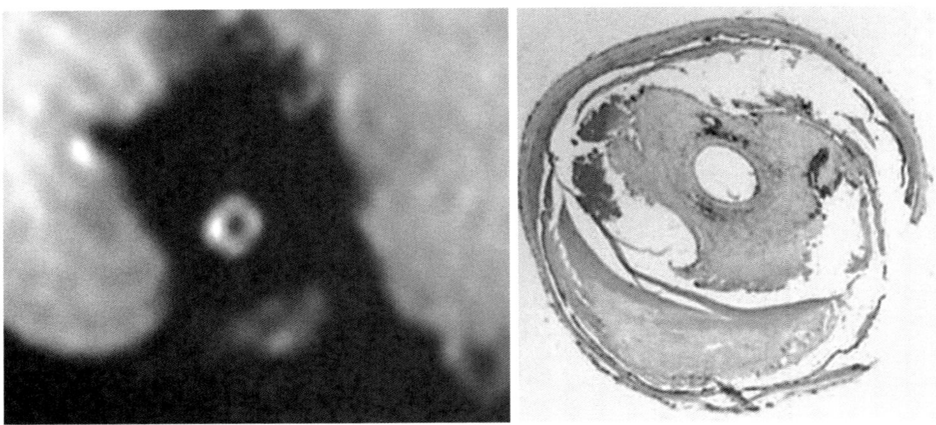

Fig. 5. 1.5T magnetic resonance imaging (MRI) (T1 sequence) shows hyperintense signal; histological demonstration of the haemorrhage within the plaque (haematoxylin and eosin (H&E) staining, magnification 1.6 × 1.6×). With permission [95].

showed a correlation between atherosclerotic plaque components visualized on in-vivo 3T HRMRI images and pathological findings in postmortem artery specimens. Majidi et al. [71]also performed an in vitro comparative study and showed that virtual histology-intravascular ultrasonography and HRMRI are reliable imaging tools to detect atherosclerotic plaques within the intracranial arterial wall, although both imaging modalities have some limitations in accurate characterization of plaque components (fig. 6). A more recent study attempted to adopt 7T HRMRI to establish the clinical indications of HRMRI sequences by scanning five specimens of the circle of Wills [72]. This analysis showed that 7.0T MRI has the capability to identify focal intracranial vessel wall thickening and distinguish areas of different signal intensities spatially corresponding to plaque components within more advanced atherosclerotic plaques (fig. 7). Considering that signal intensity changes on HRMRI vessel wall images have not been well-interpreted, additional studies that further validate signal characteristics will improve in vivo characterization of intracranial atherosclerotic plaques and determine the clinical utility of defining plaque morphology and composition.

The development of proper animal models simulating human cerebral atherosclerosis is required to further explore the pathogenesis of ICAS and to assess various strategies to prevent or treat ICAS-related stroke [73–75]. Various species, including swine, chickens, dogs, rabbits, rats, and monkeys [73–80] have been used to evaluate atherosclerosis in intracranial arteries. Although systemic atherosclerosis can be produced in rabbits taking an atherogenic diet [81] or in Watanabe heritable hyperlipidemic (WHHL) rabbits [82], it is difficult to induce atherosclerosis in intracranial arteries. In homozygous WHHL rabbits that are known to have hypercholesterolemia and severe coronary atherosclerosis, Ito et al. [83] described spontaneously developing cerebral atherosclerosis beginning at 9 months of age. To produce cerebral artery atherosclerosis, additional application of hypertension was more effective than inducing hyperlipidemia alone [82–88], which was found to be successful in a cynomolgus monkey [85]. Aside from high blood pressure, hemodynamic derangement was also found to be effective for the development of fat deposition in cerebral arteries. Yamori et al. [89] successfully produced fat deposition in the posterior commu-

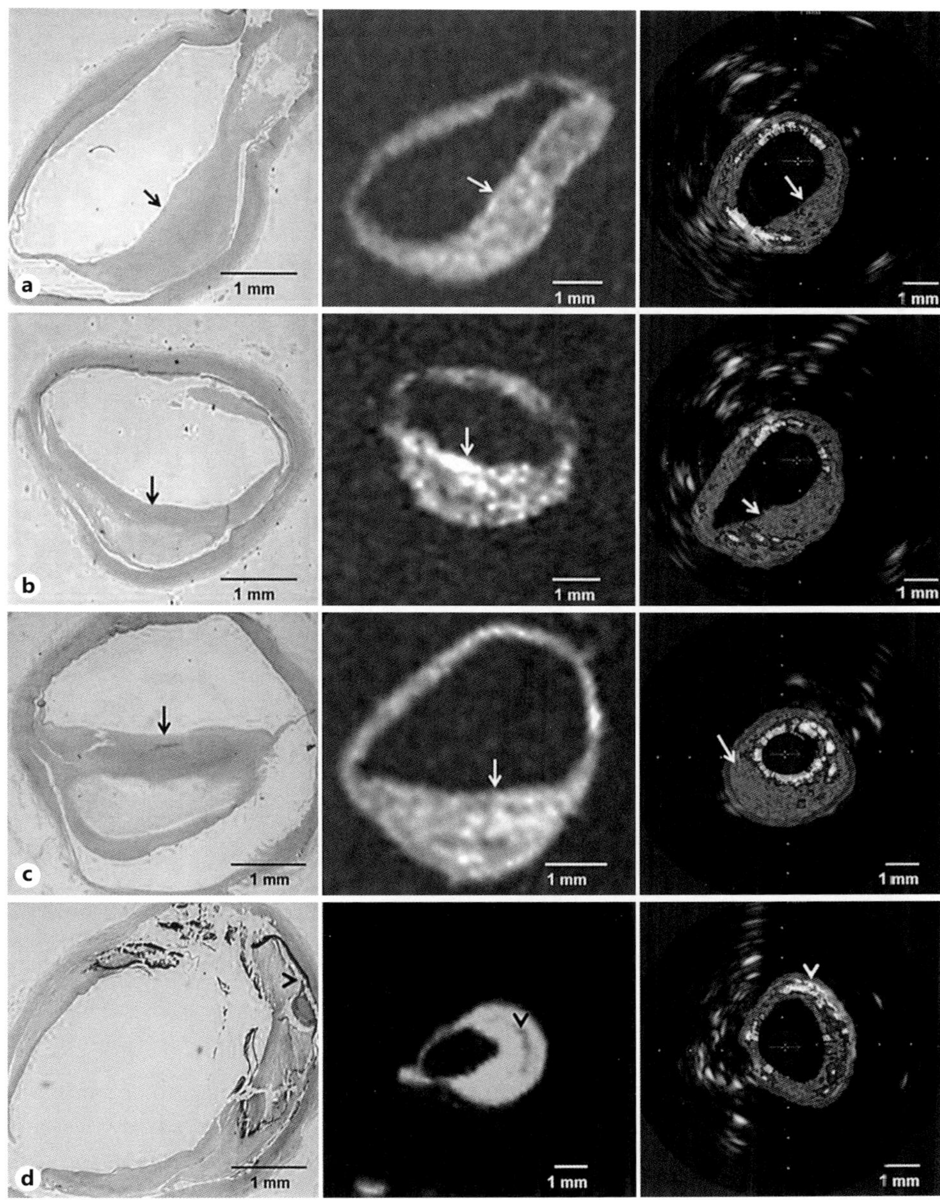

Fig. 6. a–d Four different histopathologic sections of intracranial vessels with atherosclerotic plaque and their corresponding 3D SPACE MR imaging (in the middle) and VH-IVUS (on the right) images. With permission [96]. SPACE = Sampling perfection with application-optimized contrasts by use of different flip angle evolutions; VH-IVUS = virtual histology-intravascular ultrasonography.

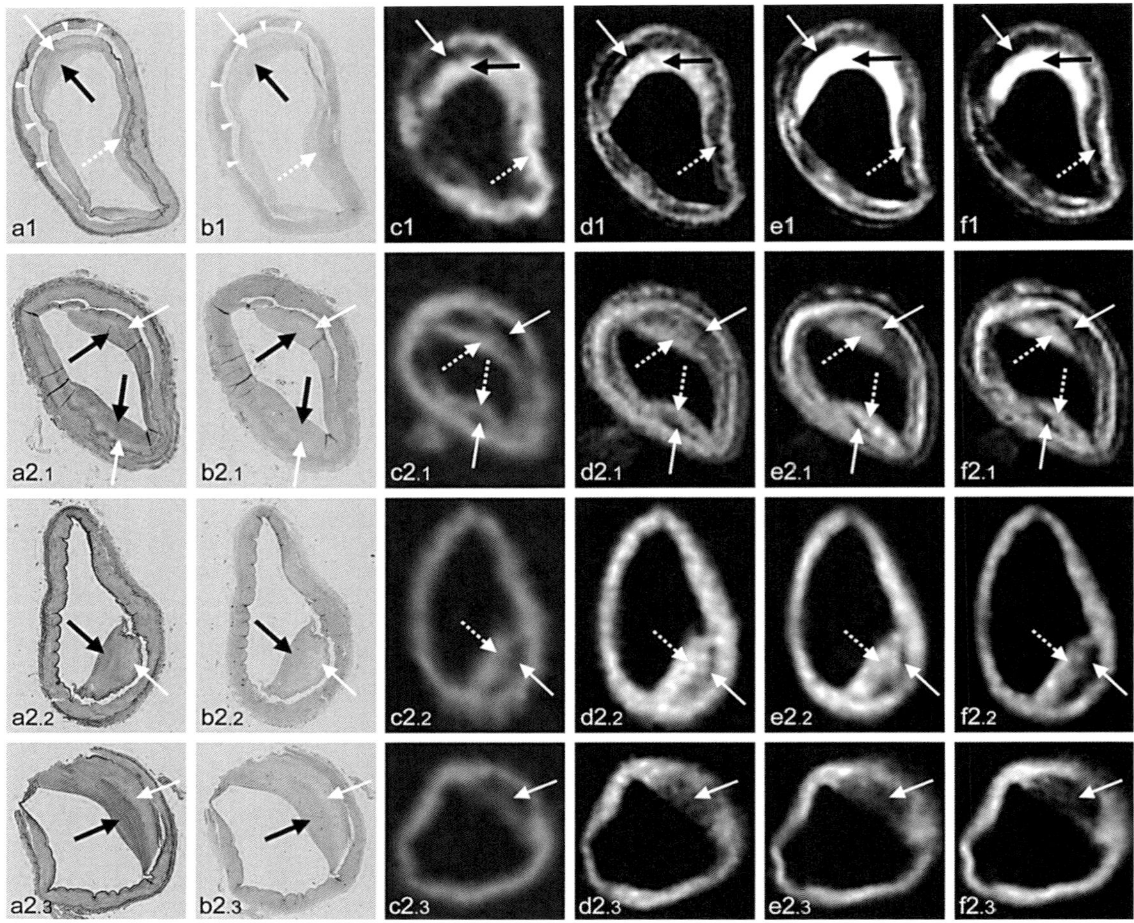

Fig. 7. Four examples of atherosclerotic plaques with corresponding signal heterogeneity on 7T MR images. With permission [97].

nicating arteries in normotensive rats by 10 weeks' feeding with high-fat cholesterol, following ligation of one or both ICAs or the BA.

Successful animal models of cerebral atherosclerosis have shown morphological features of ICAS. In hypertensive WHHL rabbits [82], atherosclerotic lesions developed near the vertebral-basilar arterial confluence and the circle of Willis 6 months after hypertension-inducing surgery; the lesions remained less severe than in the aorta and coronary arteries and also had qualitative morphologic differences from extracranial atherosclerosis. Another study of experimental rabbits also produced early lesions of ICAS [84] with widespread thickening and contraction in almost all intracranial small arteries. Imai et al. [78] investigated diet-induced cerebral atherosclerosis in swine and observed the progression of lesions from proliferative to atheromatous stages. Animal models can also be used to study stroke mechanisms. For example, an animal model of cerebral athero-embolism was established by injecting human atheromatous material into the brain vasculature of rabbits via the common carotid artery [90]. Signs of neurologic deficit such as motor dysfunction were seen in some surviving animals; ischemic lesions were predominantly localized to ipsilateral cortical and subcortical areas within the territory of the MCA.

Acknowledgements

Supported by NIH R01 NS 20989 (Dr. Fisher).

References

1 Gorelick PB, Mazzone T: Plasma lipids and stroke. J Cardiovasc Risk 1999;6: 217–221.
2 Mathur KS, Kashyap SK, Kumar V: Correlation of the extent and severity of atherosclerosis in the coronary and cerebral arteries. Circulation 1963;27:929–934.
3 Sadoshima S, Kurozumi T, Tanaka K, Ueda K, Takeshita M, Hirota Y, et al: Cerebral and aortic atherosclerosis in hisayama, japan. Atherosclerosis 1980; 36:117–126.
4 McGarry P, Solberg LA, Guzman MA, Strong JP: Cerebral atherosclerosis in New Orleans. Comparisons of lesions by age, sex, and race. Lab Invest 1985;52: 533–539.
5 Gorelick PB: Distribution of atherosclerotic cerebrovascular lesions. Effects of age, race, and sex. Stroke 1993;24:I16–I19; discussion I20–I21.
6 Napoli C, Witztum JL, de Nigris F, Palumbo G, D'Armiento FP, Palinski W: Intracranial arteries of human fetuses are more resistant to hypercholesterolemia-induced fatty streak formation than extracranial arteries. Circulation 1999;99:2003–2010.
7 Moossy J: Cerebral infarcts and the lesions of intracranial and extracranial atherosclerosis. Arch Neurol 1966;14:124–128.
8 Caplan LR, Gorelick PB, Hier DB: Race, sex and occlusive cerebrovascular disease: a review. Stroke 1986;17:648–655.
9 Moossy J: Pathology of cerebral atherosclerosis. Influence of age, race, and gender. Stroke 1993;24:I22–I23; I31–I32.
10 Leung SY, Ng TH, Yuen ST, Lauder IJ, Ho FC: Pattern of cerebral atherosclerosis in hong kong chinese. Severity in intracranial and extracranial vessels. Stroke 1993;24:779–786.
11 Sacco RL, Kargman DE, Zamanillo MC: Race-ethnic differences in stroke risk factors among hospitalized patients with cerebral infarction: the northern Manhattan stroke study. Neurology 1995;45: 659–663.
12 Ingall TJ, Homer D, Baker HL Jr, Kottke BA, O'Fallon WM, Whisnant JP: Predictors of intracranial carotid artery atherosclerosis. Duration of cigarette smoking and hypertension are more powerful than serum lipid levels. Arch Neurol 1991;48:687–691.
13 Resch JA, Okabe N, Loewenson RB, Kimoto K, Katsuki S, Baker AB: Pattern of vessel involvement in cerebral atherosclerosis. A comparative study between a japanese and minnesota population. J Atheroscler Res 1969;9:239–250.
14 Fuster V, Badimon JJ, Chesebro JH: Atherothrombosis: Mechanisms and clinical therapeutic approaches. Vasc Med 1998; 3:231–239.
15 Yatsu FM, Fisher M: Atherosclerosis: Current concepts on pathogenesis and interventional therapies. Ann Neurol 1989;26:3–12.
16 Ross R: Atherosclerosis – an inflammatory disease. N Engl J Med 1999;340: 115–126.
17 Navab M, Fogelman AM, Berliner JA, Territo MC, Demer LL, Frank JS, et al: Pathogenesis of atherosclerosis. Am J Cardiol 1995;76:18C–23C.
18 Zarins CK, Giddens DP, Bharadvaj BK, Sottiurai VS, Mabon RF, Glagov S: Carotid bifurcation atherosclerosis. Quantitative correlation of plaque localization with flow velocity profiles and wall shear stress. Circ Res 1983;53:502–514.
19 Fisher CM GI, Okabe N, White PD: Atherosclerosis of the carotid and vertebral arteries-extracranial and intracranial. J Neuropathol Exp Neurol 1965;24:455–476.
20 Bogousslavsky J, Barnett HJ, Fox AJ, Hachinski VC, Taylor W: Atherosclerotic disease of the middle cerebral artery. Stroke 1986;17:1112–1120.
21 Feldmann E, Daneault N, Kwan E, Ho KJ, Pessin MS, Langenberg P, et al: Chinese-white differences in the distribution of occlusive cerebrovascular disease. Neurology 1990;40:1541–1545.
22 Wityk RJ, Lehman D, Klag M, Coresh J, Ahn H, Litt B: Race and sex differences in the distribution of cerebral atherosclerosis. Stroke 1996;27:1974–1980.
23 Wong KS, Li H, Chan YL, Ahuja A, Lam WW, Wong A, et al: Use of transcranial doppler ultrasound to predict outcome in patients with intracranial large-artery occlusive disease. Stroke 2000;31:2541–2647.
24 Huang YN, Gao S, Li SW, Huang Y, Li JF, Wong KS, et al: Vascular lesions in chinese patients with transient ischemic attacks. Neurology 1997;48:524–525.
25 Ritz K, Denswil NP, Stam OC, van Lieshout JJ, Daemen MJ: Cause and mechanisms of intracranial atherosclerosis. Circulation 2014;130:1407–1414.
26 Baker AB, Iannone A: Cerebrovascular disease. I. The large arteries of the circle of willis. Neurology 1959;9:321–332.
27 Chen XY, Lam WW, Ng HK, Zhao HL, Wong KS: Diagnostic accuracy of mri for middle cerebral artery stenosis: a postmortem study. J Neuroimaging 2006;16:318–322.
28 Chen XY, Wong KS, Lam WW, Ng HK: High signal on t1 sequence of magnetic resonance imaging confirmed to be intraplaque haemorrhage by histology in middle cerebral artery. Int J Stroke 2014; 9:E19.
29 Velican D, Anghelescu M, Petrescu C, Velican C: Method dependent limits in a study on the natural history of coronary and cerebral atherosclerosis. Med Interne 1982;20:215–229.
30 Resch JA, Baker AB: Etiologic mechanisms in cerebral atherosclerosis. Preliminary study of 3,839 cases. Arch Neurol 1964;10:617–628.
31 Lascelles RG, Burrows EH: Occlusion of the middle cerebral artery. Brain 1965; 88:85–96.
32 Silverstein A, Hollin S: Internal carotid vs middle cerebral artery occlusions; clinical differences. Arch Neurol 1965; 12:468–471.

33 Mathur KS, Kashyap SK, Mathur SC: Distribution and severity of atherosclerosis of aorta, coronary and cerebral arteries in persons dying without morphologic evidence of atherosclerotic catastrophe in North India. A study of 900 autopsies. J Assoc Physicians India 1968;16:113–122.
34 D'Armiento FP, Bianchi A, de Nigris F, Capuzzi DM, D'Armiento MR, Crimi G, et al: Age-related effects on atherogenesis and scavenger enzymes of intracranial and extracranial arteries in men without classic risk factors for atherosclerosis. Stroke 2001;32:2472–2479.
35 Tanaka K, Masuda J, Imamura T, Sueishi K, Nakashima T, Sakurai I, et al: A nation-wide study of atherosclerosis in infants, children and young adults in Japan. Atherosclerosis 1988;72:143–156.
36 Gorelick PB, Caplan LR, Hier DB, Parker SL, Patel D: Racial differences in the distribution of anterior circulation occlusive disease. Neurology 1984;34:54–59.
37 Wong KS, Ng PW, Tang A, Liu R, Yeung V, Tomlinson B: Prevalence of asymptomatic intracranial atherosclerosis in high-risk patients. Neurology 2007;68:2035–2038.
38 Alkan O, Kizilkilic O, Yildirim T, Atalay H: Intracranial cerebral artery stenosis with associated coronary artery and extracranial carotid artery stenosis in Turkish patients. Eur J Radiol 2009;71:450–455.
39 Moossy J: Development of cerebral atherosclerosis in various age groups. Neurology 1959;9:569–574.
40 Wong KS, Huang YN, Gao S, Lam WW, Chan YL, Kay R: Intracranial stenosis in chinese patients with acute stroke. Neurology 1998;50:812–813.
41 Bae HJ, Lee J, Park JM, Kwon O, Koo JS, Kim BK, et al: Risk factors of intracranial cerebral atherosclerosis among asymptomatics. Cerebrovasc Dis 2007;24:355–360.
42 Fuster V, Fayad ZA, Badimon JJ: Acute coronary syndromes: biology. Lancet 1999;353(suppl 2):SII5–SII9.
43 Falk E, Shah PK, Fuster V: Coronary plaque disruption. Circulation 1995;92:657–671.
44 Fuster V: Lewis A. Conner memorial lecture. Mechanisms leading to myocardial infarction: insights from studies of vascular biology. Circulation 1994;90:2126–2146.
45 Yuan C, Miller ZE, Cai J, Hatsukami T: Carotid atherosclerotic wall imaging by MRI. Neuroimaging Clin N Am 2002;12:391–401, vi.
46 Nighoghossian N, Derex L, Douek P: The vulnerable carotid artery plaque: current imaging methods and new perspectives. Stroke 2005;36:2764–2772.
47 Bornstein NM, Norris JW: The unstable carotid plaque. Stroke 1989;20:1104–1106.
48 Bornstein NM, Krajewski A, Lewis AJ, Norris JW: Clinical significance of carotid plaque hemorrhage. Arch Neurol 1990;47:958–959.
49 Narula J, Nakano M, Virmani R, Kolodgie FD, Petersen R, Newcomb R, et al: Histopathologic characteristics of atherosclerotic coronary disease and implications of the findings for the invasive and noninvasive detection of vulnerable plaques. J Am Coll Cardiol 2013;61:1041–1051.
50 Labadzhyan A, Csiba L, Narula N, Zhou J, Narula J, Fisher M: Histopathologic evaluation of basilar artery atherosclerosis. J Neurol Sci 2011;307:97–99.
51 Chen XY, Wong KS, Lam WW, Zhao HL, Ng HK: Middle cerebral artery atherosclerosis: histological comparison between plaques associated with and not associated with infarct in a postmortem study. Cerebrovasc Dis 2008;25:74–80.
52 Chen XY, Wong KS, Lam WW, Zhao HL, Ng HK: Middle cerebral artery atherosclerosis: histological comparison between plaques associated with and not associated with infarct in a postmortem study. Cerebrovasc Dis 2007;25:74–80.
53 Holmstedt CA, Turan TN, Chimowitz MI: Atherosclerotic intracranial arterial stenosis: risk factors, diagnosis, and treatment. Lancet Neurol 2013;12:1106–1114.
54 Ogata J, Masuda J, Yutani C, Yamaguchi T: Mechanisms of cerebral artery thrombosis: a histopathological analysis on eight necropsy cases. J Neurol Neurosurg Psychiatry 1994;57:17–21.
55 Droste DW, Junker K, Hansberg T, Dittrich R, Ritter M, Ringelstein EB: Circulating microemboli in 33 patients with intracranial arterial stenosis. Cerebrovasc Dis 2002;13:26–30.
56 Wong KS, Gao S, Chan YL, Hansberg T, Lam WW, Droste DW, et al: Mechanisms of acute cerebral infarctions in patients with middle cerebral artery stenosis: a diffusion-weighted imaging and microemboli monitoring study. Ann Neurol 2002;52:74–81.
57 Gao S, Wong KS, Hansberg T, Lam WW, Droste DW, Ringelstein EB: Microembolic signal predicts recurrent cerebral ischemic events in acute stroke patients with middle cerebral artery stenosis. Stroke 2004;35:2832–2836.
58 Segura T, Serena J, Molins A, Davalos A: Clusters of microembolic signals: a new form of cerebral microembolism presentation in a patient with middle cerebral artery stenosis. Stroke 1998;29:722–724.
59 Chung JW, Kim BJ, Sohn CH, Yoon BW, Lee SH: Branch atheromatous plaque: a major cause of lacunar infarction (high-resolution mri study). Cerebrovasc Dis Extra 2012;2:36–44.
60 Kim BJ, Lee DH, Kang DW, Kwon SU, Kim JS: Branching patterns determine the size of single subcortical infarctions. Stroke 2014;45:1485–1487.
61 Leng X, Wong KS, Liebeskind DS: Evaluating intracranial atherosclerosis rather than intracranial stenosis. Stroke 2014;45:645–651.
62 Bodle JD, Feldmann E, Swartz RH, Rumboldt Z, Brown T, Turan TN: High-resolution magnetic resonance imaging: an emerging tool for evaluating intracranial arterial disease. Stroke 2013;44:287–292.
63 Mossa-Basha M, Hwang WD, De Havenon A, Hippe D, Balu N, Becker KJ, et al: Multicontrast high-resolution vessel wall magnetic resonance imaging and its value in differentiating intracranial vasculopathic processes. Stroke 2015;46:1567–1573.
64 Dieleman N, van der Kolk AG, Zwanenburg JJ, Harteveld AA, Biessels GJ, Luijten PR, et al: Imaging intracranial vessel wall pathology with magnetic resonance imaging: current prospects and future directions. Circulation 2014;130:192–201.
65 Xu WH, Li ML, Gao S, Ni J, Zhou LX, Yao M, et al: Plaque distribution of stenotic middle cerebral artery and its clinical relevance. Stroke 2011;42:2957–2959.
66 van der Kolk AG, Zwanenburg JJ, Brundel M, Biessels GJ, Visser F, Luijten PR, et al: Intracranial vessel wall imaging at 7.0-t mri. Stroke 2011;42:2478–2484.
67 Li ML, Xu WH, Song L, Feng F, You H, Ni J, et al: Atherosclerosis of middle cerebral artery: evaluation with high-resolution mr imaging at 3t. Atherosclerosis 2009;204:447–452.
68 Xu WH, Li ML, Gao S, Ni J, Yao M, Zhou LX, et al: Middle cerebral artery intraplaque hemorrhage: prevalence and clinical relevance. Ann Neurol 2012;71:195–198.

69 Yuan C, Hatsukami TS, Obrien KD: High-resolution magnetic resonance imaging of normal and atherosclerotic human coronary arteries ex vivo: discrimination of plaque tissue components. J Investig Med 2001;49:491–499.
70 Turan TN, Rumboldt Z, Granholm AC, Columbo L, Welsh CT, Lopes-Virella MF, et al: Intracranial atherosclerosis: Correlation between in-vivo 3t high resolution mri and pathology. Atherosclerosis 2014;237:460–463.
71 Majidi S, Sein J, Watanabe M, Hassan AE, Van de Moortele PF, Suri MF, et al: Intracranial-derived atherosclerosis assessment: an in vitro comparison between virtual histology by intravascular ultrasonography, 7t mri, and histopathologic findings. AJNR Am J Neuroradiol 2013;34:2259–2264.
72 van der Kolk AG, Zwanenburg JJ, Denswil NP, Vink A, Spliet WG, Daemen MJ, et al: Imaging the intracranial atherosclerotic vessel wall using 7t mri: initial comparison with histopathology. AJNR Am J Neuroradiol 2015;36:694–701.
73 Robertson AL Jr, Butkus A, Ehrhart LA, Lewis LA: Experimental arteriosclerosis in dogs. Evaluation of anatomopathological findings. Atherosclerosis 1972; 15:307–325.
74 Suzuki M: Experimental cerebral atherosclerosis in the dog. I. A morphologic study. Am J Pathol 1972;67:387–402.
75 Bhardwaj JR, Kukreja RS, Banerjee AK, Datta BN, Chakravarti RN: A morphological study of experimental cerebral atherosclerosis in rhesus monkeys. Indian J Med Res 1984;79:86–92.
76 Kahn SG, Siller WG: Absence of atherosclerosis in the cerebral arteries of chickens fed an atherogenic diet. Nature 1967;213:720–721.
77 Ratcliffe HL, Luginbuhl H, Pivnik L: Coronary, aortic and cerebral atherosclerosis in swine of 3 age-groups: Implications. Bull World Health Organ 1970;42:225–234.
78 Imai H, Thomas WA: Cerebral atherosclerosis in swine: Role of necrosis in progression of diet-induced lesions from proliferative to atheromatous stage. Exp Mol Pathol 1968;8:330–357.
79 Suzuki M, Fukuuchi Y, Shimazu K, Kim HS, Meyer JS: Cerebral atherosclerosis in the dog. Ii. Cerebral circulation. Arch Pathol 1973;96:14–17.
80 Kato H: [experimental cerebral atherosclerosis in the rabbit. Scanning electron microscopic observation of initial lesion sites]. Fukuoka Igaku Zasshi 1987;78: 532–546.
81 Ooboshi H, Rios CD, Chu Y, Christenson SD, Faraci FM, Davidson BL, et al: Augmented adenovirus-mediated gene transfer to atherosclerotic vessels. Arterioscler Thromb Vasc Biol 1997;17: 1786–1792.
82 Kong J, Tamaki N, Asada M: Early lesions of cerebral atherosclerosis from induced hypertension in watanabe heritable hyperlipidemic rabbits. Kobe J Med Sci 2000;46:87–101.
83 Ito T, Shiomi M: Cerebral atherosclerosis occurs spontaneously in homozygous whhl rabbits. Atherosclerosis 2001;156: 57–66.
84 Zhang T: [an experimental study on cerebral arteriosclerosis]. Zhonghua Shen Jing Jing Shen Ke Za Zhi 1991;24: 228–230, 253.
85 Hollander W, Prusty S, Kemper T, Rosene DL, Moss MB: The effects of hypertension on cerebral atherosclerosis in the cynomolgus monkey. Stroke 1993; 24:1218–1226; discussion 1226–1227.
86 Kato H, Tokunaga O, Watanabe T, Sunaga T: Experimental cerebral atherosclerosis in the rabbit. Scanning electron microscopic study of the initial lesion site. Pathol Res Pract 1991;187:797–805.
87 Kurozumi T, Tanaka K, Yae Y: Hypertension-induced cerebral atherosclerosis in the cholesterol-fed rabbit. Atherosclerosis 1978;30:137–145.
88 Kurozumi T, Imamura T, Tanaka K, Yae Y, Koga S: Permeation and deposition of fibrinogen and low-density lipoprotein in the aorta and cerebral artery of rabbits – immuno-electron microscopic study. Br J Exp Pathol 1984;65:355–364.
89 Yamori Y, Horie R, Sato M, Fukase M: Hemodynamic derangement for the induction of cerebrovascular fat deposition in normotensive rats on a hypercholesterolemic diet. Stroke 1976;4 385–389.
90 Jeynes BJ, Warren BA: Cerebral atheroembolism. An animal model. Stroke 1982;13:312–318.
91 Ritz K, Denswil NP, Stam OC, van Lieshout JJ, Daemen MJ: Cause and mechanisms of intracranial atherosclerosis. Circulation 2014;130:1407–1414.
92 van Lammeren GW, Moll FL, De Borst GJ, de Kleijn DPV, de Vries JPPM, Pasterkamp G: Atherosclerotic plaque biomarkers: beyond the horizon of the vulnerable plaque. Curr Cardiol Rev 2011;7:22–27.
93 Chen XY, Wong KS, Lam WW, Zhao HL, Ng HK: Middle cerebral artery atherosclerosis: histological comparison between plaques associated with and not associated with infarct in a postmortem study. Cerebrovasc Dis 2008;25:74–80.
94 Chen XY, Lam WW, Ng HK, Zhao HL, Wong KS: Diagnostic accuracy of MRI for middle cerebral artery stenosis: a postmortem study. J Neuroimaging 2006;16:318–322.
95 Chen XY, Wong KS, Lam WW, Ng HK: High signal on T1 sequence of magnetic resonance imaging confirmed to be intraplaque haemorrhage by histology in middle cerebral artery. Int J Stroke 2014;9:E19.
96 Majidi S, Sein J, Watanabe M, Hassan AE, Van de Moortele PF, Suri MF, Clark HB, Qureshi AI: Intracranial-derived atherosclerosis assessment: an in vitro comparison between virtual histology by intravascular ultrasonography, 7T MRI, and histopathologic findings. AJNR Am J Neuroradiol 2013;34:2259–2264.
97 van der Kolk AG, Zwanenburg JJ, Denswil NP, Vink A, Spliet WG, Daemen MJ, Visser F, Klomp DW, Luijten PR, Hendrikse J: Imaging the intracranial atherosclerotic vessel wall using 7T MRI: initial comparison with histopathology. AJNR Am J Neuroradiol 2015;36:694–701.

Xiang-Yan Chen, MB, MM, PhD
Division of Neurology, Department of Medicine and Therapeutics
Chinese University of Hong Kong, Prince of Wales Hospital
30-32 Ngan Shing Street
Shatin, New Territory, HKSAR (China)
E-Mail fiona.xy2000@gmail.com

Kim JS, Caplan LR, Wong KS (eds): Intracranial Atherosclerosis: Pathophysiology, Diagnosis and Treatment.
Front Neurol Neurosci. Basel, Karger, 2016, vol 40, pp 34–46 (DOI: 10.1159/000448272)

Epidemiology

Philip Gorelick[a] • Ka Sing Wong[b] • Liping Liu[c]

[a]Department of Translational Science and Molecular Medicine, Michigan State University College of Human Medicine, Mercy Health Hauenstein Neurosciences, Grand Rapids, Mich., USA; [b]Chinese University of Hong Kong, Hong Kong, and [c]Department of Neurology, Beijing Tiantan Hospital, Capital Medical University, Beijing, China

Abstract

Intracranial atherosclerotic occlusive disease is an important and possibly the most common cause of stroke worldwide. Asian, Black and certain Hispanic populations have a high risk of harboring intracranial occlusive disease. In this chapter we review the epidemiology of intracranial occlusive disease by primarily focusing on studies from China, Japan, Korea, and other Asian countries. In addition, we compare and contrast the information from Asian countries with that from North America and related regions. Finally, we explore hypotheses concerning the origin of race-ethnic differences in the distribution of extracranial and intracranial atherosclerotic disease.

Intracranial atherosclerosis (ICAS) is an important cause of stroke worldwide [1–5]. Population groups which are at high risk for ICAS include US blacks, Asians and Hispanics. In the USA, it has been estimated that of the 900,000 estimated stroke or transient ischemic attacks (TIAs) annually, up to 10% are caused by ICAS and recurrence rates in these patients are 15% per year [6]. The frequency of stroke attributable to ICAS in the USA is dwarfed by corresponding statistics from Asian countries. In Chinese populations, ICAS is estimated to account for 33–50% of stroke and >50% of TIAs, in Thailand 47% of stroke, in Korea about 28–60% of stroke, and in Singapore about 48% of stroke [7–10]. The frequency of ICAS is also high in Japan although there is increasing frequency of symptomatic extracranial carotid artery stenosis. In the USA, the relative rate of stroke associated with ICAS is about 5.0 for Hispanics (mostly from Puerto Rico and the Dominican Republic) and 5.85 for blacks compared to whites. As the majority of the world's population is Asian, African or Hispanic, it seems that ICAS is the most common cerebral vascular lesion worldwide [7].

Prior hypotheses to explain racial differences in the distribution of occlusive cerebrovascular disease lesions include, for example, low lipid levels and high blood pressure predisposing to intracranial and intracerebral vascular disease, high lipids and high blood pressure predisposing to extracranial occlusive vascular lesions, and diabetes mellitus and metabolic syndrome for ICAS [1, 2, 8, 11–13]. However, the reason for racial differences in the incidence of ICAS still remains unclear. Attempts to prevent recurrence of stroke events in ICAS have focused mainly on anticoagulant therapy, antiplatelet therapy, revascularization procedures, and other medical therapy [6, 14, 15].

In this chapter, we review the epidemiology of ICAS in China, Japan, Korea and the remainder of Asian countries in which ICAS is prevalent. Ethnic differences observed in the studies from North America and related regions will also be discussed.

China, Japan, Korea and Other Asian Regions (Table 1)

Autopsy Studies

Evidence from autopsy studies has shown that African Americans and Japanese have more ICAS, whereas Caucasians have more extracranial diseases [16–18]. Masuda's autopsy series of 724 patients aged 40 or above, in the community of Hisayama, Japan, showed that ischemic stroke patients had more severe atherosclerosis of the major cerebral arteries than those without stroke or cerebral hemorrhage [19]. A more recent study showed a decrease in ICAS in the recent 28 years, in contrast with unchanged incidence of coronary artery stenosis in Japanese elderly subjects [20]. These findings might be explained by better control of cardiovascular risks.

Comparative data in Chinese populations have been relatively limited. In the early 1990s, among 114 Hong Kong Chinese autopsy patients, ICAS was found to be more severe than that of extracranial atherosclerosis [21]. Both the proximal and distal branches of the intracranial arteries were involved. Hypertension and diabetes mellitus were identified as factors associated only with ICAS, whereas ischemic heart disease was associated with atherosclerosis in both the intracranial and extracranial vessels [21]. In another autopsy study from mainland China, Liu et al. [22] showed that atherosclerotic narrowing of medium sized intracranial arteries and their primary branches was more severe than that found in the extracranial carotid arteries in stroke patients. Another autopsy study from Hong Kong featuring morphological characteristics of middle cerebral artery (MCA) atherosclerosis, luminal stenosis caused by atherosclerotic plaques, percentage of lipid area and presence of intraplaque neovasculature were independent risk factors of MCA territory infarcts [23].

Prevalence of Asymptomatic ICAS in Community-Based Populations

Wong et al. [24] published the first door-to-door study of ICAS in middle-aged, asymptomatic subjects in rural China. Five hundred and ninety villagers aged 40 or above were screened by transcranial Doppler ultrasound (TCD) and 41 subjects (prevalence 6.9%) were found to have ICAS. In a multivariate analysis, the significant risk factors for ICAS were hypertension (OR 2.53; 95% CI 1.12–5.72), glycosuria (OR 3; 1.19–7.97), heart disease (OR 4; 1.39–11.6), and family history of stroke (OR 5.2; 1.38–20). In another community-based study in Southern China involving 1,068 asymptomatic subjects over 50 years of age, MCA stenosis was shown by TCD in 63 subjects (prevalence 5.9%). Male gender, advanced age, hypertension and diabetes mellitus were independent risk factors for MCA stenosis [25]. In a sub-study aiming to determine the relationship between hyperhomocysteinemia and MCA stenosis, it was found that hyperhomocysteinemia was an independent risk factor for MCA stenosis [26].

The prevalence of asymptomatic carotid stenosis in the white population has been estimated at about 2–8% in middle age and elderly populations similar to the prevalence of ICAS in Chinese populations [27]. The presence of ICAS is an independent predictor for survival and recurrent ischemic events [28].

In relation to population based studies, Uehara et al. studied 156 Japanese subjects (37–

Table 1. Summary of clinical studies in asymptomatic and symptomatic ICAS in Asia regions

Study	Study design	Racial	Condition	Assessment	Number (%)	Risk factors/results
Thomas et al. [12], 2003	Cross-sectional (n = 2,202)	Chinese	Asymptomatic in DM patients	TCD	217 (9.9)	HT, albuminuria
Thomas et al. [13], 2004	Cross-sectional (n = 966)	Chinese	Asymptomatic in DM patients	TCD	137 (14.2)	Albuminuria may be related with ICAS in DM patients
Wong et al. [24], 2007	community-based (n = 590)	Chinese	Asymptomatic	TCD	41 (6.9)	HT, glycosuria, IHD, family history of stroke
Huang et al. [25], 2007	community-based (n = 1,068)	Chinese	Asymptomatic	TCD	63 (5.9)	Male, age, HT and DM
Wong et al. [29], 2007	Cross-sectional (n = 3,057)	Chinese	Asymptomatic in patients with vascular risk factors	TCD	385 (12.6)	Age, HT, DM and hyperlipidemia
Uehara et al. [31], 1998	Prospective (n = 156)	Japanese	Asymptomatic	MRA	23 (14.7)	Age, HT
Uehara et al. [32], 2001	Prospective (n = 151)	Japanese	Asymptomatic in CABG patients	MRA	32 (21.1)	No risk factor identified
Bae et al. [11], 2006	Retrospective (n = 246)	Korean	Asymptomatic in CABG patients	TCD MRA	71 (28.9)	Age, male, HT, DM and history of stroke/TIA
Feldmann et al. [37], 1990	Retrospective (n = 24)	Chinese Caucasian	Symptomatic stroke	DSA	2 (8) White 6 (26) Chinese	Chinese had more intracranial lesions while whites had more extracranial lesions
Thajeb [38], 1993	Prospective (n = 21)	Chinese	Symptomatic stroke	DSA	18 (85.7)	HT, hyperfibrinogenaemia, polycythaemia, and low HDL-cholesterol
Liu et al. [22], 1996	Prospective (n = 108)	Chinese	Symptomatic stroke	MRA	28 (26)	No difference in vascular risk factors between patients with intracranial and extracranial lesions
Huang et al. [51], 1997	Prospective (n = 96)	Chinese	Symptomatic TIA	TCD carotid duplex	50 (51)	Most common in terminal internal carotid artery or proximal middle cerebral artery
Wong et al. [52], 1998	Prospective (n = 100)	Chinese	Symptomatic ischemic stroke with adequate temporal windows (n = 66)	TCD	22 (33)	Intracranial occlusive disease is the most commonly found vascular lesion in our acute stroke patients
Wong et al. [53], 2000	Prospective (n = 705)	Chinese	Symptomatic stroke	TCD	258 (37%)	The risk of vascular events or death increased rapidly with rising numbers of occlusive arteries
Zhou et al. [49], 2004	Prospective (n = 300)	Chinese	Symptomatic stroke	MRA, DSA	120 (40) LAD	The incidence of LAD in Chinese patients is higher than that of the other four subtypes of stroke based on TOAST criteria

Table 1. Continued

Study	Study design	Racial	Condition	Assessment	Number (%)	Risk factors/results
Brust [35], 1975	Retrospective (n = 296)	Japanese and other population groups in Hawaii	Symptomatic stroke	DSA	5 (5.4) White 8 (9.4) Hawaii Japanese 8 (34.8) Japan Japanese	Significant difference between frequency of involvement of >50% stenosis in extracranial and intracranial vessels in Caucasian and that in the Hawaiian-born and Japan-born Japanese populations
Nishimaru et al. [34], 1984	Retrospective (n = 64)	Japanese Caucasian	Symptomatic carotid system TIA patients	DSA	Mild lesion 25 (78.1) in Japanese 29 (90.6) in Caucasians	10 of 12 severe lesions in Japanese were located intracranially, 17 of 20 severe lesions present in the American group occurred in the extracranial portion of the internal or common carotid arteries
Takahashi et al. [43], 1999	Retrospective (n = 279)	Japanese	Symptomatic stroke (n = 152) and others	MRA	36 (12.9)	HT and HbAlc
Suh et al. [10], 2003	Retrospective (n = 268)	Korean	Symptomatic stroke	DSA	37 (66) Single lesion 166 (50) Multiple lesions	Korean patients with severe atherosclerotic stenosis tend to have more intracranial stenosis
Bang et al. [8], 2005	Prospective (n = 512)	Korean	Symptomatic stroke	DSA	77 (15.0) EC-LAA 143 (27.9) IC-LAA 292 (57.0) Nonatherosclerotic	Metabolic syndrome was independently associated with intracranial atherosclerosis
Nam et al. [9], 2006	Retrospective (n = 922)	Korean	Symptomatic	DSA	245 (48)	Age, HT, smoking, IHD, history of stroke and simple aortic plaques
Kaul et al. [45], 2002	Prospective (n = 392)	Indian	Symptomatic stroke	TCD	161 (41) LAD	HT, DM and smoking
Suwanwela et al. [48], 2003	Retrospective (n = 100)	Thailand	Symptomatic stroke or TIA	TCD carotid duplex	51 (51)	DM and IHD
De Silva et al. [46], 2007	Prospective (n = 205)	South Asian	Symptomatic stroke	TCCD MRA	93 (50)	11 (79) with TACI, 14(47) PACI, 17(65) POCI and 51 (44) LACI
Wang et al. [39], 2014	Prospective (n = 2,864)	Chinese	Symptomatic stroke or TIA	MRA	1,335 (46.6) ICAS	Family history of stroke, history of cerebral ischemia or heart disease, age, NIHSS, stenosis, Heart disease, complete of circle of Willis

TCD = Transcranial doppler; HT = hypertension; IHD = ischemic heart disease; DM = diabetes mellitus; MRA = magnetic resonance angiography; CABG = coronary artery bypass grafting; EC-LAA = extracranial portion of large artery atherosclerosis; IC-LAA = intracranial portion of large artery atherosclerosis; LAD = large artery atherosclerosis; DSA = digital subtraction angiography; TCCD = transcranial color-coded doppler; TOAST = Trial of Org 10 172 in acute stroke treatment; NIHSS = National Institutes of Health Stroke Scale.

83 years, mean age of 63) with no evidence of stroke who underwent magnetic resonance angiography (MRA) for other reasons. They found that 14.7% had intracranial artery stenosis whereas 11.5% had cervical carotid artery stenosis [29]. Multiple logistic regression analysis showed that age and hyperlipidemia were independent predictors for extracranial atherosclerosis, and that age and hypertension were predictors for ICAS. Park et al. studied 835 Korean subjects (29–85 years, mean age of 53) who visited a hospital for the purpose of routine health screening. MRA showed that 3% had ICAS and 0.48% had extracranial atherosclerosis. Old age and hypertension were independent risk factors for ICAS [30]. The higher incidence of cerebral atherosclerosis in Japanese than in Koreans may be due to differences in age and other factors.

Prevalence of Asymptomatic ICAS in High-Risk Patients

Wong et al. carried out a prevalence study of MCA stenosis among high risk individuals who had vascular risk factors without history of stroke or TIA. Among 3,057 subjects who had at least one vascular risk factor (hypertension, diabetes, hyperlipidemia), 385 (12.6%) had MCA stenosis. Old age, hypertension, diabetes, and hyperlipidemia were associated risk factors. The prevalence escalated quadratically with increasing number of associated factors [31]. Two studies from Hong Kong on type 2 diabetic patients [12, 13] reported that blood pressure indices and albuminuria were closely associated with asymptomatic MCA stenosis.

In a study from Japan, 151 consecutive patients who were scheduled for coronary artery bypass graft surgery (CABG) were evaluated with MRA. Cervical carotid artery narrowing of ≥50% was detected in 16.6%, while intracranial artery stenoses of ≥50% was detected in 21.2% [32]. Previous studies found that ICAS was associated with aortic plaques, and the metabolic syndrome, factors closely related to coronary artery disease [9, 33]. However, in a Korean study of CABG patients the correlation of coronary atherosclerosis with extracranial carotid atherosclerosis was stronger than that of coronary artery atherosclerosis with ICAS [11].

Symptomatic ICAS in Stroke Patients

Conventional Cerebral Angiography-Based Studies: Japan, Korea and China Stroke Patients

In a case-control study of patients with symptomatic anterior circulation ischemia, 83% of severely stenotic lesions involved the intracranial arteries among 32 Japanese patients, whereas 85% of severe lesions involved the extracranial internal carotid artery in 32 American whites. For minor lesions, the frequency was similar between the two ethnic groups [34]. Another angiography study from Hawaii showed a more frequent involvement of the extracranial arteries in whites, and more frequent involvement of the intracranial arteries in the Hawaiian-born Japanese population [35]. Based on the study by Suh et al. [10], Korean patients with severe atherosclerotic stenoses had more intracranial than extracranial stenosis (52 vs. 48%), and 59% of intracranial lesions were located in the anterior circulation. Nam et al. [9] reported in Korean stroke patients that intracranial or extracranial atherosclerosis was found in 511 patients (55%). Simple aortic plaque was an independent predictor of ICAS.

In Taiwan Chinese patients with carotid territory TIAs, intracranial stenosis was present in 15% of 47 patients [36]. A case-control study comparing Chinese living in the USA with American whites, Chinese patients had significantly higher rates of intracranial carotid artery and MCA stenosis [37]. Of 24 Chinese patients with cerebral ischemia, 43% had symptomatic MCA stenosis, whereas the same lesion was present in only 14% of 24 age- and sex-matched white patients. In contrast, 50% of white patients had severe stenosis of the extracranial ICA, whereas only 9% of the Chinese patients had a similar lesion. A recent angiographic study of Chinese patients with acute capsular infarcts and prior ipsilateral TIA showed that intracranial stenosis was found in 67% of 21 patients [38].

MR Angiography and TCD Studies

In the CICAS (Chinese IntraCranial AtheroSclerosis) study, we evaluated 2,864 consecutive patients who experienced acute cerebral ischemia within 7 days of symptom onset. The prevalence of ICAS was 46.6% (1,335 patients, including 261 patients with co-existing extracranial carotid stenosis). Patients with ICAS had more severe stroke at admission and stayed longer in hospitals than those without intracranial stenosis (median NIHSS 3 vs. 5; median length of stay 14 vs. 16 days respectively, both $p < 0.0001$). After 12 months, recurrent stroke occurred in 3.34% of patients with no stenosis, 3.82% for 50–69% stenosis, 5.16% for 70–99% stenosis and 7.40% for total occlusion [39]. Furthermore, patients with ICAS are also at a high risk of stroke recurrence, up to 25–30% in 2 years after their first stroke [40, 41]. The authors found that the degree of stenosis is not the only independent predictor for recurrent stroke. Other factors such as diastolic blood pressure, no use of antithrombotic drug, complete circle of Willis, and history of cerebral ischemia or heart disease, and family history of stroke were also independent predictors. High blood pressure, no use of antithrombotic drugs, and significant history of stroke are well-known risk factors for recurrent stroke. Complete circle of Willis on MRA might indicate the potential for opening of the collateral circulation.

Kim et al. [42] analyzed 1,167 Korean stroke patients who underwent MRI and MRA. 491 patients (42%) showed large artery atherosclerosis which was responsible for the stroke. Symptomatic atherosclerotic lesions were most often located in the MCA (38%), followed by ICA (28%), vertebral artery (15%), posterior cerebral artery (9%), basilar artery (8%), and the anterior cerebral artery (2%). Among patients with symptomatic ICA disease proximal ICA slightly outnumbered distal ICA disease. Thus, symptomatic ICAS seems to be more common than symptomatic extracranial atherosclerosis [10].

Features may be similar in Japan and other Asian countries. Takahashi et al. [43] showed that 12.9% of Japanese stroke patients had MCA stenosis on MRA, and that hypertension and high serum HbA_{1c} levels contributed to the development of MCA lesions. An MRA study from India showed that ICAS as a cause of strokes may be more common in India than in Japan [44]. A hospital-based stroke registry in South India showed that among all ischemic stroke patients, 41, 18, 10, 4, and 27% were classified as large-artery atherosclerosis, lacunae, cardioembolism, other determined etiology and undetermined etiology, respectively [45].

Similarly, a study from Singapore showed that significant ICAS was common among all Oxfordshire Community Stroke Project subtypes [46]. The finding is consistent with the ethnic Chinese data [47]. A retrospective study in Thailand on the patients with ischemic stroke or TIA found 98% patients with extracranial stenosis had associated intracranial disease, whereas none of those with intracranial stenosis had more than 50% extracranial carotid stenosis [48].

A study from mainland China suggested that large artery atherosclerosis (40%) is the main cause of ischemic stroke [49]. In symptomatic Taiwanese patients, approximately 24% had only extracranial carotid disease, about 26% had only intracranial carotid tributary disease and 17.6% had significant lesions in both extracranial and intracranial carotid artery tributaries [50]. Ultrasonographical studies of Chinese subjects showed that ICAS occurred in 30–67% of stroke or TIA patients. One of these studies found ICAS in 51% of 96 TIA patients, while extracranial carotid disease occurred in 19% of all patients [51]. Another TCD series showed that ICAS was the most common vascular lesions, which accounted for 33% of 66 ischemic stroke patients, whereas extracranial carotid lesions were only found in 6% [52]. In another study from Hong Kong, ICAS only accounted for 37% of the patients and both intracranial and extracranial disease accounted for 10% of the patients, whereas 2% had extracranial carotid artery abnormality only. Overall, ICAS (47%) was nearly four-fold higher in frequency than extracranial carotid occlusive disease (12%) [53]. In another TCD study 75% had intracranial involvement only, 5% extracranial involvement only and 20% had both intracranial and extracranial involvement [54].

Symptomatic ICAS in Europe

Most European studies have focused on extracranial carotid artery lesions as this is the most common cause of ischemic stroke in Caucasians. The French GESICA study showed that ICAS involved the vertebral artery in 22.5%, the basilar artery in 25.5%, the MCA in 26.5%, and the internal carotid artery in 25.5%. This prospective study further suggested both a high 2-year recurrence rate of ischemic events in the stenotic cerebral artery territory (38.2%: stroke 13.7%, TIA 24.5%) and cardiovascular events (18.6%) with an 8.8% vascular death rate [55]. Olsen et al. [56] reported that 40% of patients with stroke in the carotid territory had MCA occlusion. A Spanish study found that 50% had symptomatic intracranial stenosis, and only 26.5% had significant carotid atheroma [57].

North America and Related Regions

Autopsy Studies
The early history of ICAS in North America and related areas is replete with studies that emphasized the importance of extracranial occlusive disease [58]. For example, Fisher's autopsy series of 200 patients with cerebrovascular disease did not include a single patient who had occlusion of the middle cerebral artery (MCA) [59]. In another autopsy study, Hutchinson and Yates emphasized that atherosclerosis of the vertebral artery was most prevalent in the proximal portion of this vessel [60]. Baker and Iannone, in the late 1950s, described cerebral atherosclerosis at autopsy which not only involved the origin of the internal carotid artery (ICA) but also included such areas as the distal, proximal and mid-portions of the basilar artery and the MCA [61]. Others such as Whisnant and colleagues in the US confirmed the importance of proximal ICA occlusive disease, and Swartz and Mitchell in England and Torvik and Jorgenson in Norway corroborated the importance of occlusive ICA disease at the origin and in the intracranial portion at autopsy [1]. Others suggested that intracranial MCA occlusion was predominantly embolic in origin[1]. Later, Fisher elucidated the pathological lesions underlying lacunar infarcts [62].

Racial Differences in ICAS: Autopsy Studies
In an autopsy study in 1959, Moossy showed that cerebral atherosclerosis typically involved the ICA and vertebral arteries followed by the basilar artery and MCA [63]. In a more extensive study of 2,650 brain dissections, Moossy reported the importance of intracranial arterial thrombosis in those with recent ischemic stroke [64]. In the International Atherosclerosis Project (IAP), New Orleans blacks had a higher extent of raised lesions compared to New Orleans whites, and Jamaican blacks had more raised lesions in the vertebral and other intracranial arteries. Later, McGarry et al. reported more advanced ICAS in blacks [16]. A comparison among autopsy subjects from New Orleans, Oslo and Kingston showed that blacks had more atherosclerosis intracranially and as much or more cervical atherosclerosis, but whites had more occlusive disease in the aorta and coronary arteries [65].

Sex Differences in ICAS: Autopsy Study
It has been suggested that women may have more intrinsic occlusive intracranial vascular disease [1]. Flora et al. [65] reported that the frequency of

cerebral atherosclerosis increased more rapidly in women after the 6th decade; by the 9th decade it was more common than in men; and diabetic women were particularly at risk for cerebral atherosclerosis. Caplan has suggested that persons with medium-sized ICAS and major branch disease may be disproportionately more often women, blacks or Asians, or hypertensives [1].

Conventional Cerebral Angiography-Based Studies of Racial Differences in ICAS
Caplan et al. [1] and Gorelick [2] have previously reviewed this literature. Overall, based on studies by Bauer et al., Fields et al., Russo, Heyden et al., and Heyman et al., there seems to be more surgically accessible extracranial lesions in whites than blacks and a higher frequency of intrinsic intracranial occlusive lesions among blacks [66–70].

Chicago Experience
Symptomatic Occlusive Ceerbrovascular Disease: A Series from Chicago, Illinois
This study included 26 white and 45 black patients with symptomatic occlusive cerebrovascular disease of the anterior circulation [3]. Overall, white patients had more severe disease of the extracranial carotid artery at the origin, and a clinical history of more TIAs and carotid bruits, whereas black patients had more severe disease of the MCA stem and supraclinoid ICA. This study did not include multivariable analysis. However, in a companion conventional cerebral angiographic study which included 27 whites and 24 blacks predominantly from the Chicago area, white subjects had significantly more angina pectoris, more lesions of the origin of the left vertebral artery and more severe lesions of the extracranial vertebral arteries, whereas black patients had significantly higher mean diastolic blood pressure, more diabetes mellitus, more lesions of the distal basilar artery, more severe lesions of intracranial branch vessels, and more symptomatic intracranial branch disease [4]. Logistic regression analysis showed that race was an independent predictor of the site of occlusive disease in the posterior circulation. Although the statistical power may have been low based on the small sample size in the study, there were significantly more intracranial lesions and symptomatic intracranial lesions among nondiabetic blacks than whites.

Asymptomatic Occlusive Disease
In a companion study, clinical and arteriographic characteristics in 106 subjects who had symptomatic unilateral carotid territory occlusive disease were identified to elucidate the frequency and distribution of occlusive arterial lesions in asymptomatic arterial vessels [5]. Among black patients who were younger, and more often female than the white patients, there were fewer TIAs and myocardial infarctions and less claudication by medical history, but more asymptomatic lesions of the supraclinoid carotid artery, anterior cerebral artery stem, and middle cerebral artery stem. Whereas whites who were predominantly elderly, and men, had more frequent and severe occlusive asymptomatic disease of the extracranial carotid artery and vertebral artery sites. By stepwise logistic regression analysis, predictors of asymptomatic arterial sites included white race (extracranial carotid artery), black race (major intracranial artery sites, major MCA sties), and diabetes mellitus (anterior cerebral artery sites).

Additional Observations and Perspectives
The aforementioned studies suggest that blacks may have a propensity for ICAS, whereas whites may be more predisposed to extracranial occlusive disease. Circle of Willis ICAS has been linked to hypertension in autopsy study [71], and black populations, for example, in West Africa have been shown to have little atherosclerosis of the circle of Willis when the prevalence of hypertension is low. In urban West African populations, the prevalence of ICAS is believed to increase in conjunction with raised blood pressure. Based on conventional cerebral angiographic studies,

Zambian blacks rarely had extracranial atherosclerosis, and black South African stroke patients infrequently had extracranial lesions [72].

Caplan has set forth the following hypothesis to explain racial differences in the distribution and severity of intracranial and extracranial occlusive disease [72]. He suggests that hypertension differs in blacks and whites. Blacks and Asians retain more sodium and have volume hypertension. In addition, diabetes is a disorder often accompanied by high blood volume as are certain conditions in women: menstruation, pregnancy, and sex hormone use. These conditions associated with high blood volume, female sex, diabetes, and hypertension in blacks and Asians, also are associated with intracranial occlusive disease. In contrast, hypertension in whites, for example, is associated with extracranial carotid artery and vertebral artery disease as a manifestation of a resistance form of hypertension.

In the international Extracranial/Intracranial Bypass Study entry characteristics were analyzed to determine if there were differences in the site of the lesion based on racial group [73]. In this trial, blacks more often had hypertension, diabetes or cigarette smoking, whereas whites had higher systolic blood pressure and hemoglobin levels. Asian subjects had the lowest prevalence of vascular risk factors. Multivariate analysis showed that race (black, Asian) was an independent predictor of location of cerebrovascular lesions.

In the Northern Manhattan Stroke Study (NoMASS), a greater prevalence of diabetes and hypercholesterolemia was noted among blacks and Hispanics accounting for a substantial proportion of the increased frequency of ICAS [74]. In addition, in NoMASS maximum internal carotid artery plaque thickness (MICPT) was greater in whites and blacks than in Hispanics [75]. Independent predictors of MICPT included smoking, glucose, LDL cholesterol, and hypertension. In addition, there was a significant interaction between race-ethnicity and LDL cholesterol, with a greater effect with increasing LDL cholesterol in Hispanics. Finally, in the Warfarin-Aspirin Symptomatic Intracranial Disease (WASID) trial, the metabolic syndrome was found in about 50% of subjects and was associated with higher risk of major vascular events [33]. In WASID, among persons with ICAS, the risk of subsequent stroke was predicted by stenosis ≥70%, after recent symptoms (≤17 days), and in women [76].

Burke and Howard discuss the distribution and severity of asymptomatic extracranial atherosclerosis and is reviewed elsewhere [77].

Implication of Race-Ethnic Distribution of Cerebrovascular Atherosclerosis

ICAS is a common cause of stroke in Asian, Black and Hispanic patients but not in white patients. The cause of this disparity remains uncertain. Risk factors such as hypertension, diabetes, and hyperlipidemia are also prevalent in white subjects, so that vascular risk factors alone cannot explain this difference. Whether other environmental factors such as diet, life style or genetics play a role deserves further investigation. Other studies have suggested that genetic susceptibility may play a key role. Blacks, Hispanics, and Asians might be susceptible to ICAS [5, 37]. Laboratory work has shown that genes are highly associated with phenotypic variation in carotid artery occlusive disease [78–81] as well as ICAS [82–85]. It has been suggested that metabolic syndrome and related abnormalities may explain the high prevalence of ICAS in Asians (see Chapter 4). Definitive elucidation of factors that cause or potentiate ICAS could lead to better prevention and treatment strategies.

ICAS Updates from Around the World

We provide select updates on the epidemiology of ICAS that have appeared since the 1st edition of this text in 2008. As the field of ICAS has advanced a number of *candidate biomarkers* have been identified [86]. These include a long list of potential protein, genetic and microvesicle markers that are discussed elsewhere. Furthermore, high resolution 3-tesla contrast-enhanced MRI may assist in the detection and definition of ICAS [87–89].

Community and Other Large Study Data Bases

A large Korean stroke register favored age, male sex, and hyperlipidemia as factors for extracranial disease, whereas hypertension and diabetes mellitus were factors related to ICAS, especially in the posterior circulation [90]. In primarily community-based studies in China, Tsai and colleagues concluded that there was a slightly higher overall stroke incidence and proportion of intracerebral hemorrhage in Chinese compared to white patients, but there was no clear evidence of different distributions of ischemic stroke subtypes [91]. In the population-based Rotterdam Study, over 80% of older white persons had ICA intracranial calcification [92]. Age was a predictor in men and women, whereas excessive alcohol intake and smoking were predictors in men and diabetes and hypertension in women. In another large Korean stroke register study, symptomatic steno-occlusion most frequently affected the MCA (34.6%), extracranial internal carotid artery (14%), vertebral artery (14%) and basilar artery (8.7%) [93]. Based on over 10,000 persons in a health screening program in Korea (mean age, 43 years), the risk of ICAS (TCD detection of >50% ICAS) was independently increased in participants with coronary artery calcification [94].

Kim and Bonovich draw contrasts between ICAS in the East and West [95]. They point out that ICAS occurs at younger ages in the East but at older ages in the West. In the East ICAS may be associated with branch occlusions and single subcortical infarctions, however, this has received less attention in the West. Although there has not been uniformity of findings, more women may develop ICAS in the East than men, which is similar in the West. Finally, metabolic cardiovascular risk factors may be linked to both ICAS in the East and West though the relationship may be stronger in Asia.

References

1 Caplan LR, Gorelick PB, Hier DB: Race, sex and occlusive cerebrovascular disease: a review. Stroke 1986;17:648–655.

2 Gorelick PB: Distribution of atherosclerotic cerebrovascular lesions. Effects of age, race, and sex. Stroke 1993;24:I16–I19; discussion I20–I21.

3 Gorelick PB, Caplan LR, Hier DB, et al: Racial differences in the distribution of anterior circulation occlusive disease. Neurology 1984;34:54–59.

4 Gorelick PB, Caplan LR, Hier DB, et al: Racial differences in the distribution of posterior circulation occlusive disease. Stroke 1985;16:785–790.

5 Gorelick PB, Caplan LR, Langenberg P, et al: Clinical and angiographic comparison of asymptomatic occlusive cerebrovascular disease. Neurology 1988;38: 852–858.

6 Chimowitz MI, Lynn MJ, Howlett-Smith H, et al: Comparison of warfarin and aspirin for symptomatic intracranial arterial stenosis. N Engl J Med 2005;352: 1305–1316.

7 Wong LKS: Global burden of intracranial atherosclerosis. International Journal of Stroke 2006;1:158–159.

8 Bang OY, Kim JW, Lee JH, et al: Association of the metabolic syndrome with intracranial atherosclerotic stroke. Neurology 2005;65:296–298.

9 Nam HS, Han SW, Lee JY, et al: Association of aortic plaque with intracranial atherosclerosis in patients with stroke. Neurology 2006;67:1184–1188.

10 Suh DC, Lee SH, Kim KR, et al: Pattern of atherosclerotic carotid stenosis in Korean patients with stroke: different involvement of intracranial versus extracranial vessels. AJNR Am J Neuroradiol 2003;24:239–244.

11 Bae HJ, Yoon BW, Kang DW, et al: Correlation of coronary and cerebral atherosclerosis: difference between extracranial and intracranial arteries. Cerebrovasc Dis 2006;21:112–119

12 Thomas GN, Lin JW, Lam WW, et al: Middle cerebral artery stenosis in type II diabetic Chinese patients is associated with conventional risk factors but not with polymorphisms of the renin-angiotensin system genes. Cerebrovasc Dis 2003;16:217–223.

13 Thomas GN, Lin JW, Lam WW, et al: Albuminuria is a marker of increasing intracranial and extracranial vascular involvement in Type 2 diabetic Chinese patients. Diabetologia 2004;47:1528–1534.

14 Wong KS, Chen C, Ng PW, et al: Low-molecular-weight heparin compared with aspirin for the treatment of acute ischaemic stroke in Asian patients with large artery occlusive disease: a randomised study. Lancet Neurol 2007;6:407–413.
15 Kwon SU, Cho YJ, Koo JS, et al: Cilostazol prevents the progression of the symptomatic intracranial arterial stenosis: the multicenter double-blind placebo-controlled trial of cilostazol in symptomatic intracranial arterial stenosis. Stroke 2005;36:782–786.
16 McGarry P, Solberg LA, Guzman MA, Strong JP: Cerebral atherosclerosis in New Orleans. Comparisons of lesions by age, sex, and race. Lab Invest 1985;52:533–539.
17 Nakamura M, Yamamoto H, Kikuchi Y, et al: Cerebral atherosclerosis in Japanese. I. Age related to atherosclerosis. Stroke 1971;2:400–408.
18 Resch JA, Okabe N, Loewenson RB, et al: Pattern of vessel involvement in cerebral atherosclerosis. A comparative study between a Japanese and Minnesota population. J Atheroscler Res 1969;9:239–250.
19 Masuda J, Tanaka K, Omae T, et al: Cerebrovascular diseases and their underlying vascular lesions in Hisayama, Japan – a pathological study of autopsy cases. Stroke 1983;14:934–940.
20 Koyama S, Saito Y, Yamanouchi H, et al: [Marked decrease of intracranial atherosclerosis in contrast with unchanged coronary artery stenosis in Japan]. Nippon Ronen Igakkai Zasshi 2003;40:267–273.
21 Leung SY, Ng TH, Yuen ST, et al: Pattern of cerebral atherosclerosis in Hong Kong Chinese. Severity in intracranial and extracranial vessels. Stroke 1993;24:779–786.
22 Liu F, Zhang B, Tian Y: [Morphological changes in intracranial and extracranial arteries of autopsy cases of cerebrovascular diseases]. Zhonghua Yi Xue Za Zhi 1996;76:832–835.
23 Chen XY, Wong KS, Lam WW, et al: Middle Cerebral Artery Atherosclerosis: histological comparison between plaques associated with and not associated with infarct in a postmortem study. Cerebrovasc Dis 2007;25:74–80.
24 Wong KS, Huang YN, Yang HB, et al: A door-to-door survey of intracranial atherosclerosis in Liangbei County, China. Neurology 2007;68:2031–2034.
25 Huang HW, Guo MH, Lin RJ, et al: Prevalence and risk factors of middle cerebral artery stenosis in asymptomatic residents in Rongqi County, Guangdong. Cerebrovasc Dis 2007;24:111–115.
26 Huang HW, Guo MH, Lin RJ, et al: Hyperhomocysteinemia is a risk factor of middle cerebral artery stenosis. J Neurol 2007;254:364–367.
27 Hill AB: Should patients be screened for asymptomatic carotid artery stenosis? Can J Surg 1998;41:208–213.
28 Wong KS, Li H: Long-term mortality and recurrent stroke risk among Chinese stroke patients with predominant intracranial atherosclerosis. Stroke 2003;34:2361–2366.
29 Wong KS, Ng PW, Tang A, et al: Prevalence of asymptomatic intracranial atherosclerosis in high-risk patients. Neurology 2007;68:2035–2038.
30 Park KY, Chung CS, Lee KH, Kim GM, Kim YB, Oh K: Prevalence and risk factors of intracranial atherosclerosis in an asymptomatic Korean population. J Clin Neurol 2006;2:29–33.
31 Uehara T, Tabuchi M, Mori E: Frequency and clinical correlates of occlusive lesions of cerebral arteries in Japanese patients without stroke. Evaluation by MR angiography. Cerebrovasc Dis 1998;8:267–272.
32 Uehara T, Tabuchi M, Kozawa S, Mori E: MR angiographic evaluation of carotid and intracranial arteries in Japanese patients scheduled for coronary artery bypass grafting. Cerebrovasc Dis 2001;11:341–345.
33 Ovbiagele B, Saver JL, Lynn MJ, Chimowitz M: Impact of metabolic syndrome on prognosis of symptomatic intracranial atherostenosis. Neurology 2006;66:1344–1349.
34 Nishimaru K, McHenry LC Jr, Toole JF: Cerebral angiographic and clinical differences in carotid system transient ischemic attacks between American Caucasian and Japanese patients. Stroke 1984;15:56–59.
35 Brust RW Jr: Patterns of cerebrovascular disease in Japanese and other population groups in Hawaii: an angiographical study. Stroke 1975;6:539–542.
36 Ryu SJ: Angiographic features in Chinese patients with occlusive cerebrovascular disease. Stroke 1987;18:686.
37 Feldmann E, Daneault N, Kwan E, et al: Chinese-white differences in the distribution of occlusive cerebrovascular disease. Neurology 1990;40:1541–1545.
38 Thajeb P: Large vessel disease in Chinese patients with capsular infarcts and prior ipsilateral transient ischaemia. Neuroradiology 1993;35:190–195.
39 Wang Y, Zhao X, Liu L, et al: Prevalence and outcomes of symptomatic intracranial large artery stenoses and occlusions in China: the Chinese Intracranial Atherosclerosis (CICAS) Study. Stroke 2014;45:663–669.
40 Liu L, Wong KSL, Leng X, et al: Dual antiplatelet therapy in stroke and ICAS: Subgroup analysis of CHANCE. Neurology 2015;85:1154–1162.
41 Kasner SE, Chimowitz MI, Lynn MJ, et al: Predictors of ischemic stroke in the territory of a symptomatic intracranial arterial stenosis. Circulation 2006;113:555–563.
42 Kim JT, Yoo SH, Kwon J-H, Kwon SU, Kim JS: Subtyping of ischemic stroke based on vascular imaging: analysis of 1,167 acute, consecutive patients. J Clin Neurol 2006;2:225–230.
43 Takahashi K, Kitani M, Fukuda H, Kobayashi S: Vascular risk factors for atherosclerotic lesions of the middle cerebral artery detected by magnetic resonance angiography (MRA). Acta Neurol Scand 1999;100:395–399.
44 Padma MV, Gaikwad S, Jain S, et al: Distribution of vascular lesions in ischaemic stroke: a magnetic resonance angiographic study. Natl Med J India 1997;10:217–220.
45 Kaul S, Sunitha P, Suvarna A, et al: Subtypes of Ischemic Stroke in a Metropolitan City of South India (One year data from a hospital based stroke registry). Neurol India 2002;50(suppl):S8–S14.
46 De Silva DA, Woon FP, Pin LM, et al: Intracranial large artery disease among OCSP subtypes in ethnic South Asian ischemic stroke patients. J Neurol Sci 2007;260:147–149.
47 Li H, Wong KS: Racial distribution of intracranial and extracranial atherosclerosis. J Clin Neurosci 2003;10:30–34.
48 Suwanwela NC, Chutinetr A: Risk factors for atherosclerosis of cervicocerebral arteries: intracranial versus extracranial. Neuroepidemiology 2003;22:37–40.
49 Zhou H, Wang YJ, Wang SX, Zhao XQ: [TOAST subtyping of acute ischemic stroke]. Zhonghua Nei Ke Za Zhi 2004;43:495–498.

50 Liu HM, Tu YK, Yip PK, Su CT: Evaluation of intracranial and extracranial carotid steno-occlusive diseases in Taiwan Chinese patients with MR angiography: preliminary experience. Stroke 1996;27: 650–653.
51 Huang YN, Gao S, Li SW, et al: Vascular lesions in Chinese patients with transient ischemic attacks. Neurology 1997; 48:524–525.
52 Wong KS, Huang YN, Gao S, et al: Intracranial stenosis in Chinese patients with acute stroke. Neurology 1998;50:812–813.
53 Wong KS, Li H, Chan YL, et al: Use of transcranial Doppler ultrasound to predict outcome in patients with intracranial large-artery occlusive disease. Stroke 2000;31:2641–2647.
54 Li H, Wong KS, Kay R: Relationship between the Oxfordshire Community Stroke Project classification and vascular abnormalities in patients with predominantly intracranial atherosclerosis. J Neurol Sci 2003;207:65–69.
55 Mazighi M, Tanasescu R, Ducrocq X, et al: Prospective study of symptomatic atherothrombotic intracranial stenoses: the GESICA study. Neurology 2006;66: 1187–1191.
56 Olsen TS, Skriver EB, Herning M: Cause of cerebral infarction in the carotid territory. Its relation to the size and the location of the infarct and to the underlying vascular lesion. Stroke 1985;16: 459–466.
57 Sanchez-Sanchez C, Egido JA, Gonzalez-Gutierrez JL, et al: [Stroke and intracranial stenosis: clinical profile in a series of 134 patients in Spain]. Rev Neurol 2004;39:305–311.
58 Caplan LR, Hennerici M: Impaired clearance of emboli (washout) is an important link between hypoperfusion, embolism, and ischemic stroke. Arch Neurol 1998;55:1475–1482.
59 Fisher M: Occlusion of the internal carotid artery. AMA Arch Neurol Psychiatry 1951;65:346–377.
60 Hutchinson EC, Yates PO: Carotico-vertebral stenosis. Lancet 1957;272:2–8.
61 Baker AB, Iannone A: Cerebrovascular disease. I. The large arteries of the circle of Willis. Neurology 1959;9:321–332.
62 Fisher CM: Lacunar strokes and infarcts: a review. Neurology 1982;32:871–876.
63 Moossy J: Development of cerebral atherosclerosis in various age groups. Neurology 1959;9:569–574.
64 Moossy J: Cerebral infarction and intracranial arterial thrombosis. Necropsy studies and clinical implications. Arch Neurol 1966;14:119–123.
65 Flora GC, Baker AB, Loewenson RB, Klassen AC: A comparative study of cerebral atherosclerosis in males and females. Circulation 1968;38:859–869.
66 Fields WS, North RR, Hass WK, et al: Joint study of extracranial arterial occlusion as a cause of stroke. I. Organization of study and survey of patient population. JAMA 1968;203:955–960.
67 Heyden S, Heyman A, Goree JA: Nonembolic occlusion of the middle cerebral and carotid arteries – a comparison of predisposing factors. Stroke 1970;1: 363–369.
68 Heyman A, Karp HR, Heyden S, et al: Cerebrovascular disease in the biracial population of Evans County, Georgia. Arch Intern Med 1971;128:949–955.
69 Russo LS Jr: Carotid system transient ischemic attacks: clinical, racial, and angiographic correlations. Stroke 1981; 12:470–473.
70 Bauer RB, Sheehan S, Wechsler N, Meyer JS: Arteriographic study of sites, incidence, and treatment of arteriosclerotic cerebrovascular lesions. Neurology 1962;12:698–711.
71 Kuller LH: Introduction and overview commentary; in Gillum R, Gorelick PB, Cooper ES (eds): Stroke in Blacks. A guide to Management and Prevention. S. Karger AG, Basel, 1999, pp 1–6.
72 Caplan LR: Cerebral ischemia and infarction in blacks. Clinical, autopsy and angiographic studies; in Gillum R, Gorelick PB, Cooper ES (eds): Stroke in Blacks. A guide to Management and Prevention. S. Karger AG, Basel, 1999, pp 7–18.
73 Inzitari D, Hachinski VC, Taylor DW, Barnett HJ: Racial differences in the anterior circulation in cerebrovascular disease. How much can be explained by risk factors? Arch Neurol 1990;47:1080–1084.
74 Sacco RL, Kargman DE, Gu Q, Zamanillo MC: Race-ethnicity and determinants of intracranial atherosclerotic cerebral infarction. The Northern Manhattan Stroke Study. Stroke 1995;26:14–20.
75 Sacco RL, Roberts JK, Boden-Albala B, et al: Race-ethnicity and determinants of carotid atherosclerosis in a multiethnic population. The Northern Manhattan Stroke Study. Stroke 1997;28:929–935.
76 Kasner SE, Chimowitz MI, Lynn MJ, et al: Predictors of ischemic stroke in the territory of a symptomatic intracranial arterial stenosis. Circulation 2006;113: 555–563.
77 Burke GL, Howard G: Ethnic differences in cerebral atherosclerosis. In: Gillum R, Gorelick PB, Cooper ES (eds): Stroke in Blacks. A guide to Management and Prevention. S. Karger AG, Basel, 1999, pp 94–105.
78 Oda K, Tanaka N, Arai T, et al: Polymorphisms in pro- and anti-inflammatory cytokine genes and susceptibility to atherosclerosis: a pathological study of 1,503 consecutive autopsy cases. Hum Mol Genet 2007;16:592–599.
79 Robinet P, Vedie B, Chironi G, et al: Characterization of polymorphic structure of SREBP-2 gene: role in atherosclerosis. Atherosclerosis 2003;168:381–387.
80 Markus HS, Labrum R, Bevan S, et al: Genetic and acquired inflammatory conditions are synergistically associated with early carotid atherosclerosis. Stroke 2006;37:2253–2259.
81 Fiotti N, Altamura N, Fisicaro M, et al: MMP-9 microsatellite polymorphism and susceptibility to carotid arteries atherosclerosis. Arterioscler Thromb Vasc Biol 2006;26:1330–1336.
82 Wang L, Gu Y, Wu G, et al: [A case control study on the distribution of apolipoprotein AI gene polymorphisms in the survivors of atherosclerosis cerebral infarction]. Zhonghua Liu Xing Bing Xue Za Zhi 2000;21:22–25.
83 Sertic J, Hebrang D, Janus D, et al: Association between deletion polymorphism of the angiotensin-converting enzyme gene and cerebral atherosclerosis. Eur J Clin Chem Clin Biochem 1996;34:301–304.
84 Liu ZZ, Lv H, Gao F, et al: Polymorphism in the human C-reactive protein (CRP) gene, serum concentrations of CRP, and the difference between intracranial and extracranial atherosclerosis. Clin Chim Acta 2007, Nov 29. [Epub ahead of print].
85 Abboud S, Karhunen PJ, Lutjohann D, et al: Proprotein Convertase Subtilisin/Kexin Type 9 (PCSK9) Gene Is a Risk Factor of Large-Vessel Atherosclerosis Stroke. PLoS One 2007;2:e1043.
86 Kim SJ, Moon GH, Bang OY: Biomarkers for stroke. Journal of Stroke 2013;15: 27–37.

87 Swartz RH, Buhta SS, Farb RI, Agid R, Willinsky RA, et al: Intracranial arterial wall imaging using high-resolution 3-tesla contrast-enhanced MRI. Neurology 2009;72:627–634.
88 Ahn S-H, Lee J, Kim Y-J, Kwon SU, Lee D, Jung S-C, et al: Isolated MCA disease in patients without significant atherosclerotic risk factors. A high-resolution magnetic resonance imaging study. Stroke 2015;46:697–703.
89 Mossa-Basha M, Hwang WD, De Havenon A, Hippe D, Balu N, Becker KJ, et al: Multicontrast high-resolution vessel wall magnetic resonance imaging and its value in differentiating intracranial vasculopathic processes. Stroke 2015;46: 1567–1573.
90 Kim JS, Nah H-W, Park SM, Kim S-K, Cho KH, Lee J, et al: Risk factors and stroke mechanisms in atherosclerotic stroke. Intracranial compared with extracranial and anterior compared with posterior circulation disease. Stroke 2012;43:3313–3318.
91 Tsai C-F, Thomas B, Sudlow CLM: Epidemiology of stroke and its subtypes in Chinese vs. white populations. A systematic review. Neurology 2013;81:264–272.
92 Bos D, Maggee Van der Rijk MJM, Geeraedts TEA, Hofman A, Krestin GP, Witteman JCM, et al: Intracranial carotid artery atherosclerosis. Prevalence and risk factors in the general population. Stroke 2012;43:1878–1884.
93 Kang K, Park TH, Lee KB, Park J-M, Ko Y, Lee SJ, et al: Symptomatic steno-occlusion in patients with acute cerebral infarction: prevalence, distribution, and functional outcome. Journal of Stroke 2014;16:36–43.
94 Oh H-G, Chung P-W, Rhee E-J: Increased risk for intracranial arterial stenosis in subjects with coronary artery calcification. Stroke 2015;46:151–156.
95 Kim JS, Bonovich D: Research on intracranial atherosclerosis from the East and West: why are the results different? Journal of Stroke 2014;16:105–113.

Prof. Philip Gorelick, MD, MPH
Department of Translational Science and Molecular Medicine
Michigan State University College of Human Medicine
Mercy Health Hauenstein Neurosciences, 220 Cherry Street SE
Grand Rapids, MI 49503 (USA)
E-Mail pgorelic@mercuhealth.com

Kim JS, Caplan LR, Wong KS (eds): Intracranial Atherosclerosis: Pathophysiology, Diagnosis and Treatment.
Front Neurol Neurosci. Basel, Karger, 2016, vol 40, pp 47–57 (DOI: 10.1159/000448301)

Risk Factors

T. Uehara[a] • O.Y. Bang[b] • J.S. Kim[c] • K. Minematsu[d] • R. Sacco[e]

[a]Hyogo Brain and Heart Center at Himeji, Himeji, Japan; [b]Sungkyunkwan University, Samsung Medical Center, and [c]Department of Neurology, Asan Medical Center, University of Ulsan, Seoul, Korea; [d]Department of Cerebrovascular Medicine, National Cerebral and Cardiovascular Center, Osaka, Japan; [e]Jackson Memorial Miller School of Medicine, University of Miami, Miami, Fla., USA

Abstract

Studies investigating risk factors for intracranial atherosclerosis (ICAS) have been infrequent. However, due to recent availability of non-invasive vascular imaging techniques that can assess intracranial cerebral arteries, there are a growing number of studies on risk factors for ICAS. Conventional vascular risk factors such as hypertension, diabetes, hypercholesterolemia and cigarette smoking are risk factors for ICAS. However, it remains uncertain whether there is a difference in risk factors between ICAS and extracranial atherosclerosis (ECAS). It also remains unclear why ICAS is more common in Asians and Blacks than in Caucasians. Although we reviewed available evidences on these differences, the review was limited because studies were heterogeneous in the definition of risk factors, diagnostic method, and characteristics of study subjects (hospitalized vs. community) or cerebral vessels (symptomatic vs. asymptomatic). Nevertheless, it seems that hypercholesterolemia is more closely associated with ECAS than ICAS. The difference in hypercholesterolemia prevalence is one of the main reasons for racial differences in the location of cerebral atherosclerosis. Intracranial arteries contain higher antioxidant level than extracranial arteries and may be more vulnerable to risk factors that deplete antioxidants (e.g., metabolic syndrome and diabetes mellitus). Intracranial arteries may be more vulnerable to factors associated with hemodynamic stress (e.g., advanced, salt-retaining hypertension and arterial tortuosity) because of a smaller diameter, thinner media and adventitia, and fewer elastic medial fibers than extracranial arteries. Additionally, non-atherosclerotic arterial diseases (e.g., moyamoya disease) that commonly occur in the intracranial arteries of East Asians may contaminate the reports of ICAS cases. Various genes, including *RNF 213,* might also explain racial differences in atherosclerotic location. Prospective, well-designed risk factor and genetic studies should be performed in a homogeneous group of patients with diverse ethnicities. These efforts are essential in the prevention of atherosclerotic diseases based on adequate knowledge of the risk factors and pathogenesis.

Studies investigating risk factors for intracranial atherosclerosis (ICAS) have been infrequent as compared to those for extracranial carotid atherosclerosis (ECAS). This may be attributable to the limited availability of non-invasive vascular imaging techniques assessing intracranial cerebral arteries. During the past couple of decades, a variety of imaging technologies have become available to evaluate the status of the intracranial vascular system, including transcranial doppler ultrasonography (TCD), magnetic resonance angiography (MRA), and computed tomography angiography (CTA). These improvements in vascular imaging technologies have yielded a growing number of studies on risk factors for ICAS.

The distribution of atherosclerotic lesions in the cervicocephalic vascular systems varies among different race-ethnic groups [1–7]. In Caucasians, atherosclerosis develops frequently in the extracranial carotid arteries, while ICAS is the common cause of stroke in Asians, Africans, and Hispanics. Several studies have demonstrated that hypercholesterolemia, atrial fibrillation, and ischemic heart disease (IHD) are more frequent, while hypertension and diabetes mellitus are less prevalent in Caucasians than in African-Americans and Hispanics [4, 5, 8]. It still remains elusive, however, whether race-ethnicity is an independent determinant of ICAS or is confounded by differences in the prevalence and control of stroke risk factors among different ethnic groups.

In this chapter, various risk factors for ICAS including conventional and nonconventional risk factors are reviewed. The reasons for East-West differences in the distribution of cerebral atherosclerosis will also be discussed.

Conventional Stroke Risk Factors for Intracranial Atherosclerosis

A number of clinical studies have assessed conventional risk factors for ICAS mainly in Asian populations. Table 1 summarizes the results.

(1) Age
Several autopsy and imaging studies showed that advanced age is associated with increasing prevalence and severity of ICAS [9–16].

(2) Gender
The relationship of ICAS and gender remains controversial. Several studies have shown a female predominance in ICAS [1, 9, 17–19]. Clinical [14, 20] and autopsy studies [21, 22] mainly on asymptomatic subjects, however have reported a male predominance for ICAS. Progression of atherosclerosis with age may be different between men and women [15]. In one study, ICAS developed earlier in men than in women; however, it progressed faster in women than in men [1]. It was speculated that post-menopausal hormonal changes may influence the progression rate of ICAS [23].

(3) Hypertension
One of the most important risk factors for atherosclerosis, especially ICAS, is hypertension [24]. Early autopsy studies reported that hypertension was strongly associated with atherosclerosis particularly in the intracranial cerebral arteries [21, 25]. Many clinical studies [9–14, 26–28] have confirmed the close correlation between hypertension and ICAS. Moreover, hypertension has been correlated to the severity of ICAS [12, 17, 19].

(4) Diabetes Mellitus
Autopsy-based studies demonstrated that the risk of ICAS was increased among those with diabetes mellitus [29, 30]. In clinical studies, diabetes mellitus has also been found to be a significant risk factor for ICAS in symptomatic [3, 18, 31–34] and asymptomatic cohorts [11–14, 16, 19, 30, 34]. In Koreans, diabetes mellitus was an independent risk factor for intracranial lesions only after 50 years of age [35] and only in posterior, not anterior, circulation atherosclerosis in a prospective study [17]. Diabetes mellitus has been correlated to progression of ICAS [36].

(5) Dyslipidemia
Dyslipidemia is an established risk factor for ECAS. However, its role in ICAS remains unclear. In the Northern Manhattan Stroke Study, the

Table 1. Clinical studies on risk factors for intracranial atherosclerosis

Author, year	Country	Sym/Asym	Evaluation method	Evaluation sites	Significant risk factors
Yasaka et al. [26], 1993	Japan	Sym	CA	MCA, BA	*MCA:* advanced HT *BA:* DM, HL, IHD
Uehara et al. [10], 1998	Japan	Asym	MRA	ICA, MCA, BA	Age, HT
Kim and Choi-Kwon [31], 1999	Korea	Sym	CA, MRA	MCA, ACA, BA, PCA	HT, DM
Takahashi et al. [27], 1999	Japan	Sym + Asym	MRA	MCA	HT, HbA1c
Arenillas et al. [32], 2004	Spain	Sym	MRA, CTA, TCD	ICA, MCA, ACA VA, BA, PCA	DM, Lp(a)
Bang et al. [44], 2005	Korea	Sym	CA, MRA	MCA, VA, BA	MetS
Uehara et al. [11], 2005	Japan	Asym	MRA	ICA, MCA, VA, BA	*ICA:* Age, HT, DM, IHD *MCA:* Age, HT *BA:* HT, DM *VA:* HL, IHD
Bae et al. [12], 2007	Korea	Asym	TCD	ICA, MCA, ACA VA, BA, PCA	Age, HT, DM
Park et al. [45], 2007	Korea	Sym	MRA	MCA, ACA, BA, PCA	MetS
Wong et al. [28], 2007	Hong Kong	Asym	TCD	ICA, MCA, ACA VA, BA, PCA	HT, glycosuria, heart disease Family history of stroke
Wong et al. [13], 2007	Hong Kong	Asym	TCD	MCA	Age, HT, DM, HL
Huang et al. [14], 2007	Hong Kong	Asym	TCD	MCA	Age, male, HT, DM
Bang et al. [46], 2007	Korea	Sym	CA, MRA, CTA	ICA, MCA	low Adiponectin
Kim et al. [9], 2009	Korea	Sym	CA, MRA	n.d.	Age, HT
Rincon et al. [34], 2009	USA	Sym	TCD	MCA, ACA, BA, PCA	DM, MetS
Park et al. [38], 2011	Korea	Sym	CA, MRA, CTA	ICA, MCA, ACA VA, BA, PCA	MetS, high apoB/apoAI
Kim et al. [35], 2011	Korea	Asym	TCD	n.d.	Male (≥50 years): Age, DM, HL Female (<50 years): HT Female (≥50 years): DM
Kim et al. [17], 2012	Korea	Sym	CA, MRA, CTA	MCA, ACA, BA, PCA	MetS (in posterior circulation)
Kim et al. [39], 2012	Korea	Sym	MRA	MCA, BA VA, BA, PCA	low HDL-C, high apoB/apoAI
Lopez-Cancio et al. [19], 2012	Spain	Asym	MRA	ICA, MCA, ACA	DM, MetS
Qian et al. [40], 2013	China	Sym	MRA	ICA, MCA, ACA VA, BA, PCA	low HDL-C
Lei et al. [18], 2014	China	Sym	MRA	ICA, MCA, ACA VA, BA, PCA	DM, high LDL-C

Sym = Symptomatic; Asym = asymptomatic; CA = conventional angiography; CTA = CT angiography; MRA = MR angiography; TCD = transcranial Doppler; ICA = internal carotid artery; MCA = middle cerebral artery; ACA = anterior cerebral artery; VA = vertebral artery; BA = basilar artery; PCA = posterior cerebral artery; HT = hypertension; DM = diabetes mellitus; HL = hyperlipidemia; IHD = ischemic heart disease; Lp(a) = lipoprotein (a); MetS = metabolic syndrome; n.d. = no data.

higher prevalence of diabetes mellitus and hypercholesterolemia among African-Americans and Hispanics accounted for the much higher frequency of stroke related to ICAS when compared to white individuals [3]. High LDL cholesterol level was associated mainly with ECAS [24], whereas a high ratio of apolipoprotein B to apolipoprotein I and low levels of apolipoprotein AI, the major protein component of high-density lipoprotein (HDL), correlated with intracranial lesions [37–39]. Cohort studies of acute ischemic stroke showed that low HDL-cholesterol level was associated with the development of intracranial artery stenosis [39, 40].

(6) Cigarette Smoking
Cigarette smoking is a well-established risk factor for ischemic stroke [41]. A few studies suggested that smoking, especially duration of smoking, is a risk factor for ICAS [16, 37]. Smoking has been correlated to the severity of ICAS [42] and progression of ICAS [36].

(7) Metabolic Syndrome
Metabolic syndrome is a constellation of risk factors including abdominal obesity, elevated triglyceride level, low high-density-lipoprotein cholesterol level, hypertension, and impaired fasting glucose level [43]. Two hospital-based studies showed that metabolic syndrome was independently associated with strokes with ICAS, while individual conventional risk factors were not [44, 45]. Patients with 1–2, 3, and 4–5 components of metabolic syndrome were about 2.5–3.8, 4.4, and 5.9–6.4 times more likely to have ICAS, respectively, as compared to those who had no components [44]. By contrast, such associations were not observed in patients with ECAS [44, 45]. The frequency of multiple, tandem ICAS lesions increased as the number of syndrome components increased [45, 46]. Metabolic syndrome may also predict higher risk of major vascular events in patients with ICAS [47].

Adiponectin, one of adipose tissue-specific cytokines [48], may be one of the mediators connecting metabolic syndrome with ICAS. Adiponectin may have a protective effect against atherosclerosis through various mechanisms: suppression of neointimal formation, inhibiting the expression of inflammatory cytokines and adhesion molecules [49, 50]. Hypoadiponectinemia was reported to be associated with endothelial dysfunction [51], and was found in adults with early [52] and advanced [53, 54] atherosclerosis. It was reported that symptomatic ICAS was associated with the lower serum adiponectin level when compared to other ischemic stroke subtypes [46].

In addition, metabolic syndrome is associated with systemic inflammation, sleep apnea and increased oxidative stress. Oxidative stress has been suggested to play a role in endothelial dysfunction and subsequent atherosclerosis [55, 56]; adults with metabolic syndrome had suboptimal concentrations of several antioxidants [57]. An autopsy study revealed that intracranial arteries responded with accelerated atherogenesis to the greater degree than extracranial arteries when the antioxidant protection was decreased [58]. The progression of atherosclerosis within intracranial arteries may therefore be attributable to the failure of the intracellular defense system against free radical-mediated processes.

Non-Conventional Stroke Risk Factors in Intracranial Atherosclerosis

Beside conventional risk factors and metabolic syndrome, several nonconventional risk factors may be involved in the development and progression of ICAS.

(1) Inflammation
Progression of symptomatic ICAS was reportedly associated with pro-inflammatory state, as reflected by high levels of inflammatory markers

(e.g., C-reactive protein), and with defective fibrinolysis [59]. In addition, lipoprotein-associated phospholipase A2 was increased in patients with ICAS and predicted patients at higher risk of recurrent stroke [60, 61]. Lipoprotein (a), a lipid-protein complex with proatherogenic and prothrombotic properties, is associated with inflammatory markers in patients with metabolic syndrome [62] and also with ICAS [63]. Lastly, autopsy studies showed that certain infectious agents, such as Chlamydia pneumonia may invade the endothelium and possibly be associated with development of ICAS [64].

(2) Endothelial Dysfunction
Endothelial dysfunction may be associated with ICAS [65]. Asymmetric-dimethylarginine, a marker of endothelial dysfunction, was independently associated with ICAS [19]. Jung et al. [66] evaluated phenotypes of endothelial microparticle from patients with intracranial and extracranial atherosclerosis and showed that endothelial activation is related to plaque instability in extracranial atherosclerosis, whereas endothelial apoptosis is related to vascular narrowing in ICAS.

(3) Sleep Apnea
Sleep apnea may be involved in the relationship between the metabolic syndrome and ICAS. The relationship between obstructive sleep apnea and metabolic syndrome [67–71] and chronic inflammation [72] has been demonstrated. Vgontzas and colleagues [73] even suggested that sleep apnea may be a manifestation of the metabolic syndrome; (a) there is a high prevalence of symptomatic sleep apnea in patients with insulin resistance [69] and in women with polycystic ovarian syndrome (a disorder in which insulin resistance is the primary pathogenetic mechanism) [74], (b) the metabolic syndrome and insulin resistance are stronger determinants of sleepiness compared to apnea/hypopnea index, (c) similar age distribution between symptomatic sleep apnea and the metabolic syndrome [75], and (d) the beneficial effect of exercise on both sleep apnea and insulin resistance [76]. Sleep apnea was found to be associated with a lesser degree of obesity in Asians than in white people [77]. This different prevalence or severity of sleep apnea syndrome among different ethnic groups might in part explain the ethnic differences in the location of cerebral atherosclerosis.

(4) Genetic Factors
In Japanese individuals with metabolic syndrome, several genetic polymorphisms (e.g., 2445→A (Ala54Thr) polymorphism of FABP2) were associated with atherosclerotic stroke, suggesting the effects of these polymorphisms on both insulin resistance and lipid metabolism may account for their association with atherothrombotic cerebral infarction [78]. In addition, genetic polymorphisms on the C-reactive protein gene have been tested in patients with symptomatic ICAS, but the results were inconsistent [79, 80].

Risk Factors for Subtypes of Intracranial Atherosclerosis

Intracranial atherosclerotic stroke can be caused by various mechanisms of stroke, including branch occlusive disease (BOD), artery-to-artery embolism, and hemodynamic impairment [81, 82]. Recent studies showed that risk factors and vessel wall pathology may differ among subtypes of intracranial atherosclerotic stroke [30, 83–87]. Specifically, current smoking and hypertension were more prevalent [83], and rupture-prone positive remodeling and enhancing plaque are more frequently observed in non-BOD type ICAS, compared to BOD-type ICAS [87]. Similarly, an autopsy study of patients with fatal stroke showed that history of myocardial infarction was associated with intracranial plaques [30].

Differences between East and West, and Intra- and Extracranial Atherosclerosis

ICAS is more prevalent in Asians and Blacks whereas ECAS is more common in Caucasians [1–6, 17, 88]. The reasons for the racial differences in the location of cerebral atherosclerosis remain uncertain, but the following facts have been considered [89].

Differences in Risk Factors

Hypertension

Studies from West [1, 2] and the East [10] have found that ICAS is more strongly related to hypertension than ECAS, although the results were not reproduced in other studies [5, 20]. Considering the fact that genetic polymorphisms associated with high salt-sensitivity (e.g. genes coding α-adducin, angiotensinogen and aldosterone synthase) are more prevalent in Asians than in Caucasians [90], Asians may more often have high-volume hypertension. Because intracranial arteries have a thinner media and adventitia and fewer elastic medial fibers than extracranial arteries [24], intracranial arteries may be more vulnerable to hemodynamic stress in this situation.

Diabetes mellitus

Diabetes mellitus was more closely associated with ICAS than with ECAS in previous studies [18, 19, 34]. However, because diabetes mellitus is not more frequent in East Asians than Caucasians, this cannot explain the high prevalence of ICAS in East Asia. The different controllability of diabetes mellitus [29], or different features of diabetes across the races may matter; Asians have a lower body mass index, a young age of onset, and greater visceral adiposity that can lead to insulin resistance [91]. One study [92] showed that higher homeostasis model assessment of insulin resistance (HOMA-IR) levels were more closely associated with ICAS than ECAS in patients without diabetes.

Hypercholesterolemia

Hypercholesterolemia is a more important risk factor for ECAS than for ICAS [1, 2, 10, 17, 18, 93]. Because Asians have lower serum cholesterol levels than Caucasians, hypercholesterolemia may be an important factor explaining the racial differences in the location of cerebral atherosclerosis. Intracranial arteries may have an inherent resistance to the toxic effects of hypercholesterolemia. In monkeys [94] and rabbits [95], the development of atherosclerosis after consuming an atherogenic diet occurs significantly later in intracranial arteries than in extracranial arteries. It was suggested that a specific glycocalyx composition on luminal endothelial cells may inhibit trapping of chylomicrons and very-low-density lipoprotein, resulting in reduced deposition of apolipoproteins in the intima of intracranial vessels [94].

Cigarette Smoking

At least two studies have reported that smoking is a more important risk factor for ECAS than for ICAS [19, 29]. However, the effect of cigarette smoking on the location of atherosclerosis may differ according to age. One of the authors found that smoking was more closely associated with ICAS in young men, but not in old men (unpublished data). Perhaps, intracranial arteries may be more vulnerable to the harmful effect (e.g, deletion of anti-oxidants) of smoking in young patients.

Metabolic Syndrome

Metabolic syndrome is more closely associated with ICAS than with ECAS in both Asian [44, 45, 96] and Caucasian [19] patients. As discussed above, metabolic syndrome is associated with insulin resistance, and increases patients' vulnerability to oxidative stress [97]. Because there is a greater activity of antioxidant enzymes in intracranial arteries than in extracranial arteries [58], patients with metabolic syndrome may preferentially develop ICAS. Symptomatic ICAS was found to be associated with a lower serum adiponectin level as compared to other stroke subtypes [46]. ApoAI, a marker of antioxidant properties, was found to be decreased, and apoB/apoA was increased in patients with ICAS. ApoB/apoA was closely associated with metabolic syndrome [38, 98].

Because the prevalence of metabolic syndrome is lower in Asians than in Caucasians [99], the presence of metabolic syndrome per se cannot explain the high prevalence of ICAS among Asians. There may be racial differences in the component of, or the host-response to metabolic syndrome [82]. Despite the similar age and body mass index, African-Americans [100] and Indo-Asians [101] have a lower adiponectin level and insulin sensitivity than Caucasians. In addition, there was a higher prevalence of obesity-related hypertension in African-Americans, obesity-related diabetes in Hispanics, and the glucose intolerance in lean young Asians, than in whites [102]. Racial differences in the mechanisms of metabolic syndrome-induced atherosclerotic progression were also reported [103]. Moreover, as discussed above, there have been pieces of evidence that obstructive sleep apnea is a manifestation of metabolic syndrome [73]. Sleep apnea was found to be associated with a lesser degree of obesity in Asians than in Caucasians [77]. Such racial-ethnic differences in manifestations of metabolic syndrome, possibly associated with genetic predisposition [104], may be related with the racial differences in the location of atherosclerosis [46].

Genes

Several polymorphisms of genes related to renin-angiotensin aldosterone system were also reported to be more frequent in Asians. Among them, T(–344)C polymorphism of the aldosterone system was associated with ICAS but not with ECAS [105]. A study reported that the frequency of TT genotype of phosphodiesterase (PDE4D) was significantly higher in patients with ICAS (20%) than those without ICAS (2%) [106].

A polymorphism of c.14576G>A in ring finger protein *(RNF)* 213 was found to be present in 73% of definite moyamoya disease (MMD) patients [107]. The number of patients with this genetic polymorphism was estimated to be 16.2 million in East Asian countries [108]. Interestingly, studies from Korea and Japan have shown that a significant proportion (22–24%) of patients with non-MMD ICAS have the *RNF213* variant [107, 109, 110]. Thus, *RNF213* genetic variant may not be specific for MMD, but simply a marker that increases the vascular vulnerability to hemodynamic stress, ultimately causing ICAS [111]. The different prevalence of RNF gene polymorphism may be one of the factors for the high prevalence of ICAS in East Asia.

Vascular Tortuosity and Hemodynamic Changes

Recently, the tortuosity of the middle cerebral artery was found to be higher in patients with ICAS than in patients with ECAS or control subjects [112], suggesting arterial tortuosity may a factor determining the location of atherosclerosis. The racial differences in arterial tortuosity may be one of the reasons for ethnic differences in the location of cerebral atherosclerosis. Further studies are required to compare vascular tortuosity and associated genes among different races.

Contamination of ICAS Cases with Other Non-Atherosclerotic Diseases

Imaging techniques such as magnetic resonance angiography and catheter angiography can examine luminal stenosis but not vascular wall pathology. Therefore, non-atherosclerotic etiologies such as MMD, dissection, and vasculitis can be erroneously categorized as ICAS. One diagnostic tool that can be used to examine the vessel wall is high-resolution vessel wall magnetic resonance imaging (HRMRI) [113].

A recent study from Korea assessed HRMRI findings in patients who were diagnosed as presumable ICAS, but were young (age ≤55 years) and had minimal risk factors. Of the 95 patients analyzed, only 26 (27.4%) had HRMRI findings consistent with atherosclerosis whereas others showed findings consistent with MMD, dissection, and vasculitis. These data suggest that diagnosis based solely on angiogram findings may not be accurate and that contamination of non-atherosclerosis cases have occurred in previous ICAS studies. Because MMD [114], arterial dissection [115], and vasculitis [116] are more frequent causes of intracranial disease in Asians than in Caucasians, the notion that ICAS is more common in Asians than Caucasians may at least in part be influenced by contamination.

References

1 Caplan LR, Gorelick PB, Hier DB: Race, sex and occlusive cerebrovascular disease: a review. Stroke 1986;17:648–655.

2 Kuller L, Reisler DM: An explanation for variations in distribution of stroke and arteriosclerotic heart disease among populations and racial groups. Am J Epidemiol 1971;93:1–9.

3 Sacco RL, Kargman DE, Gu Q, Zamanillo MC: Race-ethnicity and determinants of intracranial atherosclerotic cerebral infarction. The northern Manhattan stroke study. Stroke 1995;26:14–20.

4 Gorelick PB, Caplan LR, Hier DB, Parker SL, Patel D: Racial differences in the distribution of anterior circulation occlusive disease. Neurology 1984;34:54–59.

5 Inzitari D, Hachinski VC, Taylor DW, Barnett HJ: Racial differences in the anterior circulation in cerebrovascular disease. How much can be explained by risk factors? Arch Neurol 1990;47:1080–1084.

6 Nishimaru K, McHenry LC Jr, Toole JF: Cerebral angiographic and clinical differences in carotid system transient ischemic attacks between American Caucasian and Japanese patients. Stroke 1984;15:56–59.

7 White H, Boden-Albala B, Wang C, Elkind MS, Rundek T, Wright CB, et al: Ischemic stroke subtype incidence among whites, blacks, and Hispanics: the northern Manhattan study. Circulation 2005;111:1327–1331.

8 Sacco RL, Boden-Albala B, Abel G, Lin IF, Elkind M, Hauser WA, et al: Race-ethnic disparities in the impact of stroke risk factors: the northern manhattan stroke study. Stroke 2001;32:1725–1731.

9 Kim YD, Choi HY, Jung YH, Nam CM, Yang JH, Cho HJ, et al: Classic risk factors for atherosclerosis are not major determinants for location of extracranial or intracranial cerebral atherosclerosis. Neuroepidemiology 2009;32:201–207.

10 Uehara T, Tabuchi M, Mori E: Frequency and clinical correlates of occlusive lesions of cerebral arteries in japanese patients without stroke. Evaluation by mr angiography. Cerebrovasc Dis 1998; 8:267–272.

11 Uehara T, Tabuchi M, Mori E: Risk factors for occlusive lesions of intracranial arteries in stroke-free japanese. Eur J Neurol 2005;12:218–222.

12 Bae HJ, Lee J, Park JM, Kwon O, Koo JS, Kim BK, et al: Risk factors of intracranial cerebral atherosclerosis among asymptomatics. Cerebrovasc Dis 2007;24: 355–360.

13 Wong KS, Ng PW, Tang A, Liu R, Yeung V, Tomlinson B: Prevalence of asymptomatic intracranial atherosclerosis in high-risk patients. Neurology 2007;68: 2035–2038.

14 Huang HW, Guo MH, Lin RJ, Chen YL, Luo Q, Zhang Y, et al: Prevalence and risk factors of middle cerebral artery stenosis in asymptomatic residents in rongqi county, guangdong. Cerebrovasc Dis 2007;24:111–115.

15 Resch JA, Baker AB: Etiologic mechanisms in cerebral atherosclerosis. Preliminary study of 3,839 cases. Arch Neurol 1964;10:617–628.

16 Bos D, van der Rijk MJ, Geeraedts TE, Hofman A, Krestin GP, Witteman JC, et al: Intracranial carotid artery atherosclerosis: prevalence and risk factors in the general population. Stroke 2012;43: 1878–1884.

17 Kim JS, Nah HW, Park SM, Kim SK, Cho KH, Lee J, et al: Risk factors and stroke mechanisms in atherosclerotic stroke: intracranial compared with extracranial and anterior compared with posterior circulation disease. Stroke 2012;43: 3313–3318.

18 Lei C, Wu B, Liu M, Chen Y: Risk factors and clinical outcomes associated with intracranial and extracranial atherosclerotic stenosis acute ischemic stroke. J Stroke Cerebrovasc Dis 2014;23:1112–1117.

19 Lopez-Cancio E, Galan A, Dorado L, Jimenez M, Hernandez M, Millan M, et al: Biological signatures of asymptomatic extra- and intracranial atherosclerosis: the barcelona-asia (asymptomatic intracranial atherosclerosis) study. Stroke 2012;43:2712–2719.

20 Wityk RJ, Lehman D, Klag M, Coresh J, Ahn H, Litt B: Race and sex differences in the distribution of cerebral atherosclerosis. Stroke 1996;27:1974–1980.

21 Solberg LA, McGarry PA: Cerebral atherosclerosis in negroes and caucasians. Atherosclerosis 1972;16:141–154.

22 Williams AO, Resch JA, Loewenson RB: Cerebral atherosclerosis–a comparative autopsy study between Nigerian negroes and American negroes and Caucasians. Neurology 1969;19:205–210.

23 Joakimsen O, Bonaa KH, Stensland-Bugge E, Jacobsen BK: Population-based study of age at menopause and ultrasound assessed carotid atherosclerosis: the tromso study. J Clin Epidemiol 2000; 53:525–530.

24 Ritz K, Denswil NP, Stam OC, van Lieshout JJ, Daemen MJ: Cause and mechanisms of intracranial atherosclerosis. Circulation 2014;130:1407–1414.

25 Fisher CM, Gore I, Okabe N, White PD: Atherosclerosis of the carotid and vertebral arteries – extracranial and intracranial. J Neuropathol Exp Neurol 1965;24: 455–476.
26 Yasaka M, Yamaguchi T, Shichiri M: Distribution of atherosclerosis and risk factors in atherothrombotic occlusion. Stroke 1993;24:206–211.
27 Takahashi K, Kitani M, Fukuda H, Kobayashi S: Vascular risk factors for atherosclerotic lesions of the middle cerebral artery detected by magnetic resonance angiography (mra). Acta Neurol Scand 1999;100:395–399.
28 Wong KS, Huang YN, Yang HB, Gao S, Li H, Liu JY, et al: A door-to-door survey of intracranial atherosclerosis in liangbei county, china. Neurology 2007;68: 2031–2034.
29 Leung SY, Ng TH, Yuen ST, Lauder IJ, Ho FC: Pattern of cerebral atherosclerosis in hong kong chinese. Severity in intracranial and extracranial vessels. Stroke 1993;24:779–786.
30 Mazighi M, Labreuche J, Gongora-Rivera F, Duyckaerts C, Hauw JJ, Amarenco P: Autopsy prevalence of intracranial atherosclerosis in patients with fatal stroke. Stroke 2008;39:1142–1147.
31 Kim JS, Choi-Kwon S: Risk factors for stroke in different levels of cerebral arterial disease. Eur Neurol 1999;42:150–156.
32 Arenillas JF, Molina CA, Chacon P, Rovira A, Montaner J, Coscojuela P, et al: High lipoprotein (a), diabetes, and the extent of symptomatic intracranial atherosclerosis. Neurology 2004;63:27–32.
33 Gorelick PB, Caplan LR, Langenberg P, Hier DB, Pessin M, Patel D, et al: Clinical and angiographic comparison of asymptomatic occlusive cerebrovascular disease. Neurology 1988;38:852–858.
34 Rincon F, Sacco RL, Kranwinkel G, Xu Q, Paik MC, Boden-Albala B, et al: Incidence and risk factors of intracranial atherosclerotic stroke: the northern Manhattan stroke study. Cerebrovasc Dis 2009;28:65–71.
35 Kim YS, Hong JW, Jung WS, Park SU, Park JM, Cho SI, et al: Gender differences in risk factors for intracranial cerebral atherosclerosis among asymptomatic subjects. Gend Med 2011;8:14–22.
36 Miyazawa N, Akiyama I, Yamagata Z: Analysis of incidence and risk factors for progression in patients with intracranial steno-occlusive lesions by serial magnetic resonance angiography. Clin Neurol Neurosurg 2007;109:680–685.
37 Ingall TJ, Homer D, Baker HL Jr, Kottke BA, O'Fallon WM, Whisnant JP: Predictors of intracranial carotid artery atherosclerosis. Duration of cigarette smoking and hypertension are more powerful than serum lipid levels. Arch Neurol 1991;48:687–691.
38 Park JH, Hong KS, Lee EJ, Lee J, Kim DE: High levels of apolipoprotein b/ai ratio are associated with intracranial atherosclerotic stenosis. Stroke 2011;42: 3040–3046.
39 Kim DE, Kim JY, Jeong SW, Cho YJ, Park JM, Lee JH, et al: Association between changes in lipid profiles and progression of symptomatic intracranial atherosclerotic stenosis: a prospective multicenter study. Stroke 2012;43:1824–1830.
40 Qian Y, Pu Y, Liu L, Wang DZ, Zhao X, Wang C, et al: Low hdl-c level is associated with the development of intracranial artery stenosis: analysis from the Chinese intracranial atherosclerosis (cicas) study. PLoS One 2013;8:e64395.
41 Wolf PA, D'Agostino RB, Kannel WB, Bonita R, Belanger AJ: Cigarette smoking as a risk factor for stroke. The framingham study. JAMA 1988;259:1025–1029.
42 Kim DE, Lee KB, Jang IM, Roh H, Ahn MY, Lee J: Associations of cigarette smoking with intracranial atherosclerosis in the patients with acute ischemic stroke. Clin Neurol Neurosurg 2012;114: 1243–1247.
43 Executive summary of the third report of the national cholesterol education program (ncep) expert panel on detection, evaluation, and treatment of high blood cholesterol in adults (adult treatment panel iii). JAMA 2001;285:2486–2497.
44 Bang OY, Kim JW, Lee JH, Lee MA, Lee PH, Joo IS, et al: Association of the metabolic syndrome with intracranial atherosclerotic stroke. Neurology 2005;65: 296–298.
45 Park JH, Kwon HM, Roh JK: Metabolic syndrome is more associated with intracranial atherosclerosis than extracranial atherosclerosis. Eur J Neurol 2007;14: 379–386.
46 Bang OY, Saver JL, Ovbiagele B, Choi YJ, Yoon SR, Lee KH: Adiponectin levels in patients with intracranial atherosclerosis. Neurology 2007;68:1931–1937.
47 Ovbiagele B, Saver JL, Lynn MJ, Chimowitz M: Impact of metabolic syndrome on prognosis of symptomatic intracranial atherostenosis. Neurology 2006;66:1344–1349.
48 Arita Y, Kihara S, Ouchi N, Takahashi M, Maeda K, Miyagawa J, et al: Paradoxical decrease of an adipose-specific protein, adiponectin, in obesity. Biochem Biophys Res Commun 1999;257:79–83.
49 Kadowaki T, Yamauchi T, Kubota N, Hara K, Ueki K, Tobe K: Adiponectin and adiponectin receptors in insulin resistance, diabetes, and the metabolic syndrome. J Clin Invest 2006;116:1784–1792.
50 Matsuda M, Shimomura I, Sata M, Arita Y, Nishida M, Maeda N, et al: Role of adiponectin in preventing vascular stenosis. The missing link of adipo-vascular axis. J Biol Chem 2002;277:37487–37491.
51 Shimabukuro M, Higa N, Asahi T, Oshiro Y, Takasu N, Tagawa T, et al: Hypoadiponectinemia is closely linked to endothelial dysfunction in man. J Clin Endocrinol Metab 2003;88:3236–3240.
52 Pilz S, Horejsi R, Moller R, Almer G, Scharnagl H, Stojakovic T, et al: Early atherosclerosis in obese juveniles is associated with low serum levels of adiponectin. J Clin Endocrinol Metab 2005;90: 4792–4796.
53 Kumada M, Kihara S, Sumitsuji S, Kawamoto T, Matsumoto S, Ouchi N, et al: Association of hypoadiponectinemia with coronary artery disease in men. Arterioscler Thromb Vasc Biol 2003;23: 85–89.
54 Pischon T, Girman CJ, Hotamisligil GS, Rifai N, Hu FB, Rimm EB: Plasma adiponectin levels and risk of myocardial infarction in men. JAMA 2004;291: 1730–1737.
55 Cai H, Harrison DG: Endothelial dysfunction in cardiovascular diseases: the role of oxidant stress. Circ Res 2000;87: 840–844.
56 Lee KU: Oxidative stress markers in korean subjects with insulin resistance syndrome. Diabetes Res Clin Pract 2001; 54(suppl 2):S29–S33.

57 Ford ES, Mokdad AH, Giles WH, Brown DW: The metabolic syndrome and antioxidant concentrations: findings from the third national health and nutrition examination survey. Diabetes 2003;52: 2346–2352.

58 D'Armiento FP, Bianchi A, de Nigris F, Capuzzi DM, D'Armiento MR, Crimi G, et al: Age-related effects on atherogenesis and scavenger enzymes of intracranial and extracranial arteries in men without classic risk factors for atherosclerosis. Stroke 2001;32:2472–2479.

59 Arenillas JF, Alvarez-Sabin J, Molina CA, Chacon P, Fernandez-Cadenas I, Ribo M, et al: Progression of symptomatic intracranial large artery atherosclerosis is associated with a proinflammatory state and impaired fibrinolysis. Stroke 2008;39:1456–1463.

60 Massot A, Pelegri D, Penalba A, Arenillas J, Boada C, Giralt D, et al: Lipoprotein-associated phospholipase a2 testing usefulness among patients with symptomatic intracranial atherosclerotic disease. Atherosclerosis 2011;218:181–187.

61 Wang Y, Zhang J, Qian Y, Tang X, Ling H, Chen K, et al: Association of lp-pla2 mass and aysmptomatic intracranial and extracranial arterial stenosis in hypertension patients. PloS One 2015; 10:e0130473.

62 Munoz-Torrero JF, Rivas D, Alonso R, Crespo L, Costo A, Roman M, et al: Influence of lipoprotein (a) on inflammatory biomarkers in metabolic syndrome. South Med J 2012;105:339–343.

63 Kim BS, Jung HS, Bang OY, Chung CS, Lee KH, Kim GM: Elevated serum lipoprotein(a) as a potential predictor for combined intracranial and extracranial artery stenosis in patients with ischemic stroke. Atherosclerosis 2010;212:682–688.

64 Virok D, Kis Z, Karai L, Intzedy L, Burian K, Szabo A, et al: Chlamydia pneumoniae in atherosclerotic middle cerebral artery. Stroke 2001;32:1973–1976.

65 Kim JS, Lee HS, Park HY, Kim SS, Kang HG, Kim NH, et al: Endothelial function in lacunar infarction: a comparison of lacunar infarction, cerebral atherosclerosis and control group. Cerebrovasc Dis 2009;28:166–170.

66 Jung KH, Chu K, Lee ST, Park HK, Bahn JJ, Kim DH, et al: Circulating endothelial microparticles as a marker of cerebrovascular disease. Ann Neurol 2009;66: 191–199.

67 Young T, Palta M, Dempsey J, Skatrud J, Weber S, Badr S: The occurrence of sleep-disordered breathing among middle-aged adults. N Engl J Med 1993;328: 1230–1235.

68 Grunstein RR, Stenlof K, Hedner J, Sjostrom L: Impact of obstructive sleep apnea and sleepiness on metabolic and cardiovascular risk factors in the swedish obese subjects (sos) study. Int J Obes Relat Metab Disord 1995;19:410–418.

69 Ip MS, Lam B, Ng MM, Lam WK, Tsang KW, Lam KS: Obstructive sleep apnea is independently associated with insulin resistance. Am J Respir Crit Care Med 2002;165:670–676.

70 Gruber A, Horwood F, Sithole J, Ali NJ, Idris I: Obstructive sleep apnoea is independently associated with the metabolic syndrome but not insulin resistance state. Cardiovasc Diabetol 2006;5:22.

71 Coughlin SR, Mawdsley L, Mugarza JA, Calverley PM, Wilding JP: Obstructive sleep apnoea is independently associated with an increased prevalence of metabolic syndrome. Eur Heart J 2004; 25:735–741.

72 Vgontzas AN, Papanicolaou DA, Bixler EO, Hopper K, Lotsikas A, Lin HM, et al: Sleep apnea and daytime sleepiness and fatigue: relation to visceral obesity, insulin resistance, and hypercytokinemia. J Clin Endocrinol Metab 2000;85:1151–1158.

73 Vgontzas AN, Bixler EO, Chrousos GP: Sleep apnea is a manifestation of the metabolic syndrome. Sleep Med Rev 2005;9:211–224.

74 Vgontzas AN, Legro RS, Bixler EO, Grayev A, Kales A, Chrousos GP: Polycystic ovary syndrome is associated with obstructive sleep apnea and daytime sleepiness: role of insulin resistance. J Clin Endocrinol Metab 2001;86:517–520.

75 Park YW, Zhu S, Palaniappan L, Heshka S, Carnethon MR, Heymsfield SB: The metabolic syndrome: prevalence and associated risk factor findings in the us population from the third national health and nutrition examination survey, 1988–1994. Arch Intern Med 2003; 163:427–436.

76 Peppard PE, Young T: Exercise and sleep-disordered breathing: an association independent of body habitus. Sleep 2004;27:480–484.

77 Villaneuva AT, Buchanan PR, Yee BJ, Grunstein RR: Ethnicity and obstructive sleep apnoea. Sleep Med Rev 2005;9: 419–436.

78 Yamada Y, Kato K, Oguri M, Yoshida T, Yokoi K, Watanabe S, et al: Association of genetic variants with atherothrombotic cerebral infarction in Japanese individuals with metabolic syndrome. Int J Mol Med 2008;21:801–808.

79 Arenillas JF, Massot A, Alvarez-Sabin J, Fernandez-Cadenas I, del Rio-Espinola A, Chacon P, et al: C-reactive protein gene c1444t polymorphism and risk of recurrent ischemic events in patients with symptomatic intracranial atherostenoses. Cerebrovasc Dis 2009;28:95–102.

80 Liu ZZ, Lv H, Gao F, Liu G, Zheng HG, Zhou YL, et al: Polymorphism in the human c-reactive protein (crp) gene, serum concentrations of crp, and the difference between intracranial and extracranial atherosclerosis. Clin Chim Acta 2008;389:40–44.

81 Caplan LR: Intracranial branch atheromatous disease: a neglected, understudied, and underused concept. Neurology 1989;39:1246–1250.

82 Bang OY: Intracranial atherosclerosis: current understanding and perspectives. J Stroke 2014;16:27–35.

83 Ryoo S, Park JH, Kim SJ, Kim GM, Chung CS, Lee KH, et al: Branch occlusive disease: clinical and magnetic resonance angiography findings. Neurology 2012;78:888–896.

84 Xu WH, Li ML, Gao S, Ni J, Zhou LX, Yao M, et al: Plaque distribution of stenotic middle cerebral artery and its clinical relevance. Stroke 2011;42:2957–2959.

85 Nah HW, Kang DW, Kwon SU, Kim JS: Diversity of single small subcortical infarctions according to infarct location and parent artery disease: analysis of indicators for small vessel disease and atherosclerosis. Stroke 2010;41:2822–2827.

86 Turan TN, Derdeyn CP, Fiorella D, Chimowitz MI: Treatment of atherosclerotic intracranial arterial stenosis. Stroke 2009;40:2257–2261.

87 Ryoo S, Lee MJ, Cha J, Jeon P, Bang OY: Differential vascular pathophysiologic types of intracranial atherosclerotic stroke: a high-resolution wall magnetic resonance imaging study. Stroke 2015; 46:2815–2821.

88 Conklin J, Silver FL, Mikulis DJ, Mandell DM: Are acute infarcts the cause of leukoaraiosis? Brain mapping for 16 consecutive weeks. Ann Neurol 2014;76: 899–904.
89 Kim JS, Kim YJ, Ahn SH, Kim BJ: Location of cerebral atherosclerosis: why is there a difference between east and west? Int J Stroke 2016 [Epub ahead of print].
90 Kokubo Y: Prevention of hypertension and cardiovascular diseases: a comparison of lifestyle factors in westerners and East Asians. Hypertension 2014;63:655–660.
91 Rhee EJ: Diabetes in asians. Endocrinol Metab (Seoul) 2015;30:263–269.
92 Park HY, Kyeong H, Park DS, Lee HS, Chang H, Kim YS, et al: Correlation between insulin resistance and intracranial atherosclerosis in patients with ischemic stroke without diabetes. J Stroke Cerebrovasc Dis 2008;17:401–405.
93 Heyden S, Heyman A, Goree JA: Nonembolic occlusion of the middle cerebral and carotid arteries – a comparison of predisposing factors. Stroke 1970;1: 363–369.
94 Weber G: Delayed experimental atherosclerotic involvement of cerebral arteries in monkeys and rabbits (light, sem and tem observations). Pathol Res Pract 1985;180:353–355.
95 Kurozumi T, Imamura T, Tanaka K, Yae Y, Koga S: Permeation and deposition of fibrinogen and low-density lipoprotein in the aorta and cerebral artery of rabbits – immuno-electron microscopic study. Br J Exp Pathol 1984;65:355–364.
96 De Silva DA, Woon FP, Lee MP, Chen CL, Chang HM, Wong MC: Metabolic syndrome is associated with intracranial large artery disease among ethnic Chinese patients with stroke. J Stroke Cerebrovasc Dis 2009;18:424–427.
97 Palmieri VO, Grattagliano I, Portincasa P, Palasciano G: Systemic oxidative alterations are associated with visceral adiposity and liver steatosis in patients with metabolic syndrome. J Nutr 2006; 136:3022–3026.
98 Li MM, Lin YY, Huang YH, Zhuo ST, Yang ML, Lin HS, et al: Association of apolipoprotein a1, b with stenosis of intracranial and extracranial arteries in patients with cerebral infarction. Clin Lab 2015;61:1727–1735.
99 Hoang KC, Le TV, Wong ND: The metabolic syndrome in east asians. J Cardiometab Syndr 2007;2:276–282.
100 Lee S, Bacha F, Gungor N, Arslanian SA: Racial differences in adiponectin in youth: relationship to visceral fat and insulin sensitivity. Diabetes Care 2006; 29:51–56.
101 Valsamakis G, Chetty R, McTernan PG, Al-Daghri NM, Barnett AH, Kumar S: Fasting serum adiponectin concentration is reduced in Indo-Asian subjects and is related to hdl cholesterol. Diabetes Obes Metab 2003;5: 131–135.
102 Cossrow N, Falkner B: Race/ethnic issues in obesity and obesity-related comorbidities. J Clin Endocrinol Metab 2004;89:2590–2594.
103 Li S, Chen W, Srinivasan SR, Tang R, Bond MG, Berenson GS: Race (black-white) and gender divergences in the relationship of childhood cardiovascular risk factors to carotid artery intima-media thickness in adulthood: The bogalusa heart study. Atherosclerosis 2007;194:421–425.
104 Oguri M, Kato K, Yoshida T, Fujimaki T, Horibe H, Yokoi K, et al: Association of a genetic variant of btn2a1 with metabolic syndrome in east asian populations. J Med Genet 2011;48:787–792.
105 Munshi A, Sharma V, Kaul S, Rajeshwar K, Babu MS, Shafi G, et al: Association of the -344c/t aldosterone synthase (cyp11b2) gene variant with hypertension and stroke. J Neurol Sci 2010;296:34–38.
106 Kalita J, Somarajan BI, Kumar B, Kumar S, Mittal B, Misra UK: Phosphodiesterase 4 d gene polymorphism in relation to intracranial and extracranial atherosclerosis in ischemic stroke. Dis Markers 2011;31:191–197.
107 Miyawaki S, Imai H, Takayanagi S, Mukasa A, Nakatomi H, Saito N: Identification of a genetic variant common to moyamoya disease and intracranial major artery stenosis/occlusion. Stroke 2012;43:3371–3374.
108 Liu W, Hitomi T, Kobayashi H, Harada KH, Koizumi A: Distribution of moyamoya disease susceptibility polymorphism p.R4810k in rnf213 in east and southeast Asian populations. Neurol Med Chir 2012;52:299–303.
109 Bang OY, Ryoo S, Kim SJ, Yoon CH, Cha J, Yeon JY, et al: Adult moyamoya disease: a burden of intracranial stenosis in east asians? PLoS One 2015; 10:e0130663.
110 Miyawaki S, Imai H, Shimizu M, Yagi S, Ono H, Mukasa A, et al: Genetic variant rnf213 c.14576g>a in various phenotypes of intracranial major artery stenosis/occlusion. Stroke 2013;44:2894–2897.
111 Fujimura M, Sonobe S, Nishijima Y, Niizuma K, Sakata H, Kure S, et al: Genetics and biomarkers of moyamoya disease: significance of rnf213 as a susceptibility gene. J Stroke 2014;16:65–72.
112 Kim BJ, Kim SM, Kang DW, Kwon SU, Suh DC, Kim JS: Vascular tortuosity may be related to intracranial artery atherosclerosis. Int J Stroke 2015;10: 1081–1086.
113 Choi YJ, Jung SC, Lee DH: Vessel wall imaging of the intracranial and cervical carotid arteries. J Stroke 2015 17: 238–255.
114 Kuroda S, Houkin K: Moyamoya disease: current concepts and future perspectives. Lancet Neurol 2008;7:1056–1066.
115 Huang YC, Chen YF, Wang YH, Tu YK, Jeng JS, Liu HM: Cervicocranial arterial dissection: experience of 73 patients in a single center. Surg Neurol 2009;72(suppl 2):S20–S27; discussion S27.
116 Cheng MK: A review of cerebrovascular surgery in the people's republic of China. Stroke 1982;13:249–255.

Toshiyuki Uehara, MD
Department of Neurology, Hyogo Brain and Heart Center at Himeji
520 Saisho-ko, Himeji
Hyogo 670-0981 (Japan)
E-Mail tuehara@hbhc.jp

Kim JS, Caplan LR, Wong KS (eds): Intracranial Atherosclerosis: Pathophysiology, Diagnosis and Treatment.
Front Neurol Neurosci. Basel, Karger, 2016, vol 40, pp 58–71 (DOI: 10.1159/000448302)

Stroke Mechanisms

Ka Sing Wong[a] · Louis R. Caplan[b] · Jong S. Kim[c]

[a]Department of Medicine and Therapeutics, Chinese University of Hong Kong, Shatin, Hong Kong, SAR, China; [b]Department of Neurology, Beth Israel Deaconess Medical Center, Harvard Medical School, Boston, Mass., USA; [c]Department of Neurology, Asan Medical Center, University of Ulsan, Seoul, Korea

Abstract

Recent advances in neuroimaging technologies, such as diffusion weighted magnetic resonance imaging (MRI), perfusion weighted computed tomography (CT)/MRI, MR/CT angiography and Doppler ultrasonography allow us to determine the mechanisms of stroke and transient ischemic attack. In addition, high-resolution vessel wall MRI is nowadays increasingly used to understand the stroke mechanism in patients with intracranial atherosclerosis. Artery to artery embolism, hypoperfusion and the combination of the two are the important stroke mechanisms in patients with extracranial atherosclerosis. In addition to the above two, branch occlusion and in-situ thrombotic occlusion are important stroke mechanisms in patients with intracranial atherosclerosis. Branch occlusion leads to subcortical or brainstem infarcts indistinguishable from infarcts caused by small artery disease. In-situ thrombotic occlusion leads to larger territorial infarcts. However, whole territory infarcts are uncommon due to relatively well developed collateral circulation in these patients. The treatment strategy should be based on the correct understanding of the stroke mechanism in individual patients.

Atherosclerotic disease of the intracranial large artery, especially the middle cerebral artery (MCA), is the commonest cause of stroke and transient ischemic attack (TIA) in most part of the world, except in Europe and North America. The pathology of intracranial atherosclerosis is not much different from atherosclerosis in other part of the circulation such as the aorta, coronary and carotid arteries. Lipid-laden plaques with various thickness of capsule are commonly found in intracranial atherosclerosis. The details of the pathological features are covered in Chapter 2.

Yet, the stroke mechanisms may vary in different patients. Artery to artery embolism, in-situ thrombosis, hemodynamic insufficiency, branch occlusive diseases or the combination of these mechanisms leads to brain ischemia. Coexisting causes such as small vessel disease and cardioembolism are also commonly found in the same patient. Recently, advances in neuroimaging technologies such as high resolution magnetic resonance imaging (HRMRI) vessel wall imaging,

Table 1. Mechanisms of brain infarction and TIA in patients with intracranial atherosclerosis

Stroke mechanism	Frequency	Pattern of infarcts	Number of infarct
In situ thrombotic occlusion	Uncommon	Large subcortical Sometimes with borderzone Rarely, whole territory	Single Sometimes enlarging
Artery to artery embolism*	Common	Small cortical and subcortical	Multiple
Impaired clearance of emboli*	Common	Small, scattered, alongside the borderzone region	Multiple
Branch occlusive disease	Common	Small subcortical, lacune-like	Single
Hemodynamic	Uncommon	Borderzone May be without lesion	Multiple None

* These mechanisms frequently co-exist.

computer flow dynamic, microembolic signal (MES) detection, diffusion weighted imaging (DWI) and various blood flow measurement have provided insights into various aspects of stroke mechanism in patients with intracranial atherosclerosis. It is important to delineate the stroke mechanism since treatment and prevention strategies should be based on the correct understanding of pathophysiological mechanism in an individual patient.

Neuroimaging Investigations to Study Stroke Mechanisms

Advances in neuroimaging have provided new insights into the stroke mechanisms of intracranial atherosclerosis. Newer generation CT angiography and MR angiography easily depict the location and severity of intracranial stenosis. DWI is the most sensitive tool to detect tiny, symptomatic or asymptomatic cerebral ischemic lesions and can differentiate recent infarcts from old ones [1]. Using DWI, the characteristic topographic patterns of cerebral infarcts may be individually assessed. On the other hand, fluid-attenuated inversion recovery (FLAIR) sequences offer advantages in detection of infarcts affecting the cortical ribbon because cortical infarcts may be hard to detect given the similarly high signal of cortical gray matter and adjacent cerebrospinal fluid, and the complex convolutional geometry of the surface of the brain [2]. In addition, transcranial Doppler (TCD) can non-invasively identify narrowing and collateralization of major intracranial large arteries in patients with good temporal windows. MES detected by TCD is likely to represent artery to artery embolus passing through the insonated artery [3]. The application of these advanced imaging technologies is described in detail in Chapters 8 and 9.

Stroke Mechanisms in Intracranial Atherosclerosis

Possible mechanisms for brain infarction or TIA arising from intracranial atherosclerosis include thrombosis leading to complete occlusion, artery-to-artery embolism, hemodynamic compromise (hypoperfusion), local branch occlusion of the orifice of a deep perforator, or the combination of these mechanisms [4, 5] (table 1).

In situ Thrombotic Occlusion

Acute thrombosis begins with fissuring of the fibrous cap of the atherosclerotic plaque, which disrupts the endothelial surface of the artery. Release of tissue factors promotes the development of a clot adjacent to the plaque [6]. Local occlusion and secondary artery to artery embolism can then result [7]. Occlusive mural thrombosis can be formed at the site of severe stenosis with or without plaque rupture/intraplaque haemorrhage [8]. Plaque instability can be related to factors such as inflammation, autoimmunity, or genetic predisposition, and these conditions may play a role in acceleration of atherosclerosis in addition to traditional risk factors [9].

In patients with intracranial atherosclerosis, in-situ thrombotic occlusion usually produces infarcts that are larger than those caused by other mechanisms. However, unlike patients with cardiogenic embolism, the in-situ thrombotic occlusion rarely produces whole territory infarction because of the relatively well developed collateral circulation in patients with chronic atherosclerotic disease. In patients with MCA steno-occlusion, the initial lesions are usually restricted to the striatocapsular area, borderzone area or the combination of both. Occasionally, an initial infarct evolves to a larger lesion along with progressive neurological worsening. Thus, the ultimate size of the infarct may vary according to the development of collateral circulation, the speed of arterial occlusion and hemodynamic stability after the occurrence of stroke. With sufficient collaterals, total thrombotic intracranial occlusion may remain asymptomatic, or produce only minor brain infarcts or TIAs. With the availability of high resolution MRI, it is now feasible to show lumen thrombosis in clinical practice [10].

Artery to Artery Embolism

Apart from occlusion at the site of thrombosis, forceful blood flow can break up a portion of the thrombus and carry it to distal branches. Besides, ulceration of the surface of the plaque can be the source of atherosclerotic debris (cholesterol embolism) that migrates to distal vessels. Blockage of the distal branches by embolism causes cerebral infarction. MES monitoring is now an established method to detect symptomatic or asymptomatic embolism in patients with MCA disease [3, 11].

For MCA occlusion, cardiac diseases especially atrial fibrillation is the most frequent cause. The resultant stroke is usually quite large and disabling [12]. Internal carotid artery (ICA) atherosclerotic disease is another important source of embolism, leading to MCA occlusion and brain infarcts [13]. Cerebral angiography within the first 6 h after the onset of ischemic symptoms shows intracranial occlusion in about 80% of the cases that is usually caused by emboli [14, 15]. Cardioembolic stroke is commonly associated with a bigger infarct than an embolic stroke of arterial origin partly because the clots are larger and partly because of the insufficient development of collateral circulation.

In patients with intrinsic intracranial atherosclerosis, artery to artery embolism (i.e., proximal MCA to distal MCA) is also an important mechanism of stroke (fig. 1). DWI is particularly useful in assessing the embolic mechanism of stroke because it can reliably detect small, scattered, infarcts occasionally along the borderzone regions (fig. 1 in Chapter 6). Moreover, the artery-to-artery embolism is often associated with perfusion deficits in the territory of the stenosed vessel [16]. Perhaps, underlying perfusion deficits may contribute to the development of embolic infarction through impaired clearance of emboli [12].

Branch Occlusive Disease

Atherosclerotic plaque in the intracranial artery can protrude into the orifice of the perforators and occlude the lumen causing a subcortical infarct [17]. This so-called atheromatous branch occlusion is different from lipohyalinosis, a hypertensive change of the media of small vessels. Lipohyalinosis causes segmental disorganization of penetrating arteries along the course of the

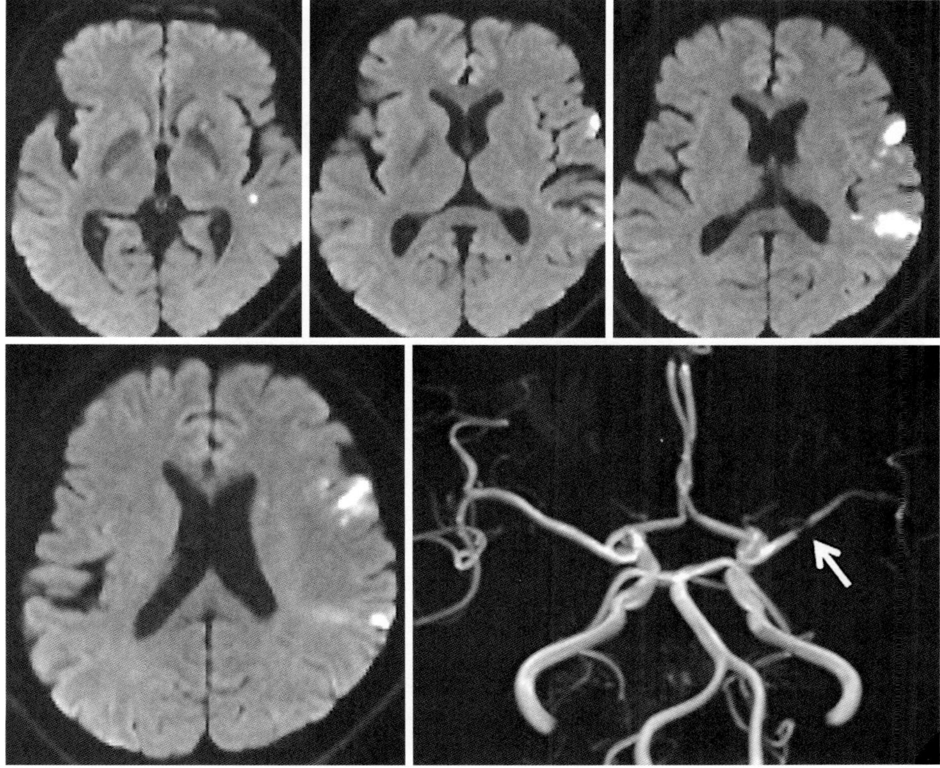

Fig. 1. A 64-year-old man with hypertension and diabetes mellitus developed mild mixed aphasia and right arm weakness. Diffusion weighted MRI showed several scattered, embolic infarcts in the left MCA territory. MR angiography showed severe atherosclerotic narrowing of the left MCA (arrow, right lower image). He did not have an embolic heart disease such as atrial fibrillation.

vessel, whereas atheromatous branch disease affects the vessel orifice. Pathological features of this type of branch occlusion were previously described by Lhermitte et al. [18] and Fisher [19–21]. The pathology includes microdissection, plaque hemorrhage, and platelet and platelet-fibrin materials.

The concept of atheromatous branch occlusive disease has broadened our understanding on the pathogenesis of deep, subcortical (lacunar) infarcts. Traditionally accepted pathological hallmarks of lacunar infarction are 15–20 mm, irregular cavities deep in the cerebral hemisphere, brain stem, and cerebellum [19, 22–28]. However, true lacunar infarcts are usually smaller than 0.5–1 cm when they are detected by brain imaging studies. If the lesion is larger than 1 cm, the diagnosis of small artery occlusive disease may have to be questioned. Although lipohyalinosis or fibrinoid necrosis of a small artery is still an important cause of these small, deep subcortical infarcts [29], Caplan [17] argued that (1) deep infarcts may also be caused by large cerebral artery diseases or even embolization from proximal artery or the heart [30, 31]; (2) the clinical diagnosis of lacune is difficult to make and not easily be differentiated from symptoms caused by large artery occlusive disease; and (3) many patients with lacunar infarction do not have hypertension nor have a history of high blood pressure.

Thus, lacunar infarcts are actually caused by intracranial branch atheromatous disease in many patients [17]. Nevertheless, atheromatous branch disease has been documented uncommonly because of the rarity of careful neuropathologic studies of intracranial arteries. Branch pathology can be accurately assessed only by meticulous analysis of serial sections of intracranial vascular specimens at necropsy. Although branch disease is a pathologic entity that can only be diagnosed with certainty at postmortem, following clinical or imaging features may support the diagnosis of atheromatous branch disease; (1) the infarcts are small, deep and confined to the territory of one or a few penetrating branches and (2) gradual or stepwise progression or fluctuation of symptoms and signs suggesting intrinsic 'thrombotic' disease rather than embolism, (3) vascular studies and cardiac evaluation show no significant extracranial large artery occlusive disease or emboligenic heart disease (4) there is no past or present hypertension and no evidence of end organ damage of hypertension such as retinopathy or left ventricular cardiac hypertrophy [17].

With the advances of imaging technologies such as MR angiogram or CT angiogram, intracranial atherosclerosis producing branch occlusion is nowadays more easily recognized. Recent literatures from Asian countries that used such imaging tools have shown that perforating branch occlusion is an important stroke mechanism of intracranial atherosclerosis and that many of the so-called lacunar infarcts are actually caused by intracranial large artery disease rather than lipohyalinosis [32–34].

The infarction resulting from occlusion of the orifice of the branch tends to extend to the basal surface and is vertically long (fig. 2, and fig. 2 in Chapter 6) while a lacune caused by lipohyalinosis usually produces an island of small ischemic tissue within the parenchyma. The subcortical infarcts caused by branch atheromatous disease are expected to be larger in size and associated with more unstable clinical course than those caused by lipohyalinosis [32, 33]. However, other studies argued that the size and clinical presentations are not different between these two groups of subcortical infarction [35].

One of the problems in investigating this issue is the sensitivity and specificity of existing imaging techniques in detecting mild atherosclerosis. As discussed above, the arterial stenosis producing branch occlusion is usually less severe than that producing artery to artery embolism or hemodynamic stroke [36]. In patients with very mild intracranial stenosis, the stenotic lesion cannot be detected by TCD, and remains often questionable even when MR angiography is used. Moreover, because the imaging diagnosis of atherosclerosis is based on findings of luminal narrowing of an artery, atherosclerotic thickening of the vessel walls without causing intraluminal narrowing cannot be identified with current technologies. In this sense, it seems likely that atheromatous branch disease is still underestimated even in this era of MRI and MR angiography. Vessel wall imaging using HRMRI improves our understanding of branch atheromatous disease [37] (fig. 3). Branch atheromatous disease on HRMRI without lumen stenosis has been shown to be associated with capsular warning syndrome [38].

Hypoperfusion

Before the onset of acute thromboembolism formation, atherosclerotic plaque gradually increases over years. The vessel can remodel to expand outward initially [39] but later the plaque grows slowly and impinges on the vascular lumen; consequently, blood flow becomes disturbed [40]. The narrowing leads to turbulence of blood flow and finally hypoperfusion distal to the stenosis. Severe stenosis or occlusion leads to failure of perfusion to one or more regions of the brain. In addition, turbulence and fast flow velocity increase the shear stress on the endothelium and encourage fissuring of the plaque which in turn activates platelets and clotting factors. Recent observations [41, 42] showed a close correlation

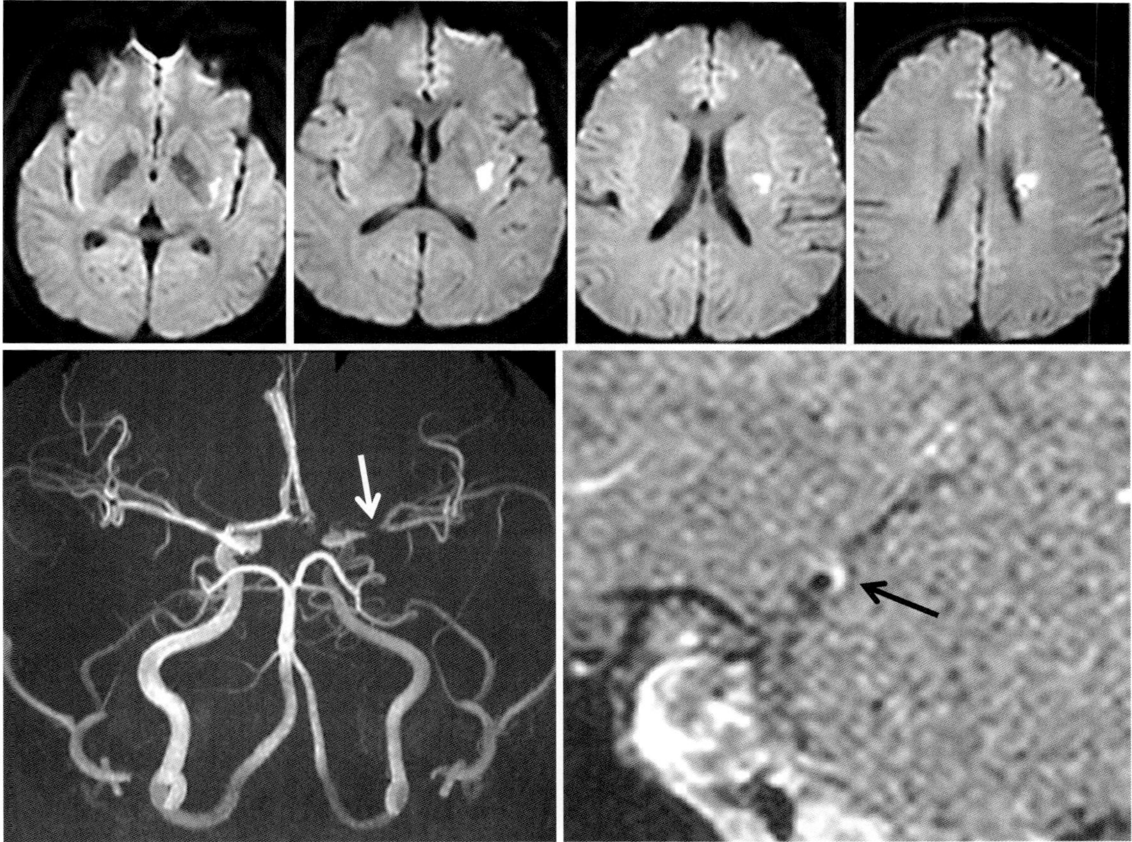

Fig. 2. A 55-year-old hypertensive man developed right hemiparesis and dysarthria. Diffusion weighed MRI showed a subcortical infarct that involves the right corona radiata and internal capsule (upper row). MR angiography showed a focal, right middle cerebral artery stenosis that probably occluded the orifice of the perforating artery (arrow, Left lower image). High resolution vessel wall MRI showed enhanced plaque in the stenosed vessel (arrow, right lower image).

between the recurrence of ischemic stroke and the severity of occlusive disease producing hypoperfusion. Chronic intracranial atherosclerosis of the MCA stenosis with borderzone infarcrtion is associated with increased Oxygen Extraction Fraction on PET scan indicating hemodynamic compromise may be an important factor [43].

In clinical practice, hypoperfusion caused by a process occurring at a distance from the brain (for example, the heart or neck arteries) rarely produces major brain infarction [44]. On the contrary, decreased blood flow caused by a lesion directly at the site of vulnerable brain tissue is not so benign. Occlusion of penetrating arteries by a lipohyalinotic process or by atheromatous branch disease [17, 19, 20, 37] often causes an infarct directly in the center of perfusion of the obstructed artery. Similarly, severe intracranial arterial occlusive disease seems more likely to cause brain infarction than extracranial occlusive disease [45–47]. While the Circle of Willis serves as a collateral supply in patients with extracranial diseases, it may take more time to develop cortical collaterals in those with intracranial arterial diseases.

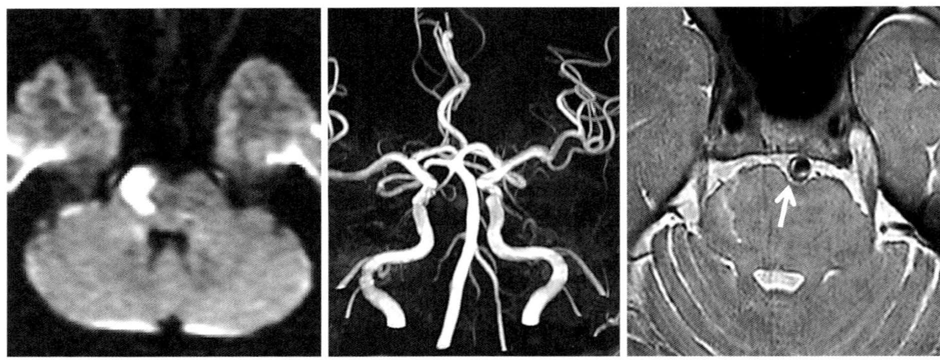

Fig. 3. A 61-year-old hypertensive and diabetic woman developed left hemiparesis and dysarthria. Diffusion weighed MRI showed a right pontine infarction (left image). MR angiography showed a normal-looking basilar artery (middle image). High resolution vessel wall MRI showed enhanced plaque in the right lateral and dorsal part of the vessel wall (arrow, right image) that probably caused branch occlusion.

Although hypoperfusion to a specific region of the brain is clearly an important factor for the development of infarct, the status of the collateral circulation can influence the size of the lesion. Insufficient collaterals and blood flow may be a factor predicting future strokes as well. According to Han et al. [48] who measured the extracranial arterial blood flow volume by color velocity imaging quantification ultrasound (CVIQ) in a cohort of 210 acute stroke patients, total cerebral blood flow was an independent predictor for future ischemic events; the mean extracranial blood flow volume was significantly lower for patients who had a recurrent stroke than those without.

In patients with insufficient collaterals, so-called hemodynamic strokes or TIAs may occur. Typically, TIA symptoms such as hemiparesis, dysarthria, aphasia (in anterior circulation disease) or dizziness, diplopia, visual disturbances (in posterior circulation disease) occur briefly and stereotypically when the patients are dehydrated, exhausted or at the time when they suddenly stand up. When stroke occurs, the symptoms may fluctuate widely according to the degree of hydration and head position. Adequate hydration and cerebral blood flow maintenance is important in the management of these patients. Occasionally, interventional revascularization therapies such as by-pass surgery or angiography/stenting relieve the patients' symptoms dramatically (fig. 4).

Traditionally, hypoperfusion and embolism are considered independent mechanisms of stroke in patients with arterial occlusive diseases. However, very often they co-exist in patients with severe occlusive lesions. This is explained in part by the fact that both mechanisms are related to shared pathologic features: a complicated atherosclerotic plaque easily protrudes into the lumen leading to hypoperfused status in the distal area and also tends to produce plaque fissuring resulting in embolism to distal arteries. In addition, recent imaging studies have shown that hypoperfusion and embolism interacts complementarily. For instance, Sedlaczek et al. [49] described patients with arterial occlusive diseases who had subcortical embolization within the borderzone areas. Caplan and Hennerici [50] analyzed the pattern of small infarcts detected by DWI in patients with large artery occlusive disease, and realized that many of these tiny infarcts were located in the borderzone regions (fig. 1 in Chapter 6). They proposed that in the region with poor perfusion (borderzone area), emboli cannot be washed out and therefore ultimately result in small

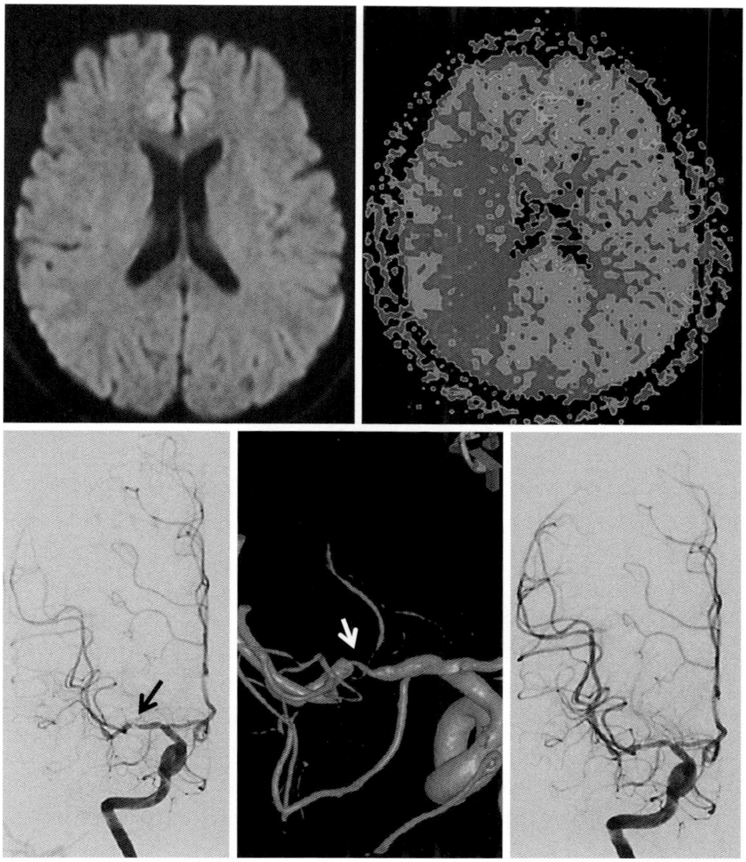

Fig. 4. A 71-year-old woman with hypertension and diabetes mellitus developed brief and stereotypical episodes of left hemiparesis that developed when she stood up suddenly or when she was exhausted and dehydrated. Diffusion weighted MRI showed no lesions (left image, upper row) while perfusion weighted MRI showed decreased perfusion in the right MCA territory (right image, upper row). Angiogram showed severe stenosis of the right MCA (arrow, left image, lower row), which was more clearly visualized in three dimensional angiogram (arrow, middle image, lower row). After angioplasty and stenting, the stenosis improved (right image, lower row). The patient no longer developed neurological symptoms afterwards.

infarcts. Thus, embolism and hypoperfusion synergistically contribute to development of stroke in patients with severe large artery occlusive disease [12] including intracranial atherosclerotic disease. A more recent study using 3D DSA and MES monitoring also suggests that impaired washout of emboli at border zones may be an important mechanism in stroke recurrence [51].

Finally, there is a phenomenon called Bernoulli's principle, which may contribute to low flow to the perforating artery even without actual branch occlusion. This principle states that for any flow, an increase in the velocity occurs simultaneously with a decrease in pressure. Progressive narrowing in arterial stenosis invariably increases the flow velocity in the MCA which is the hallmark for diagnosis of stenosis by Doppler. Sometimes the flow velocity in the MCA exceeds 300 m/s. According to the Bernoulli's principle, the higher the flow velocity in the MCA, the lower the pressure in the perforating arteries, which often arise from the MCA perpendicularly. The potential importance of this mechanical cause of low perfusion remains unknown in clinical practice.

Stroke Mechanisms in Different Vascular Territories

In patients with intracranial atherosclerosis, Kim et al. [5] reported that artery-to-artery embolism occurred in 59.7%, local branch occlusion in

14.9%, in situ thrombo-occlusion in 13.7%, hemodynamic impairment in 0.9%, and mixed in 10.8%. There are major difference between the mechanisms of stroke between the anterior and posterior circulation. Branch occlusive disease was more frequently associated with posterior circulation whereas artery to artery embolism was more frequent in the anterior circulation. Branch occlusive disease was observed in 64% of the basilar artery, 27% of the distal VA, 23% of the posterior cerebral artery, and 16% of the MCA. Artery to artery embolism was observe in 70% of the distal ICA, 51% of the MCA, 53% of the distal VA, 39% of the anterior cerebral artery, 37% of the posterior cerebral artery, and 17% of the basilar artery [5].

Anterior Circulation Disorders

MCA Territory Infarction

Although embolic occlusion of MCA either from the heart or the atherosclerotic ICA has been considered the main cause of MCA territory infarction, intrinsic atherosclerosis is an important cause of stroke at least in Asian population (see Chapter 6 for detail). MCA atherosclerosis produces diverse topographic patterns of infarction depending on the variability in blood supply, degree of primary and secondary collateralization, and pathogenesis of infarcts [52]. Secondary ischemic lesions visualized by brain imaging include small deep infarcts, large striatocapsular lesions, branch cortical strokes, or a combination of these lesions [53, 54].

Histopathologically observed fibrin-platelet microembolism has been found in patients with MCA stenosis presenting with TIA [55]. Using MES detection by TCD together with DWI to explore the pathophysiology of cerebral infarct in acute stoke patients with moderate to severe MCA stenosis, Wong et al. [4] found that common stroke mechanisms in these patients are the occlusion of a single penetrating artery to produce a small subcortical infarction and artery-to-artery embolism with impaired clearance of emboli producing multiple, small cerebral infarcts especially along the border zone region. Thus, small scattered infarcts along the border zone are common with severe MCA stenosis. Other studies using DWI and MR angiography, also showed that perforating artery infarcts, whether single or occurring in addition to pial or border-zone infarcts, are the most common lesion pattern in patients with MCA stenosis [36].

The severity of MCA stenosis is an independent predictor of future stroke, suggesting the importance of hypoperfusion in the pathogenesis of infarction [56]. Droste el al. [57] reported that more severe MCA stenosis, as evidenced by very high flow velocity (>210 cm/s) in TCD, was associated with detection of MES and clinical symptoms. The presence and the frequency of MES predicts further risk of stroke and TIAs [58]. In addition, Wong et al. [59, 60] reported that involvement of multiple vessels is more likely to cause further stroke both in short-term and long-term.

On the other hand, in subjects with chronic, asymptomatic MCA stenosis (lasting more than 12 months), MES are rarely detectable regardless of the patients' medication [57, 61, 62]. Therefore, chronic, asymptomatic MCA stenosis does not seem to represent a significant embolic source. Follow-up studies of patients with asymptomatic stenosis also confirmed the low risk of stroke in these patients [46]. However, as discussed earlier, severe MCA occlusive disease with insufficient collateralization may produce recurrent hemodynamic TIAs (fig. 4). In addition, the patients with severe MCA occlusive disease may have disabling cognitive impairment especially when they have bilateral MCA diseases.

Finally, sudden thrombotic MCA occlusion may produce relatively large infarction in the MCA territory. However, as compared to cardiogenic infarction the so-called malignant MCA infarction involving the whole MCA territory is definitely uncommon in patients with intrinsic

MCA atherosclerotic disease due to relatively well developed collateral circulation in these patients. Thus, even in patients with acute thrombotic occlusion, the infarct may be limited to the part of the MCA territory, usually at the striatocapsular region or borderzone areas. In some of these patients, the relatively small initial lesion may progressively enlarge along with neurological deterioration. Revascularization procedures such as stenting and angioplasty, if performed early enough, may be of help in these patients.

Anterior Cerebral Artery (ACA) Territory Infarction

ACA territory infarction is rare, occurring in less than 3% of all strokes [63–65]. As in patients with MCA territory infarction, embolism either from the heart or the proximal ICA atherosclerotic disease has been considered the most important cause of ACA territory infarction [63, 64]. However, intrinsic atherosclerotic disease seems to be the more important cause of ACA territory infarction in Asian population [65, 66] (see Chapter 6 for details). As in intrinsic MCA disease, ACA atherosclerosis produces infarction by way of insitu thrombotic occlusion, local branch occlusion, artery to artery embolization and the combination of these mechanisms. Collateral circulation and hemodynamic factors also play a role in determining the location and size of the final infarct. Unlike the MCA territory infarction, however, embolism from the diseased heart or ICA disease does not necessarily produce massive ACA territory infarction, probably due to the presence of abundant collaterals connecting both ACA systems.

Posterior Circulation Disorders

Vertebral Artery (VA) Atherosclerosis

In the western hemisphere, the most common location for atherosclerosis of the VA is the extracranial first segment. Less commonly, atherosclerotic disease can cause stenosis of the second, third segments of the VA or the distal intracranial segment adjacent to the origin of the posterior inferior cerebellar artery [67, 68]. However, intracranial VA atherosclerosis was slightly more common than extracranial VA atherosclerosis (6% versus 4%) in a Korean study [5]. Intracranial VA atherosclerosis can produce occlusion of the branches supplying the medulla, which is the most important pathogenic mechanism for medullary (either lateral or medial) infarction [69, 70] (see Chapter 6 for detail).

In patients with relatively severe atherosclerosis, either at extracranial or extracranial VA, mural thrombosis can lead to artery-to-artery emboli that cause occlusion of distal branches such as the posterior cerebral artery, the superior cerebellar artery, the posterior inferior cerebellar artery, the basilar artery or the combination of some of them [71–74]. In patients with bilateral, severe atherosclerosis or in those with unilateral VA disease with contralateral hypoplasic VA, hemodynamic disturbances may contribute to ischemic symptoms. However, lesion pattern of hemodynamic stroke is less well established in posterior circulation disease as compared to anterior circulation diseases. It seems that hemodynamic insufficiency plays an additive role in development of artery-to-artery embolism in many patients. Although rare, patients have repeated episodes of hemodynamic TIAs, which may be improved by revascularization such as angioplasty and stenting. In patients with severe and longstanding hemodynamic compromise, MRI may reveal atrophic changes in the posterior fossa.

Basilar Artery (BA) Atherosclerosis

The low-middle portion of the BA is relatively common site for advanced atherosclerosis. Patients with high-grade BA stenosis are at risk for a local thrombosis. Acute basilar artery thrombotic occlusion may occlude multiple perforators producing bilateral pontine infarcts, resulting in coma, quadriparesis, and ocular motor disturbances. In many occasion, the patients' neurological deficits progress from unilateral to bilateral ones as the steno-occlusive process continues. The resultant stroke and consequent neuralgic deficits (locked-in-syndrome) are one of the most devastating sequelae of stroke. However, chronic occlusion with the presence of sufficient collaterals, especially from the posterior communicating arteries, may not produce any significant neurologic deficits.

More often, a milder degree of BA stenosis and resultant local thrombus produces occlusion of one or a few perforating branches (branch occlusion) producing more benign unilateral pontine infarction (fig. 6 in Chapter 6). In these cases, patients usually present with lacunar syndromes. Occlusion of the anterior inferior cerebellar artery also results from BA atherothrombosis. In addition, embolization arising from the clot formed in the basilar artery can migrate to the distal basilar artery, the posterior cerebral artery, the superior cerebellar arteries or some of these vessels resulting in relevant clinical syndromes. Combined branch artery occlusion and artery-to-artery embolization is also commonly observed. Acute, multiple brain infarcts due to distal embolization are more clearly observed when DWI is used, which helps us understand the embolic nature of strokes [75]. Finally, basilar artery dolichoectesia is a vascular anomaly related to atherosclerosis, which may cause brainstem ischemia by multiple mechanisms, including thrombosis, embolism, and occlusion of deep penetrating arteries [76].

Posterior Cerebral Artery (PCA) Atherosclerosis

The frequency and stroke mechanism of intrinsic PCA atherosclerosis has been rarely studied. Literatures have shown that the leading etiology of PCA territory infarcts is the embolism from the heart or proximal vertebobasilar atherosclerotic disease, while intrinsic atherosclerosis of the PCA has been considered an uncommon occurrence [77–79]. As in anterior circulation disease, however, the importance of intrinsic PCA atherosclerotic disease as a cause of PCA territory infarction seems to greater in Asians than in Caucasians.

In a recent study from Korea using DWI and MR angiography [80], out of 205 patients with PCA territory infarction, large artery atherosclerosis was the cause of stroke in 87 patients in whom 38 patients had intrinsic PCA atherosclerotic disease. In these patients, the most frequent stroke mechanism was atheromatous branch occlusion (19 patients) followed by in situ thrombo-occlusion (11 patients) and artery-to-artery embolism (8 patients). Although embolic PCA occlusion most frequently damages the occipital lobe, intrinsic PCA atherothrombosis produces subcortical lesions (i.e., ventrolateral thalamus) more frequently. The branch occlusion due to atheromatous PCA disease is an important mechanism of stroke occurring in the midbrain and thalamus [81] (fig. 7 and 8 in Chapter 6). Although uncommon, patients with PCA stenosis may have recurrent TIAs as in those with MCA stenosis [82].

References

1 Warach S, Gaa J, Siewert B, Wielopolski P, Edelman RR: Acute human stroke studied by whole brain echo planar diffusion-weighted magnetic resonance imaging. Ann Neurol 1995;37:231–241.

2 Brant-Zawadzki M, Atkinson D, Detrick M, Bradley WG, Scidmore G: Fluid-attenuated inversion recovery (flair) for assessment of cerebral infarction. Initial clinical experience in 50 patients. Stroke 1996;27:1187–1191.

3 Markus H: Transcranial Doppler detection of circulating cerebral emboli. A review. Stroke 1993;24:1246–1250.

4 Wong KS, Gao S, Chan YL, Hansberg T, Lam WW, Droste DW, Kay R, Ringelstein EB: Mechanisms of acute cerebral infarctions in patients with middle cerebral artery stenosis: a diffusion-weighted imaging and microemboli monitoring study. Ann Neurol 2002;52:74–81.

5 Kim JS, Nah HW, Park SM, Kim SK, Cho KH, Lee J, Lee YS, Kim J, Ha SW, Kim EG, Kim DE, Kang DW, Kwon SU, Yu KH, Lee BC: Risk factors and stroke mechanisms in atherosclerotic stroke: Intracranial compared with extracranial and anterior compared with posterior circulation disease. Stroke 2012;43:3313–3318.

6 Badimon JJ, Lettino M, Toschi V, Fuster V, Berrozpe M, Chesebro JH, Badimon L: Local inhibition of tissue factor reduces the thrombogenicity of disrupted human atherosclerotic plaques: effects of tissue factor pathway inhibitor on plaque thrombogenicity under flow conditions. Circulation 1999;99:1780–1787.
7 Sitzer M, Muller W, Siebler M, Hort W, Kniemeyer HW, Jancke L, Steinmetz H: Plaque ulceration and lumen thrombus are the main sources of cerebral microemboli in high-grade internal carotid artery stenosis. Stroke 1995;26:1231–1233.
8 Ogata J, Masuda J, Yutani C, Yamaguchi T: Mechanisms of cerebral artery thrombosis: a histopathological analysis on eight necropsy cases. J Neurol Neurosurg Psychiatry 1994;57:17–21.
9 Rothwell PM, Villagra R, Gibson R, Donders RC, Warlow CP: Evidence of a chronic systemic cause of instability of atherosclerotic plaques. Lancet 2000; 355:19–24.
10 Xu WH, Li ML, Niu JW, Feng F, Jin ZY, Gao S: Luminal thrombosis in middle cerebral artery occlusions: a high-resolution mri study. Ann Transl Med 2014; 2:75.
11 Caplan LR: Brain embolism, revisited. Neurology 1993;43:1281–1287.
12 Caplan LR, Wong KS, Gao S, Hennerici MG: Is hypoperfusion an important cause of strokes? If so, how? Cerebrovasc Dis 2006;21:145–153.
13 Ringelstein EB, Zeumer H, Angelou D: The pathogenesis of strokes from internal carotid artery occlusion. Diagnostic and therapeutical implications. Stroke 1983;14:867–875.
14 Fieschi C, Argentino C, Lenzi GL, Sacchetti ML, Toni D, Bozzao L: Clinical and instrumental evaluation of patients with ischemic stroke within the first six hours. J Neurol Sci 1989;91: 311–321.
15 Furlan A, Higashida R, Wechsler L, Gent M, Rowley H, Kase C, Pessin M, Ahuja A, Callahan F, Clark WM, Silver F, Rivera F: Intra-arterial prourokinase for acute ischemic stroke. The proact ii study: a randomized controlled trial. Prolyse in acute cerebral thromboembolism. JAMA 1999;282:2003–2011.
16 Chen H, Hong H, Liu D, Xu G, Wang Y, Zeng J, Zhang R, Liu X: Lesion patterns and mechanism of cerebral infarction caused by severe atherosclerotic intracranial internal carotid artery stenosis. J Neurol Sci 2011;307:79–85.
17 Caplan LR: Intracranial branch atheromatous disease: A neglected, understudied, and underused concept. Neurology 1989;39:1246–1250.
18 Lhermitte F, Gautier JC, Derouesne C: Nature of occlusions of the middle cerebral artery. Neurology 1970;20:82–88.
19 Fisher CM, Caplan LR: Basilar artery branch occlusion: a cause of pontine infarction. Neurology 1971;21:900–905.
20 Fisher CM: Bilateral occlusion of basilar artery branches. J Neurol Neurosurg Psychiatry 1977;40:1182–1189.
21 Fisher CM: Capsular infarcts: the underlying vascular lesions. Arch Neurol 1979;36:65–73.
22 Fisher CM: A lacunar stroke. The dysarthria-clumsy hand syndrome. Neurology 1967;17:614–617.
23 Fisher CM: Lacunar strokes and infarcts: a review. Neurology 1982;32:871–876.
24 Fisher CM: Ataxic hemiparesis. A pathologic study. Arch Neurol 1978;35:126–128.
25 Fisher CM, Curry HB: Pure motor hemiplegia. Trans Am Neurol Assoc 1964;89: 94–97.
26 Fisher CM, Cole M: Homolateral ataxia and crural paresis: a vascular syndrome. J Neurol Neurosurg Psychiatry 1965;28: 48–55.
27 Fisher CM: Pure sensory stroke involving face, arm, and leg. Neurology 1965; 15:76–80.
28 Fisher CM: Lacunes: small, deep cerebral infarcts. Neurology 1965;15:774–784.
29 Mohr JP: Lacunes. Stroke 1982;13:3–11.
30 Sacco SE, Whisnant JP, Broderick JP, Phillips SJ, O'Fallon WM: Epidemiological characteristics of lacunar infarcts in a population. Stroke 1991;22:1236–1241.
31 Mast H, Thompson JL, Voller H, Mohr JP, Marx P: Cardiac sources of embolism in patients with pial artery infarcts and lacunar lesions. Stroke 1994;25:776–781.
32 Adachi T, Kobayashi S, Yamaguchi S, Okada K: Mri findings of small subcortical 'lacunar-like' infarction resulting from large vessel disease. J Neurol 2000; 247:280–285.
33 Bang OY, Heo JH, Kim JY, Park JH, Huh K: Middle cerebral artery stenosis is a major clinical determinant in striatocapsular small, deep infarction. Arch Neurol 2002;59:259–263.
34 Mok VC, Fan YH, Lam WW, Hui AC, Wong KS: Small subcortical infarct and intracranial large artery disease in chinese. J Neurol Sci 2003;216:55–59.
35 Cho AH, Kang DW, Kwon SU, Kim JS: Is 15 mm size criterion for lacunar infarction still valid? A study on strictly subcortical middle cerebral artery territory infarction using diffusion-weighted mri. Cerebrovasc Dis 2007;23:14–19.
36 Lee DK, Kim JS, Kwon SU, Yoo SH, Kang DW: Lesion patterns and stroke mechanism in atherosclerotic middle cerebral artery disease: Early diffusion-weighted imaging study. Stroke 2005;36: 2583–2588.
37 Klein IF, Lavallee PC, Schouman-Claeys E, Amarenco P: High-resolution mri identifies basilar artery plaques in paramedian pontine infarct. Neurology 2005; 64:551–552.
38 Zhou L, Ni J, Xu W, Yao M, Peng B, Li M, Cui L: High-resolution mri findings in patients with capsular warning syndrome. BMC Neurol 2014;14:16.
39 Lam WW, Wong KS, So NM, Yeung TK, Gao S: Plaque volume measurement by magnetic resonance imaging as an index of remodeling of middle cerebral artery: Correlation with transcranial color Doppler and magnetic resonance angiography. Cerebrovasc Dis 2004;17: 166–169.
40 Caplan LR, Gorelick PB, Hier DB: Race, sex and occlusive cerebrovascular disease: a review. Stroke 1986;17:648–655.
41 Chambers BR, Norris JW: Outcome in patients with asymptomatic neck bruits. N Engl J Med 1986;315:860–865.
42 Beneficial effect of carotid endarterectomy in symptomatic patients with high-grade carotid stenosis. North American symptomatic carotid endarterectomy trial collaborators. N Engl J Med 1991;325:445–453.
43 Yamauchi H, Nishii R, Higashi T, Kagawa S, Fukuyama H: Hemodynamic compromise as a cause of internal border-zone infarction and cortical neuronal damage in atherosclerotic middle cerebral artery disease. Stroke 2009;40: 3730–3735.

44 Halliday A, Mansfield A, Marro J, Peto C, Peto R, Potter J, Thomas D: Prevention of disabling and fatal strokes by successful carotid endarterectomy in patients without recent neurological symptoms: randomised controlled trial. Lancet 2004;363:1491–1502.
45 Thijs VN, Albers GW: Symptomatic intracranial atherosclerosis: outcome of patients who fail antithrombotic therapy. Neurology 2000;55:490–497.
46 Kern R, Steinke W, Daffertshofer M, Prager R, Hennerici M: Stroke recurrences in patients with symptomatic vs asymptomatic middle cerebral artery disease. Neurology 2005;65:859–864.
47 Klijn CJ, Kappelle LJ, Algra A, van Gijn J: Outcome in patients with symptomatic occlusion of the internal carotid artery or intracranial arterial lesions: a meta-analysis of the role of baseline characteristics and type of antithrombotic treatment. Cerebrovasc Dis 2001;12:228–234.
48 Han JH, Ho SS, Lam WW, Wong KS: Total cerebral blood flow estimated by color velocity imaging quantification ultrasound: a predictor for recurrent stroke? J Cereb Blood Flow Metab 2007;27:850–856.
49 Sedlaczek O, Caplan L, Hennerici M: Impaired washout – embolism and ischemic stroke: further examples and proof of concept. Cerebrovasc Dis 2005;19:396–401.
50 Caplan LR, Hennerici M: Impaired clearance of emboli (washout) is an important link between hypoperfusion, embolism, and ischemic stroke. Arch Neurol 1998;55:1475–1482.
51 Leung TW, Wang L, Soo YO, Ip VH, Chan AY, Au LW, Fan FS, Lau AY, Leung H, Abrigo J, Wong A, Mok VC, Ng PW, Tsoi TH, Li SH, Man CB, Fong WC, Wong KS, Yu SC: Evolution of intracranial atherosclerotic disease under modern medical therapy. Ann Neurol 2015;77:478–486.
52 Min WK, Park KK, Kim YS, Park HC, Kim JY, Park SP, Suh CK: Atherothrombotic middle cerebral artery territory infarction: topographic diversity with common occurrence of concomitant small cortical and subcortical infarcts. Stroke 2000;31:2055–2061.
53 Lyrer PA, Engelter S, Radu EW, Steck AJ: Cerebral infarcts related to isolated middle cerebral artery stenosis. Stroke 1997;28:1022–1027.
54 Caplan L, Babikian V, Helgason C, Hier DB, DeWitt D, Patel D, Stein R: Occlusive disease of the middle cerebral artery. Neurology 1985;35:975–982.
55 Adams HP Jr, Gross CE: Embolism distal to stenosis of the middle cerebral artery. Stroke 1981;12:228–229.
56 Kasner SE, Chimowitz MI, Lynn MJ, Howlett-Smith H, Stern BJ, Hertzberg VS, Frankel MR, Levine SR, Chaturvedi S, Benesch CG, Sila CA, Jovin TG, Romano JG, Cloft HJ: Predictors of ischemic stroke in the territory of a symptomatic intracranial arterial stenosis. Circulation 2006;113:555–563.
57 Droste DW, Junker K, Hansberg T, Dittrich R, Ritter M, Ringelstein EB: Circulating microemboli in 33 patients with intracranial arterial stenosis. Cerebrovasc Dis 2002;13:26–30.
58 Gao S, Wong KS, Hansberg T, Lam WW, Droste DW, Ringelstein EB: Microembolic signal predicts recurrent cerebral ischemic events in acute stroke patients with middle cerebral artery stenosis. Stroke 2004;35:2832–2836.
59 Wong KS, Li H, Chan YL, Ahuja A, Lam WW, Wong A, Kay R: Use of transcranial doppler ultrasound to predict outcome in patients with intracranial large-artery occlusive disease. Stroke 2000;31:2641–2647.
60 Wong KS, Li H: Long-term mortality and recurrent stroke risk among chinese stroke patients with predominant intracranial atherosclerosis. Stroke 2003;34:2361–2366.
61 Sliwka U, Klotzsch C, Popescu O, Brandt K, Schmidt P, Berlit P, Noth J: Do chronic middle cerebral artery stenoses represent an embolic focus? A multirange transcranial Doppler study. Stroke 1997;28:1324–1327.
62 Wong KS, Gao S, Lam WW, Chan YL, Kay R: A pilot study of microembolic signals in patients with middle cerebral artery stenosis. J Neuroimaging 2001;11:137–140.
63 Gacs G, Fox AJ, Barnett HJ, Vinuela F: Occurrence and mechanisms of occlusion of the anterior cerebral artery. Stroke 1983;14:952–959.
64 Bogousslavsky J, Regli F: Anterior cerebral artery territory infarction in the Lausanne stroke registry. Clinical and etiologic patterns. Arch Neurol 1990;47:144–150.
65 Kang SY, Kim JS: Anterior cerebral artery infarction: stroke mechanism and clinical-imaging study in 100 patients. Neurology 2008;70:2386–2393.
66 Kazui S, Sawada T, Naritomi H, Kuriyama Y, Yamaguchi T: Angiographic evaluation of brain infarction limited to the anterior cerebral artery territory. Stroke 1993;24:549–553.
67 Muller-Kuppers M, Graf KJ, Pessin MS, DeWitt LD, Caplan LR: Intracranial vertebral artery disease in the new england medical center posterior circulation registry. Eur Neurol 1997;37:146–156.
68 Shin HK, Yoo KM, Chang HM, Caplan LR: Bilateral intracranial vertebral artery disease in the new england medical center, posterior circulation registry. Arch Neurol 1999;56:1353–1358.
69 Kim JS, Kim HG, Chung CS: Medial medullary syndrome. Report of 18 new patients and a review of the literature. Stroke 1995;26:1548–1552.
70 Kim JS: Pure lateral medullary infarction: clinical-radiological correlation of 130 acute, consecutive patients. Brain 2003;126:1864–1872.
71 Witvk RJ, Chang HM, Rosengart A, Han WC, DeWitt LD, Pessin MS, Caplan LR: Proximal extracranial vertebral artery disease in the new england medical center posterior circulation registry. Arch Neurol 1998;55:470–478.
72 Pessin MS, Daneault N, Kwan ES, Eisengart MA, Caplan LR: Local embolism from vertebral artery occlusion. Stroke 1988;19:112–115.
73 Caplan LR, Amarenco P, Rosengart A, Lafranchise EF, Teal PA, Belkin M, DeWitt LD, Pessin MS: Embolism from vertebral artery origin occlusive disease. Neurology 1992;42:1505–1512.
74 Levine SR, Quint DJ, Pessin MS, Boulos RS, Welch KM: Intraluminal clot in the vertebrobasilar circulation: clinical and radiologic features. Neurology 1989;39:515–522.
75 Koch S, Amir M, Rabinstein AA, Reyes-Iglesias Y, Romano JG, Forteza A: Diffusion-weighted magnetic resonance imaging in symptomatic vertebrobasilar atherosclerosis and dissection. Arch Neurol 2005;62:1228–1231.
76 Kumral E, Kisabay A, Atac C, Kaya C, Calli C: The mechanism of ischemic stroke in patients with dolichoectatic basilar artery. Eur J Neurol 2005;12:437–444.

77 Yamamoto Y, Georgiadis AL, Chang HM, Caplan LR: Posterior cerebral artery territory infarcts in the New England medical center posterior circulation registry. Arch Neurol 1999;56: 824–832.

78 Brandt T, Steinke W, Thie A, Pessin MS, Caplan LR: Posterior cerebral artery territory infarcts: clinical features, infarct topography, causes and outcome. Multicenter results and a review of the literature. Cerebrovasc Dis 2000;10:170–182.

79 Kumral E, Bayulkem G, Atac C, Alper Y: Spectrum of superficial posterior cerebral artery territory infarcts. Eur J Neurol 2004;11:237–246.

80 Lee E, Kang DW, Kwon SU, Kim JS: Posterior cerebral artery infarction: diffusion-weighted mri analysis of 205 patients. Cerebrovasc Dis 2009;28: 298–305.

81 Kim JS, Kim J: Pure midbrain infarction: clinical, radiologic, and pathophysiologic findings. Neurology 2005;64:1227–1232.

82 Kim JS: Pure or predominantly sensory transient ischemic attacks associated with posterior cerebral artery stenosis. Cerebrovasc Dis 2002;14:136–138.

Ka Sing Wong, MD
Division of Neurology, Department of Medicine and Therapeutics
Chinese University of Hong Kong, Prince of Wales Hospital
30-32 Ngan Shing Street
Shatin, New Territory, HKSAR (China)
E-Mail ks-wong@cuhk.edu.hk

Kim JS, Caplan LR, Wong KS (eds): Intracranial Atherosclerosis: Pathophysiology, Diagnosis and Treatment.
Front Neurol Neurosci. Basel, Karger, 2016, vol 40, pp 72–92 (DOI: 10.1159/000448303)

Clinical Stroke Syndromes

Jong S. Kim[a] · Louis R. Caplan[b]

[a]Department of Neurology, Asan Medical Center, University of Ulsan, Seoul, Korea; [b]Department of Neurology, Beth Israel Deaconess Medical Center, Boston, Mass., USA

Abstract

The main mechanism of stroke in patients who have extracranial atherosclerosis is artery to artery embolism, occasionally associated with hemodynamic disturbances. Although these mechanisms are also important in patients with intracranial atherosclerosis, branch occlusion and in-situ thrombotic occlusion play a relatively more important role in these patients. Accordingly, clinical stroke syndromes differ between extracranial atherosclerosis and intracranial atherosclerosis. In anterior circulation, middle cerebral artery atherosclerosis frequently produces subcortical infarction by way of branch occlusion. The clinical syndromes are similar to lacunar syndromes classically associated with small perforator artery diseases, although a larger size infarction can be accompanied by cortical dysfunction such as aphasia or neglect. In-situ thrombotic occlusion of the large intracranial anterior circulation arteries leads to larger infarction that results in cortical symptoms – however, parts of the cortex are usually spared due to relatively well developed collateral circulation associated with prolonged perfusion impairment. In the posterior circulation, intracranial atherosclerosis is common in the distal vertebral artery and basilar artery that often causes medullary and pontine infarction syndromes, mostly by way of branch occlusion. Posterior cerebral artery atherosclerosis produces pure midbrain or thalamic infarction through branch occlusion. Artery to artery embolisms from posterior fossa intracranial atherosclerosis lead to cortical infarction – cerebellar or temporo-occipital lobe infarction, producing ataxic syndromes, and visual field defects and associated neurobehavioral syndromes, respectively.

Introduction

Symptomatic atherosclerosis is known to occur most often in the proximal internal carotid artery (ICA). However, in East Asians, middle cerebral artery (MCA) atherosclerosis is more prevalent. In a large hospital study performed in Korea, the location of the lesions that caused atherosclerotic ischemic stroke were: the MCA

(34%), proximal ICA (23%) and basilar artery (BA) (8%), in the order of frequency. Overall, intracranial atherosclerosis (ICAS) was more common than extracranial atherosclerosis with the ratio of 7:3 [1].

The main mechanism of stroke associated with extracranial atherosclerosis is artery to artery embolism, occasionally associated with hemodynamic disturbances. Although these mechanisms are also important in patients with ICAS, branch occlusions and in-situ thrombotic occlusions play a relatively more important role in these patients (see Chapter 5). Accordingly, clinical stroke syndromes in ICAS differ from those in patients with extracranial atherosclerosis.

In patients with acute intracranial artery occlusion, intravenous thrombolysis, endovascular therapy or the combination of the two are tried [2]. In patients with arterial occlusion associated with ICAS, residual stenosis and re-occlusion are relatively common after clot-retrieving therapy. Therefore, intravenous antiplatelet agents, and balloon angioplasty with or without stenting are more often used during or after the procedure in patients with ICAS than in those with embolic occlusion [3].

In this chapter, clinical syndromes that are often associated with ICAS are described.

Anterior Circulation Disease

Middle Cerebral Artery Diseases

General Clinical Syndromes

The MCA is the largest cerebral artery and supplies most of the outer surface of the cerebral cortex, basal ganglia, internal capsule and corona radiata. Occlusion of the main MCA trunk produces contralateral hemiparesis, hemisensory deficit, deviation of eyes toward the side of the infarct, and hemianopia. Global aphasia occurs when the dominant hemisphere is severely damaged, while hemineglect occurs when the infarct develops in the right hemisphere. Divisional or branch occlusion results in partial or minor neurological deficits. Occlusion of perforating arteries produces subcortical infarction sparing the cortex and typically yields lacunar syndrome such as pure motor, sensori-motor, ataxic-hemiparesis, or dysarthria clumsy syndromes. Patients with MCA atherosclerosis rarely present with a total MCA syndrome; they tend to have lacunar syndromes associated with deep infarcts whereas cortical symptoms are less common and less severe than in patients with embolism to the MCA from proximal sources.

Significance of MCA Atherosclerosis in MCA Territory Infarction

Occlusion of the MCA due to embolism arising from the atherosclerotic ICA, the diseased heart or aorta has traditionally been regarded as the most important cause whereas MCA atherosclerosis has been considered an uncommon cause of MCA territory infarction. About 50 years ago, LHermitte et al. [4] studied 122 patients with MCA territory infarction, 94 assessed by cardiac and angiographic examination and 28 patients by post-mortem examination. MCA occlusion was identified in 40 cases (41.7%), and atherosclerotic MCA occlusive disease accounted for 11 cases (27.5% of MCA occlusion). In 6 of them, there remained the possibility of embolic occlusion from atherosclerotic proximal ICA disease. There were only 5 instances in which firm evidence of atherosclerotic MCA occlusion was documented. When 2 patients with MCA stenosis were added, atherosclerosis of MCA disease with sufficient evidence was found in 7 (16.6%) patients with MCA territory infarction. In a subsequent study [5], they reported post-mortem findings in 41 patients with MCA territory infarction. Again, only 2 patients had atherothrombotic MCA occlusion.

With the advances in techniques such as TCD, MRA, and CTA, we can now more easily detect stenosis of intracranial vessels that produce less severe clinical symptoms and signs. Later studies showed that MCA atherosclerosis was a more important cause of MCA territory infarction in Blacks and Asians than in Caucasians [6–8]. Recent series of studies from Asian countries using advanced imaging technologies confirmed these findings.

Min et al. [9] studied 42 Korean patients with MCA territory infarction who underwent MRI and angiographic studies (either conventional angiograms or MRA). Patients with potential cardiogenic embolism were excluded. They found that intrinsic MCA atherosclerosis was the cause of infarction in as many as 30 patients (71%). More recently, Lee et al. [10] studied 185 Korean patients with MCA territory infarction diagnosed by diffusion weighted MRI (DWI) and MRA. Vascular disease was considered significant when there was stenosis of ≥50% or occlusion. There were 63 patients with MCA atherosclerotic disease (34%), 38 with ICA disease (21%), and 84 with cardiac embolism (45%).

Studies have shown that lesion patterns and consequent stroke syndromes of MCA territory infarction are different according to different etiologies. The difference was suggested by Caplan et al. [11] more than 30 years ago. They compared 20 patients with angiographically proven MCA atherosclerotic disease with 25 patients with MCA territory infarction caused by embolism from proximal ICA disease. Patients with MCA atherosclerosis were more often black, female, and younger, more often had hypertension, and had fewer transient ischemic attacks (TIA) and a lower incidence of subsequent cardiac death. In the following year, Bogousslavsky et al. [12] analyzed 352 patients with intrinsic MCA disease recruited from the patient pool of EC/IC Bypass Study, and found that they tended to have (approximately 30%) deep infarcts in the lenticulostriate artery territory. Lyrer et al. [13] studied 22 stroke patients with intrinsic MCA stenosis. CT scan showed small deep infarcts in 10 (46%), large striatocapsular infarcts in 2 (9%), pial MCA branch infarction in 3 (14%), and striatocapsular plus pial territory infarcts in 4 patients (18%). Only one patient (5%) had a large territorial infarction. Clinical features included lacunar syndrome in 10 (46%), while 12 (54.4%) had non-lacunar syndromes such as aphasia or neglect. Subsequently, Yoo et al. [14] analyzed 89 patients with MCA territory infarction from the New England Stroke Registry. There were 28 patients with intrinsic MCA diseases, 17 with embolism, and 44 patients with significant ICA disease. Infarcts in patients with intrinsic MCA disease mostly involved the striatocapsular area (61%), while those due to embolism more often involved the parietal lobe.

With the advent of MRI, the lesion patterns of MCA territory infarction could be defined more clearly. Lee et al. [15] compared DWI-identified lesion patterns between 76 infarcts attributable to MCA atherosclerosis and 31 due to cardiac origin embolism. The lesion patterns produced by MCA atherosclerosis were subcortical in 53 (83%) patients, cortical (involving one M2 branch territory) in 8 (13%), and territorial in 3 (5%) patients. The locations of MCA infarcts associated with cardiac embolism were subcortical in 6 (19%), cortical in 10 (32%), and territorial in 15 (48%) patients. Borderzone infarction was also more common in the atherosclerosis group than in the embolism group (24 vs. 1) (fig. 1). Clinical features were also different. In patients with MCA atherosclerosis, there were lacunar syndrome in 31 (48%), partial MCA syndrome in 25 (39%), and total MCA syndrome in 8 (13%), while those with cardiac embolism included lacunar syndrome in 6 (20%), partial syndrome in 3 (10%), and total syndrome in 21 (70%). Patients with embolism showed more abrupt onset of disease, higher initial NIHSS scores (9.7 vs. 4.6), and shorter onset-to-admission time than those with MCA atherosclerosis.

Subcortical infarcts are significantly more common in patients with MCA atherosclerosis than in the embolism group, while cortical or territorial infarcts are more common in patients with embolism. The frequent sparing of the cor-

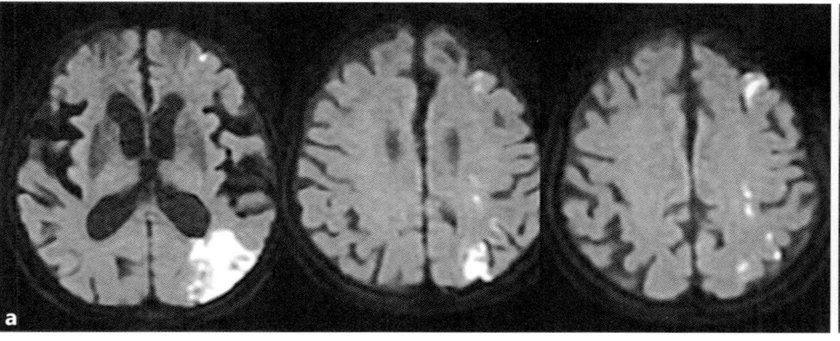
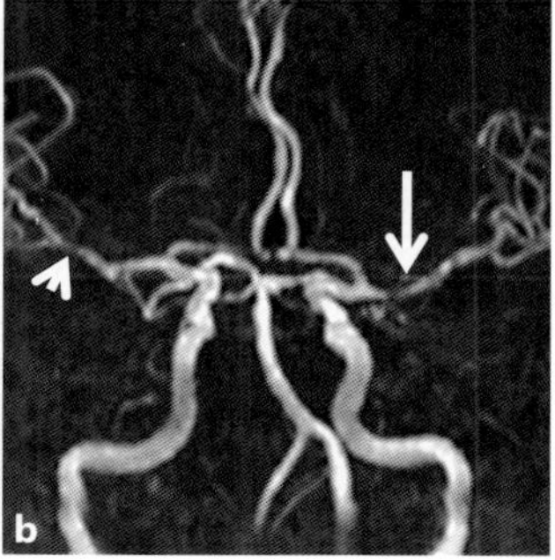

Fig. 1. 92-year-old female who had hypertension and diabetes mellitus developed aphasia, dysarthria and mild right hemiparesis. Diffusion weighted MRI showed a territorial infarction in the parietal area and additional dot like infarcts in the internal borderzone areas (**a**). MR angiogram showed focal severe stenosis in left proximal middle cerebral artery (MCA) (**b**, long arrow). The presumed stroke mechanism was artery to artery embolism combined with hemodynamic impairment. There also were multifocal atherosclerotic stenoses in intracranial arteries including right MCA (short arrow).

tex in patients with MCA atherosclerosis is probably related to pre-existing, well-developed collateral circulation. The less frequent cortical damage in patients with MCA atherosclerosis explains less frequent cortical symptoms such as aphasia, eye deviation, and post-stroke seizures (2% according to Bogousslavsky et al. [12]). Due to the sparing of the cortex, so-called 'malignant' MCA infarction is rare in MCA atherosclerosis.

Table 1 summarizes the differences in MCA territory infarction according to different etiologies.

Subcortical Infarction Associated with MCA Atherosclerosis

Because subcortical infarction sparing the cerebral cortex is one of the important stroke patterns caused by MCA atherosclerosis at least in Asia, this topic deserves a separate description. Bang et al. [16] studied 102 Korean patients with lacunar syndrome and relevant small (<1.5 cm), MRI-identified subcortical infarcts. Angiograms (conventional or MRA) were performed in all the patients. They detected responsible MCA atherosclerosis in 37 (36%) patients. Embolic sources were found in 25 patients (25%), while small vessel occlusion was considered to be the cause of infarcts in the other patients. MCA disease was an important cause of subcortical infarction even in those with small sized lesions. A study from Hong Kong, China, [17] analyzed 71 patients who had small (0.2–2.0 cm in diameter) subcortical infarcts identified by DWI, that were attributable to relevant intracranial large artery disease in 12 (16.9%) and ipsilateral ICA disease in 3 patients (4.2%). None had cardiac origin embolism. Cho et al. [18] studied 118 Korean patients with acute, strictly subcortical infarction assessed by DWI and angiograms (mostly MRA). They found that 33 patients (28%) had MCA atherosclerosis, five (4%) had emobligenic heart disease, and seven (6%) had significant ICA disease.

In patients with strictly subcortical infarction assessed with DWI, embolism either from the heart or ICA is a rare cause of stroke in East Asia. The maximal diameter of infarction caused by MCA disease was not significantly larger than that caused by small vessel disease. Single subcortical infarction associated with MCA disease tends to involve the lower portion of the basal ganglia and abuts on the MCA (fig. 2). The lesion has been occasionally called proximal single subcortical infarction (pSSI). The pSSI is more often associated with atherosclerosis characteristics,

Table 1. Differences in MCA territory infarction according to difference etiologies

	Intrinsic MCA disease	Cardiac embolism	ICA disease
Ethnicities	Asian, Black, Hispanics	Variable	Caucasian
Onset	Gradual	Abrupt	Variable
Precedence by TIAs	++	+	+++
Important risk factors	Advanced hypertension Metabolic syndrome	Emboligenic heart disease	Hyperlipidemia
Degree of arterial stenosis	Either severe or mild	none	Usually severe
Coronary heart disease	++	++	+++
Peripheral artery disease	++	+	+++
Lesion pattern	Subcortical Combined cortical and subcortical	Cortical Territorial	Cortical Internal borderzone
Lacunar syndrome	+++	+	+
Cortical symptoms	+	+++	++
Neurological progression	+++	+	++
Acute herniation	+	+++	++

MCA = Middle cerebral artery; ICA = internal carotid artery.

larger volume and worse neurologic outcome than subcortical infarction caused by distal small vessel disease [19].

Anterior Cerebral Artery Disease

General Clinical Features

ACA territory infarction accounts for less than 3% of ischemic stroke [20–23]. Clinically, ACA infarction is characterized by limb weakness, worse in the leg than in the arm. A small lesion may produce isolated lower limb weakness. Decreased shoulder shrug and proximal arm weakness often accompany leg weakness in the early stage. Sensory dysfunction is usually less severe and occurs almost always in the paretic limbs. Hypobulia/apathy characteristically occurs and has been shown to be related to callosal [24, 25] or antero-medial frontal lobe damage [26]. This finding is more severe and persistent in patients with bilateral than in those with unilateral lesions [26]. Other symptoms include urinary incontinence, alien hand sign, and limb apraxia. When the infarct involves the left brain, aphasia may develop, transcortical motor aphasia being the most common [27, 28]. Other miscellaneous symptoms include emotional lability/incontinence [29], drowsiness/somnolence, acute confusion/agitation, motor perseveration, amnesia, and parkinsonian symptoms [30, 31].

Significance of ACA Atherosclerosis in ACA Territory Infarction

Intrinsic ACA atherosclerosis has been considered to be a rare etiology of ACA territory infarction. Bogousslavsky and Regli [21] reported that, among 27 patients with ACA territory infarction, embolism from either the ICA disease or the heart was found in 17 patients (63%), while in situ thrombotic occlusion of ACA was detected in only one.

Studies from Asia report different results. Kazui et al. [22] reported 17 Japanese patients

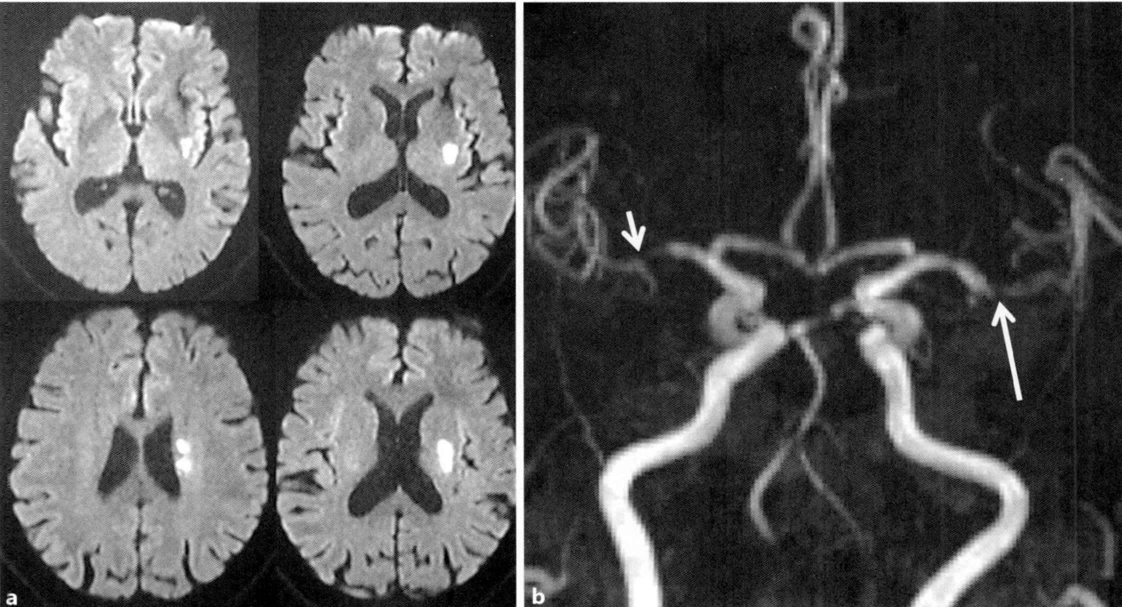

Fig. 2. A 78-year-old woman who had hypertension and dyslipidemia developed right hemiparesis. Her initial motor symptoms (arm II/V, leg III/V) progressed (arm 1/V, leg II/V) during admission. Diffusion weighted MRI showed an infarct that involved areas from the lower portion of the basal ganglia up to the corona radiata (**a**). MR angiogram showed severe stenosis in the left middle cerebral artery (MCA) (**b**, long arrow). Asymptomatic right MCA stenosis was also observed (short arrow).

assessed by CT and angiography. The majority (10 patients, 59%) were caused by intrinsic ACA atherosclerosis, while cardiogenic infarction occurred in only 3 patients (18%). Kang and Kim [26] studied 100 Korean patients with ACA territory infarction assessed by MRI and angiography (mostly MRA). Presumed etiologies were large artery atherosclerosis in 73, cardiogenic embolism in 10, and unknown cause in 17 patients. Among the patients with large artery atherothrombosis, there were local ACA atherosclerotic abnormalities in 61, ICA lesions in 6, and either ICA or ACA disease in 6 patients. The responsible atherosclerotic change occurred most frequently in the A2 portion of the ACA (n = 38).

Intrinsic ACA atherothrombosis is the most frequent etiology of ACA territory infarction at least in East Asia. A study from Turkey revealed intermediate results [23]. Regarding the detailed mechanism of stroke, Kang and Kim [26] reported that among the 61 patients with ACA atherosclerosis, local branch occlusion (LBO) occurred in 20, in situ thrombotic occlusion (ITO) in 20, artery to artery embolism (AAE) in 12, and combined mechanism in 9 patients. Figure 3 represents a patient who developed infarction through in situ thrombotic occlusion of the ACA. Since the lesions tend to involve the anterior frontal cortex or the anterior part of the corpus callosum, patients with LBO and ITO more often had hypobulia/apathy than those with AAE. In patients with AAE, embolism tends to produce small, scattered lesions in the distal ACA territory or in the MCA/ACA borderzone area, usually producing monoparesis (weakness in the lower extremity) without significant hypobulia/apathy. Nowadays, ACA dissection has been recognized as another important cause of ACA infarction [32].

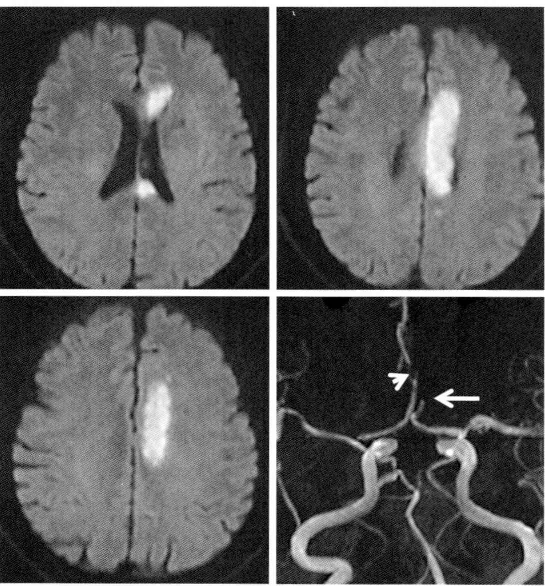

Fig. 3. A 69-year-old woman who had hypertension and diabetes developed mild right hemiparesis. Examination showed that she was alert but apathic and had transcortical motor aphasia. Initially, she had mild (IV/V) right hemiparesis, that progressed over time to more severe leg weakness (arm IV/V and leg II/V). Diffusion weighted MRI showed left anterior cerebral artery (ACA) infarction. MR angiogram showed total occlusion of left proximal A2 (long arrow) and severe asymptomatic stenosis of right A2 (short arrow) portion of the ACA.

Intracranial Internal Carotid Artery Disease

In contrast to proximal ICA disease, atherosclerosis occurring at the intracranial ICA has not drawn much interest. In the Joint Study of Extracranial Arterial Occlusion, carotid bifurcation disease was six times more common than intracranial ICA disease [33]. Although pathologic studies have found occasional cases with distal ICA thrombotic occlusion associated with either anterograde or retrograde thrombus extension, whether the thrombosis was caused by embolic occlusion or by intrinsic atherosclerosis remained often uncertain [34, 35].

Studies have shown that intracranial ICA atherosclerosis is relatively common in blacks and Asians [15]. As in patients with proximal ICA disease, intracranial ICA disease may produce stroke or TIA by way of artery-to-artery embolism, hemodynamic insufficiency or the combination of the two [36] (fig. 4). Thrombi that develop at the site of intracranial ICA atherosclerosis may extend distally to occlude the MCA or ACA, causing MCA and ACA territory infarcts, respectively [20]. Severe intracranial ICA disease at or proximal to the origin of the ophthalmic artery has been posited to cause ocular ischemia with transient or permanent monocular blindness. According to Craig et al. [37], who reviewed 47 symptomatic patients with angiographically documented intracranial ICA stenosis, there were 15 (26%) patients presenting with major stroke, 7 (12%) with partial non-progressing stroke, 9 (15%) with reversible ischemic neurologic deficits, and 16 (28%) with TIAs.

Clinical studies have shown that the prognosis of significant intracranial ICA stenosis is not favorable, and may even be worse than that of proximal ICA stenosis. Previous studies on patients with significant (>50%) stenosis have shown that ischemic symptoms occurred in 27–40% (stroke ipsilateral to the stenosed artery in 17–33%) during the average follow-up period of 30–51 months [36–38]. The presence of tandem extracranial ICA stenosis significantly increased the risk. The mortality rate was also high ranging from 33% to 50%, approximately half of them being related to cardiac events. Intracranial ICA disease not only produces embolic or hemodynamic strokes per se but also serves as an important marker for generalized atherosclerosis, carrying a high risk of recurrent stroke and other vascular events.

Anterior Choroidal Artery Territory Infarction

The Anterior chordoidal artery (AchA) supplies the lower part of the internal capsule, lateral geniculate body, crus cerebri, and the medial temporal lobe. Although the internal capsule is the most frequently involved, when the infarcts are restricted to the internal capsule, it often remains

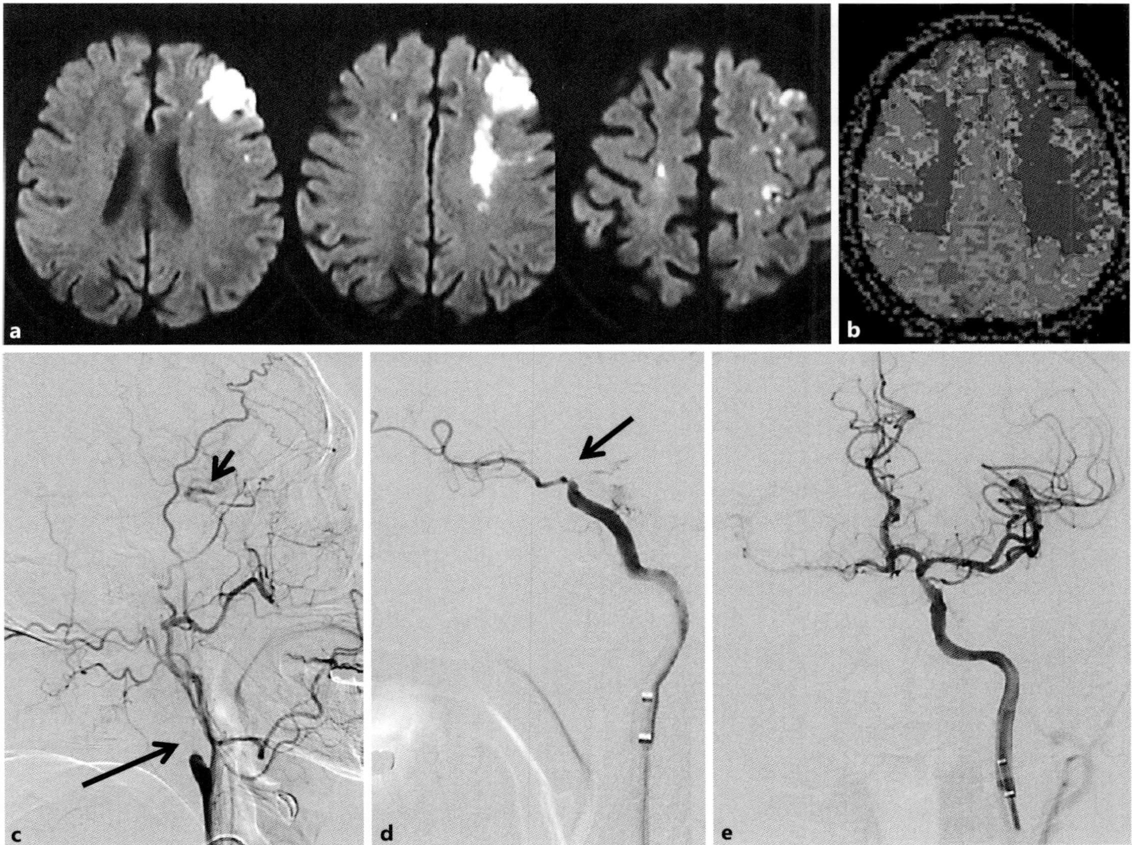

Fig. 4. A 61-year-old male smoker experienced transient episodes of right hemiparesis followed by progressive limb weakness (I/IV in the arm and IV/V in the leg) associated with global aphasia. Diffusion weighted MRI showed acute infarction in left anterior cerebral artery (ACA)-middle cerebral artery (MCA) border zone areas, and a small infarct in the right ACA territory (**a**). MTT map showed decreased perfusion at both internal carotid artery (ICA) territory (**b**). Right carotid arteriogram showed complete occlusion of proximal ICA (**c**, long arrow). A part of distal ICA was shown through transorbital collateral from external carotid artery system (**c**, short arrow). The right ICA territory was also supplied by posterior cerebral artery through posterior communicating artery (not shown). Left carotid angiogram showed sluggish flow and contrast filling to the cavernous portion. There was complete occlusion of distal ICA just above ophthalmic branch (**d**, arrow). Thrombi in the distal ICA was retrieved from Solitaire clot retriever, but there remain severe segmental, eccentric stenosis, which suggests underlying arteriosclerosis. Balloon angioplasty and self-expanding stent was applied. Final angiogram showed improved antegrade flow that perfuse left hemisphere and a part of the right ICA territory through anterior communicating artery (**e**).

uncertain whether this is caused by AchA or lenticular perforator occlusion. In a recent series that studied 127 patients with pure AchA territory infarction [39], clinical features included dysarthria (85%), hemparesis (81%), facial palsy (73%), ataxia (31%), hemisensory deficits (28%), visual field defect (14%) and aphasia (8%). Angiograms showed ipsilateral distal ICA steno/occlusion in 12% and proximal ICA disease in 8%. Patients with ICA disease tend to have lesions beyond the internal capsule. Intracranial ICA atherosclerosis is an important cause of AchA territory infarction. This finding is consistent with the fact that in 75% of the subjects, AchA arises from the distal ICA. Distal ICA atherosclerosis probably leads to infarction by way of blocking the orifice of the AchA.

Posterior Circulation Disease

In the posterior circulation, atherosclerosis is prone to occur in the proximal vertebral artery (VA), distal intracranial VA, lower-middle portion of the BA, and proximal PCA [1, 40]. Thrombus formed within the intracranial VA occasionally extends into the proximal BA [41]. Within the BA, atherosclerotic stenosis is common in the proximal 2 cm of the vessel, more often seen on the ventral than in the dorsal side [41, 42]. Intracranial (distal VA, BA and PCA) atherosclerosis leads to stroke or TIA by way of artery to artery embolism, branch occlusion, hypoperfusion and in situ atherothrombotic occlusion.

Intracranial VA Diseases
Clinical Features

Lateral Medullary Infarction Syndrome. Dizziness and gait instability, attributed either to vestibular or cerebellar system dysfunction, occur in more than 90% of the patients. Whirling vertigo occurs in approximately 60% [43], usually accompanied by nystagmus and nausea/vomiting. Gait ataxia is usually more severe than limb incoordination [43, 44]. The nystagmus is mostly horizontal-rotational to the side opposite to the lesions [45, 46]. Skew deviation, with the isilateral eye going down, is also frequent. Ptosis and meiosis (components of a Horner syndrome), is caused by involvement of the descending sympathetic fibers in the lateral reticular substance, occurs in about 90% of patients.

Involvement of the nucleus ambiguous results in dysphagia, dyarthria and hoarseness. Dysphagia is present in approximately 2/3 of LMI patients, among whom about 60% require nasogastric tube feeding [43, 44]. Dysphagia is distinctly more severe in patients with rostral than in caudal lesions [43, 47]. Approximately 1/4 of patients develop hiccup [43, 44], often days after the stroke onset. Headache, most often occurring in the ipsilateral occipital or upper nuchal area, occurs in approximately a half of the patients [43, 44]. Prominent and persistent neck pain may be a manifestation of arterial dissection. Facial palsy, usually mild and upper neuron type, is present in 1/5 to 1/4 of patients [43].

Sensory symptoms/signs are common, and sensory function remains intact in only 4% of the patients [43]. A selective loss of spinothalamic sensation is a rule [48]. Crossed (ipsilateral trigeminal-contralateral limb/body) sensory changes are characteristic, but recent studies have identified more diverse sensory pattern [48]. In one study [43], the patterns included ipsilateral trigeminal-contralateral limb/body in 26%, contralateral trigeminal-contralateral limb/body in 25%, bilateral trigeminal-contralateral limb/body in 14%, limb/body involvement without trigeminal involvement in 21% and trigeminal involvement without limb/body involvement in 10%. In addition, approximately 7% of LMI patients have additional ipsilateral tingling sensation often associated with lemniscal sensory deficits [49] due to involvement of yet uncrossed lemniscal sensory fibers in the caudal medulla.

Medial Medullary Infarction (MMI) Syndrome. Dejerine proposed a triad of medial medullary syndrome: contralateral hemiplegia sparing the face, contralateral loss of deep sensation, and ipsilateral hypoglossal paralysis [50]. Recent studies using MRI showed that MMI lesions are mostly unilateral, located in the rostral medulla, and usually present with relatively benign, sensori-motor stroke [51]. Definite ipsilateral hypoglossal paresis is rare [52].

Contralateral hemiparesis sparing the face is the most characteristic sign of MMI [53]. Quadriparesis occurs in less than 10% of patients [43,

52]. Facial paresis, usually slight, occurs in 1/4 to 1/2 [44, 52] of the patients. In patients with quadriparesis, dysarthria and dysphagia are severe while in those with unilateral lesion, a nasogastric tube is required in less than 10%.

Sensory dysfunction is the second most important symptom/sign of MMI. Unlike LMI patients, MMI patients typically complain of tingling sensation from the onset, and show decreased perception of position and vibration due to selective involvement of the lemniscal sensory fibers. The involved area is usually hemibody/limbs below the ear or neck sparing the face. Limb incoordination is occasionally observed [52, 54].

Vertigo/dizziness, nystagmus and ocular motor disturbances are closely related to involvement of dorsal medulla [52, 55], that contain vestibular nuclei and the nucleus prepositus hypoglossi. In contrast to LMI, nystagmus is mostly ipsilesional, and ocular lateropulsion is to the contralateral side (contrapulsion) [56]. Upbeat nystagmus is found in 1/10 to 1/5 of patients [52, 55].

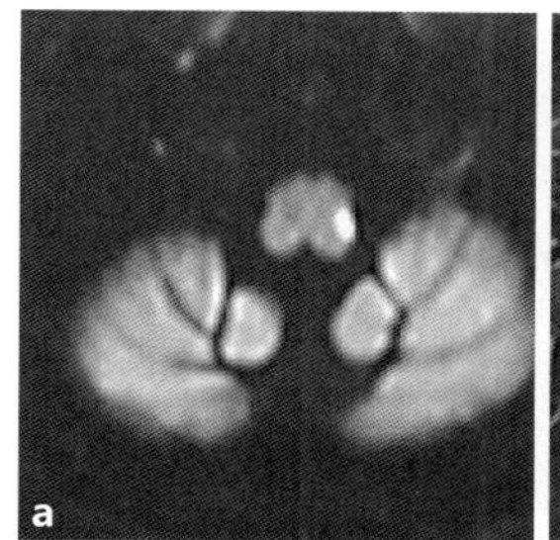

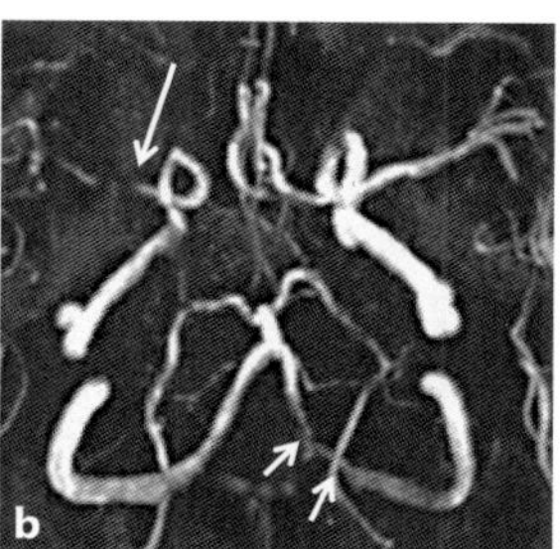

Fig. 5. A 88-year-old hypertensive woman developed dizziness and gait instability. Examination showed left Horner sign, nystagmus, severe gait ataxia and decreased pinprick sensation in the right leg. Diffusion weighted MRI showed an acute infarction in the left medulla (**a**). MR angiogram showed irregular stenosis in the left intradural vertebral artery (**b**, short arrows) that probably caused branch occlusion and lateral medullary infarction. There also were severe stenosis in the right middle cerebral artery (long arrow) and posterior cerebral artery irregularity.

Significance of Intracranial Vertebral Artery Disease in Medullary Syndromes

The medulla is mainly supplied by a number of penetrating arteries arising from the intracranial vertebral arteries (ICVAs). The dorsal area is also supplied by branches arising from the posterior inferior cerebellar artery (PICA). The most rostral part is also supplied by branches from the BA or anterior inferior cerebellar artery (AICA). The caudal part of the anterior medulla is supplied by penetrating arteries arising from the anterior spinal artery (ASA). Atherothrombosis occurring in the ICVA or its penetrators is the most important cause of medullary infarction (fig. 5).

Wallenberg initially considered PICA disease as a cause of lateral medullary infarction [57]. Half a century later, Fisher et al. [45] identified sole involvement of the PICA in only two of their 17 cases of lateral medullary infarction; 14 patients showed ICVA steno-occlusion. Since then, the most common cause of LMI has been recognized as occlusion of penetrating branches associated with ICVA steno-occlusive disease [45]. In a large series investigating 123 LMI patients [43], ipsilateral VA steno-occlusive disease was present in 83 (67%) (33, ICVA disease, 34, whole VA disease and 5 proximal VA disease) and PICA disease in 12 (10%) patients. Altherothrombosis is the dominant pathology, while dissection of the VA or PICA is the cause of steno-occlusive lesion in approximately 14–33% of patients [43, 58, 59]. In patients with normal angiographic findings, atherothrombotic occlusion of a perforating artery itself seems to be the mechanism of infarction. Embolic occlusion of the PICA or ICVA from diseased heart or a proximal vessel (e.g., extracranial VA) atherosclerosis may also produce LMI [41, 60], but concomitant brainstem or cerebellar infarcts are usually present in these patients.

Regarding the medial medullary syndrome, ASA occlusion was initially considered an important stroke mechanism [50, 61, 62]. However, more recent studies reported that MMI is most often caused by occlusion of penetrating branches associated with atherosclerotic ICVA or VA-BA junction steno-occlusion [63]. In one series, relevant VA atherosclerotic disease was present in 62% of patients while perforator occlusion without VA disease (small artery disease) occurred in 28% patients [52]. Dissection of the ICVA may result in MMI, but is less common than in LMI.

Basilar Artery (BA) Diseases

The lower/middle portion of the BA is relatively common site for advanced atherosclerosis. In some patients atherostenosis in the distal portion of the ICVA near the BA origin leads to clot formation that propagates into the BA from the ICVA. The most important clinical syndromes associated with BA disease are those caused by pontine infarction.

Clinical Features (Pontine Infarction Syndromes)

Pontine infarct may occur in isolation or in association with other posterior fossa infarction. Hospital registry studies showed that the patients with isolated pontine infarcts account for 2.6–3% of ischemic strokes and 12–15% of patients with posterior circulation infarcts [64–66]. One study from Asia showed a higher prevalence; 7.6% of cerebral infarcts and 28% of vertebrobasilar artery territory infarcts [67].

Motor Dysfunction (Including Dysarthria and Ataxia). The pontine base contains fibers regulating motor function including descending corticospinal, corticopontocerebellar, and corticobulbar tracts. Although limb weakness is the most common symptom/sign, the clinical features depend upon the degree of involvement of each fiber tract and may manifest as pure motor stroke [63], ataxic-hemiparesis [68], and dysarthria clumsy hand syndromes [69].

Sensory Dysfunction. Tegmental pontine infarcts involving the sensory tracts (medial lemnscus and spinothalamic tract) produce a hemisensory deficit [70, 71]. Small infarcts often produce sensory symptoms in restricted body parts, most frequently in the pattern of cheiro-oral syndrome [70].

Ocular Motor Dysfunction. Structures related to ocular motor function are located in the dorsal paramedian pontine tegmentum that include: abducens nucleus/fascicles, paramedian pontine reticular formation (PPRF) and MLF. Lesions affecting these structures produce various ocular motor dysfunctions than include 6th nerve palsy, internuclear ophthalmoplegia (INO): paralysis (or slowing) of adduction of the ipsilateral eye for conjugate eye movements, and nystagmus in the contralateral eye when this eye is in abduction [72]. A unilateral pontine lesion involving the PPRF would produce ipsilateral gaze paresis. If the lesion involves both PPRF and the MLF on the same side, the patient has ipsilateral conjugate gaze palsy and paralysis of adduction of the ipsilateral eye on conjugate gaze to the opposite side (one-and-a-half syndrome) [73].

Bilateral Infarction Syndrome. As the bilateral lesions almost always involve the ventral part, involving the corticospinal tracts, quardriparesis is usual [74–76]. The quadriparesis may start from the beginning; more often, the initial motor dysfunction is lateralized to one side and then progresses [77]. Unless successful therapy (such as recanalization) is immediately performed, asymmetrical motor disturbances often progress to severe quadriplegia. The progression usually occurs within 24 h, [78] but may be delayed up to several days.

Ataxia or incoordination is another common finding, observed in the limbs that are not severely paretic. Dysarthria and dysphagia due to bilateral bulbar muscles paresis are also common and severe. Some patients become totally unable to speak, open their mouth, or protrude their tongue. Somatosensory abnormalities should also be common, but they are usually overshadowed by motor dysfunction. Because large bilateral pontine infarcts frequently involve the dorsal tegmental area, ocular motor dysfunction is also common, including an INO and one-and-a-half syndrome.

Extensive lesions involving the abducens nucleus and PPRF produce paralysis of all horizontal eye movements. Vertical gaze is usually spared because it is mediated at a more rostral level. Ocular bobbing, ptosis and pinpoint pupils may be observed. Symptoms such as tinnitus, hearing loss and auditory hallucination are related to involvement of the central auditory tracts/nuclei or to ischemia of the 8th nerves/fascicles. Some patients develop delayed-onset palatal myoclonus.

Altered consciousness is an important sign in patients with sudden BA occlusion and is related to bilateral medial tegmental pontine ischemia. Consciousness usually improves overtime. Patients may show pathological crying and laughing spells that are triggered by minimal social-emotional stimuli. When all voluntary movements are lost, the deficit is referred to as the 'locked-in' syndrome. Intact vertical eye movements may be used in simple communications.

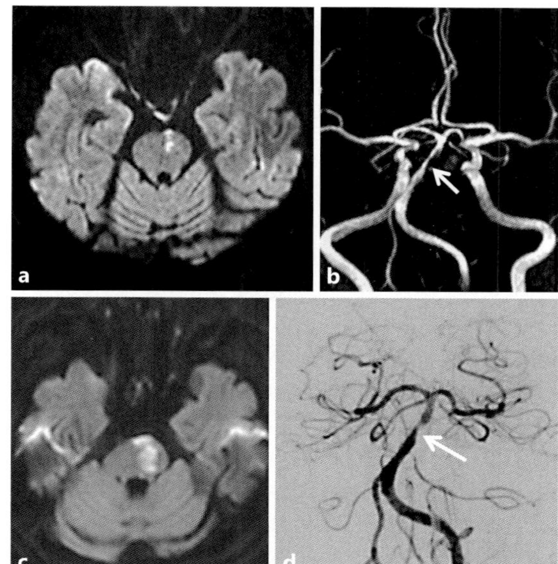

Fig. 6. A 66-year-old man who had hypertension and diabetes developed dizziness, gait instability and weakness on the right limb. Examination showed dysarthria, right facial palsy, mild (IV/V) right hemiparesis and ataxia. Diffusion weighted MRI showed paramedian pontine infarction (**a**). MR angiogram showed focal basilar artery (BA) stenosis (**b**, arrow). Despite antiplatelets and statin medication, patient's motor deficits progressed to II/IV and left internuclear ophthalamoplegia developed. Follow-up diffusion weighted MRI 7 days later showed enlarged pontine infarction (**c**). Catether angiography showed findings consistent with BA atherosclerotic stenosis (**d**, arrow).

Significance of Basilar Artery Atherosclerosis in Pontine Infarction Syndromes

The majority of pathology leading to pontine infarction is BA atherothrombosis or perforator disease. Dissection is an uncommon etiology compared to medullary infarction. Branch occlusion associated with BA stenosis is an important stroke mechanism of pontine base infarction (fig. 6); BA stenosis is present in 39–50% of patients having lesions extending to the basal surface [65, 67, 79]. Even in patients without MRA identified BA stenosis, small plaques that obliterate the orifice of perforating branches are seen occasionally if high resolution vessel wall MRI is used [80] (fig. 3 in Chapter 5). Therefore branch occlusion is actually more common than previously realized. Pontine infarcts limited to the tegmental area are mostly caused by small artery disease (lipohyalinosis), and are seldom associated with BA stenosis [64, 67, 70].

In patients with bilateral pontine infarction, significant BA steno-occlusion is usually present [75]. This may result from either embolism (from diseased heart or proximal artery [e.g., VA] diseases) or intrinsic BA thrombosis. Embolism is usually associated with infarcts in other parts of the brain, and is an uncommon cause of isolated pontine infarction. The clinical presentation of intrinsic BA diseases is less abrupt than embolism; patients often present with fluctuating or gradually progressing symptoms.

Posterior Cerebral Artery (PCA) Disease

Clinical Syndromes

The posterior cerebral arteries (PCAs) supply the midbrain, thalamus, medial temporal area, a part of the parietal lobe and the occipital lobe. Clinical syndromes are quite different according to the location of infarction.

Midbrain Infarction. In the largest series assessed by MRI [81], clinical manifestations included gait ataxia (68%), dysarthria (55%), limb ataxia (50%), sensory symptoms (43%), third nerve palsy (35%), definitive limb weakness (≤ IV/V) (23%), and INO (13%).

Although third nerve palsy has been considered a clinical hallmark of midbrain infarction, it occurs in only 35% [81] to 50% [82] of patients with pure midbrain infarction. Third nerve palsy can be caused by involvement of either the third nerve fascicles or the third nerve nucleus due to lesions involving paramedian structures. Paramedian, dorsal lower midbrain lesions involving the MLF can produce INO. Antero-lateral lesions involving the cerebral peduncle will produce various motor syndromes, i.e., pure motor stroke, ataxic-hemiparesis, dysarthria clumsy hand syndrome (fig. 7). Generally ataxia is prevalent because there are both descending (the cortico-ponto-cerebellar tract at the cerebral peduncle) and ascending (cerebello-rubro-thalamic tract, around the red nucleus) cerebellar fibers that are vulnerable to ischemic insults. Paramedian lesions may produce bilateral ataxia due to involvement of bilateral cerebello-rubro-thalamic tracts bilaterally. These patients usually have long-standing gait ataxia and dysarthria. Some patients have persistent tremor like symptoms, that may be related to concomitant involvement of cerebellar tracts and nigro-lenticular dopaminergic fibers. Tremor most often develops after a delay and is rarely evident at stroke onset. Because the trochlear nerve fascicles exit dorsally after decussation around the aqueduct, they are spared in patients with ventral midbrain lesions. Therefore, 4th nerve palsy is extremely uncommon in patients with pure midbrain infarcts [81, 82]. It may be present in patients who have SCA infarction that involve both the dorsolateral midbrain and the cerebellum.

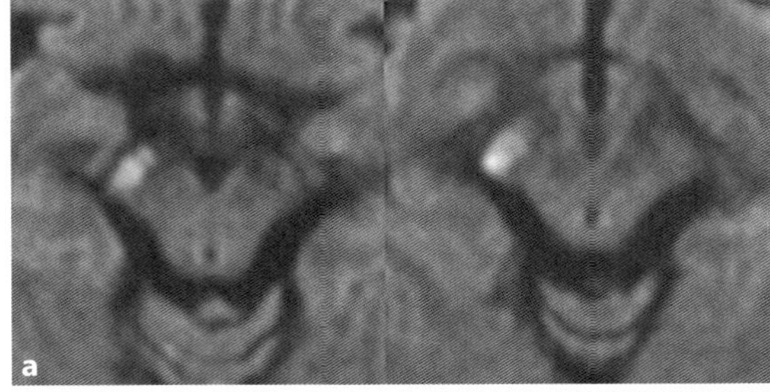

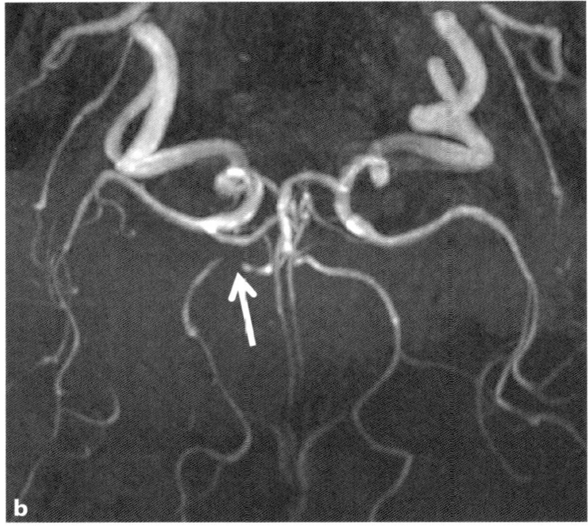

Fig. 7. A 64-year-old hypertensive woman developed left hemiparesis and dysarthria. Diffusion weighted MRI showed an infarct involving the right cerebral peduncle (**a**). MR angiogram showed a focal atherosclerotic stenosis in the right P2 portion of the posterior cerebral artery (**b**, arrow) that probably occluded the perforators supplying the cerebral peduncle.

Thalamic Infarction. The arteries that supply the thalamus branch from the P1 and P2 portions of the PCA and the posterior communication artery. Thalamic infarction generally follows the topography according to four major thalamic vascular territories: the inferolateral, tuberothalamic, paramedian, and posterior choroidal arteries [83, 84].

(a) Inferolateral (Thalamogeniculate) Artery Territory Infarction. The inferolateral (thalamogeniculate) arteries generally arise from the P2 portion of the PCA [85]. These arteries mainly supply the ventrolateral thalamus, which includes the ventrolateral (VL) and ventroposterior (VP) nuclear groups. Inferolateral artery territory infarction is the most common type of thalamic infarction (fig. 8).

The most frequent and important symptom/sign of inferolateral artery infarction is hemisensory disturbance [84, 86]. Small lateral thalamic infarcts that selectively involves the VP nucleus are the most common etiology of pure sensory stroke [87–89]. A relatively large lesion that concomitantly involves the adjacent internal capsule can result in sensorimotor stroke, and additional involvement of the cerebellothalamic fibers at the VL nucleus may result in a 'hypesthetic ataxic hemiparesis' syndrome.

(b) Tuberothalamic (Polar) Artery Territory Infarction. The tuberothalamic artery originates from the middle-third of the posterior communicating artery or occasionally from the P1 portion of the PCA [90]. The tuberothalamic arteries (also often called the polar arteries) mainly supply the ventral anterior nucleus (VA), rostral part of the VL, and the ventral pole of the medial dorsal nucleus (MD). The main clinical syndromes include neuropsychological deficits. Patients have fluctuating levels of alertness and impaired recent memory formation [90, 91]. Some patients become abulic with decreased spontaneity and delayed, brief responses to queries and conversation. Language disturbances also occur in patients with left-side infarction.

(c) Paramedian (Thalamic-Subthalamic) Artery Territory Infarction. The paramedian arteries supply the paramedian parts of the upper midbrain and thalamus, including the intralaminar nuclear group and most of the dorsomedial nucleus. Involvement of the paramedian territory is very common in patients with occlusion of the top of basilar artery). Somnolence and fluctuating levels of consciousness are a conspicuous feature during the early stages, and can last for hours or days. Confusion, agitation, aggression, and apathy may be present [84, 92, 93]. Ocular motor disturbances are also found, that include vertical gaze palsy (upgaze, downgaze or both), convergence failure, pseudo-sixth-nerve palsy, pupillary changes, and ocular tilt reaction [84, 92–94], due to involvement of rostral midbrain structures. Difficulty making new memories is another common component of the syndrome.

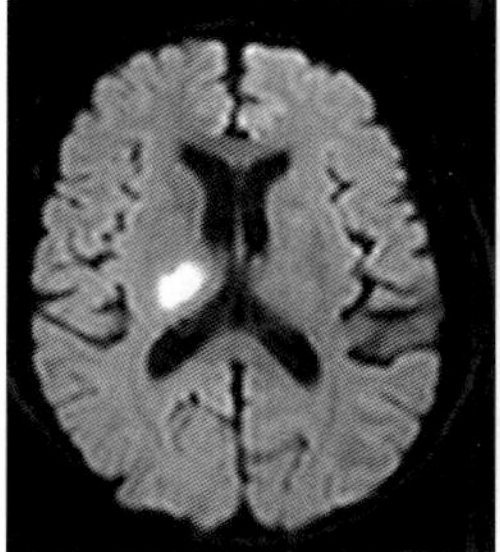
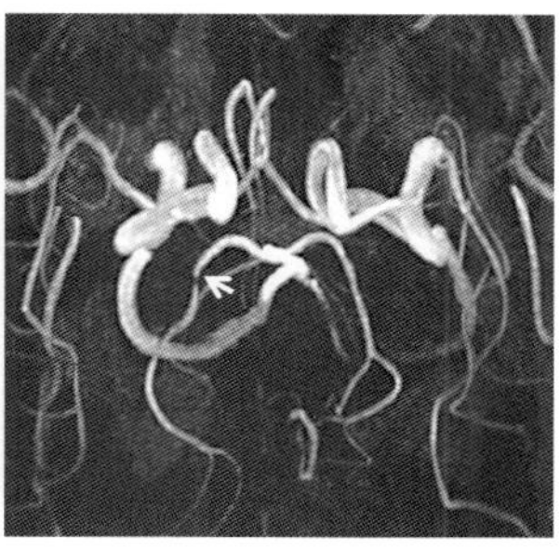

Fig. 8. A 66-year-old hypertensive man developed numb sensation in the left face and hand. Examination showed that he had sensory deficits of all sensory modality in the left face, body and limbs. In addition, he had mild left hemiparesis and ataxia. Diffusion weighted MRI showed lateral thalamic infarction. MR angiogram showed a focal atherosclerotic stenosis in the right P2 portion of the posterior cerebral artery (arrow).

(d) Posterior Choroidal Artery Territory Infarction. The posterior choroidal arteries arise from the P2 segment of the PCA distal to the origin of the posterior communicating artery. These arteries supply the lateral geniculate body (LGB), the inferolateral region of the pulvinar, the lateral dorsal nucleus, and the lateral posterior nucleus. Infarction limited to posterior choroidal artery territory area is uncommon. The two most prominent clinical manifestations are visual field defects and hemisensory deficits. Visual field defects include homonymous hemianopia (either congruent or incongruent), quadrantanopia, and sectoranopia [95]. Hemisensory dysfunction is attributed to involvement of

the VP nucleus, which is often supplied by the lateral posterior choroidal artery at least its caudal section.

Cortical (Superficial) Infarction. Hemispheric infarction due to PCA occlusion involves the occipital, posterior temporal, and parietal lobes, and clinical manifestations vary according to the location and extent of infarction. The most frequent clinical finding is a visual field defect, which occur in >90% of patients with cortical PCA territory infarction [96–98]. Various types of cognitive abnormalities have been described. According to a study on patients with only cortical PCA infarction, memory impairment and aphasia affect 18 and 15% of patients, respectively [98]. Although the cognitive deficits associated with visual dysfunction have been intensively studied, they are actually uncommon in clinical practice. In the cited study, the following frequencies were reported: visual hallucination (10%), visual neglect (9%), visual agnosia (8.5%), prosopagnosia (5.5%), color dysnomia (5%), palinopsia (3%), and color agnosia (3%).

Significance of PCA Atherosclerosis as a Cause of PCA Territory Infarction

The role of PCA atherosclerosis as a cause of PCA territory infarction remains uncertain, even though the proximal PCA is a predilection site of atherosclerosis [1]. Previous studies report a low (<10%) prevalence of intrinsic PCA disease in patients with PCA territory infarction [96, 98–100]. Recent studies from Turkey [97] and Korea [101], where MR angiograms was performed on all the patients, identified PCA atherosclerosis as a cause of PCA territory infarction in 20–25% of cases. Racial differences and the inclusion of isolated deep infarction in their studies may also explain the different prevalence of PCA disease among studies.

PCA atherosclerosis also results in either branch occlusion or artery-to-artery embolism (from the proximal PCA to distal branches) that leads to deep (midbrain or thalamus) infarction (fig. 7, 8) and cortical (temporo-occipital) infarction, respectively. In the aforementioned Koreans study [101], authors found that among 38 patients with PCA atherosclerosis, DWI-identified infarcts were located in deep structures in 53%, superficial structures in 13 and 34% had the combination. The most often affected area was the lateral thalamus (58%) followed by parieto-occipital area (45%), temporal area (26%) and midbrain (21%).

For midbrain infarction, the midbrain is mainly supplied by branches arising from the PCA, upper BA and the superior cerebellar artery (SCA). It is often affected in patients with embolic stroke occurring in the posterior circulation usually with the concomitant involvement of other structures such as the pons, thalamus, cerebellum and occipital lobe [102]. Infarcts limited to the midbrain are rare, accounting for 0.2–2.3% of admitted ischemic stroke [81, 82, 103]. Approximately 2/3 of pure midbrain infarction is caused by large artery atherosclerotic disease occurring in the proximal PCA or rostral BA. Small artery disease explains stroke in approximately 1/4 of the patients who have deep-seated lesions. Cardiac embolism is rare in patients with isolated midbrain infarction.

The frequency of PCA atherosclerosis as a cause of pure thalamic infarction is not well known. However, previous studies have shown that underlying PCA atherosclerosis was the cause of 7–22% of lateral thalamic infarcts [84, 104, 105]. Patients with lateral thalamic infarction associated with underlying PCA disease tend to have larger lesions, symptoms in addition to sensory deficits and worse clinical outcome than in those without PCA disease [105].

Cerebellar Artery Diseases

Cerebellar Infarction Syndromes

Cerebellar infarcts are uncommon, accounting for 1–4% of stroke [106–110], and usually follow the vascular topography, i.e., SCA, PICA and AICA territories, or their combination. In studies using CT or MRI [106, 107, 111], PICA infarction is slightly more common than SCA infarction. AICA infarction is distinctly uncommon.

In patients with cerebellar infarction the most common symptoms are dizziness (or less commonly vertigo) [107, 112]. Nausea/vomiting is usually accompanied by dizziness/vertigo and occurs in more than half of the patients [107]. Nystagmus is present in about half of the patients, usually horizontal, and occasionally vertical. Headache occurs usually in the ipsilateral nuchal-occipital area in 30–50% of patients [106, 107, 112], presumably related to acute distention or stretch on the intracranial pain sensitive structures including cerebral vessels. Increasing severity of headache is a sign suggesting expanding edema or hemorrhagic transformation. Severe headache localized at the nuchal area may indicate VA or PICA dissection. Limb incoordination is an important sign, occurring in 60–70% of the patients [106, 107, 112]. Dysarthria in cerebellar infarction is mainly due to involvement of the superior paravermal lesion. Therefore dysathria is more common and prominent in patients with SCA infarction than in PICA infarction.

The clinical syndrome of AICA occlusion, first described by Adams [113] is distinct from that caused by SCA or PICA occlusion. Aside from vertigo, vomiting, ataxia and dysarthria, patients have tinnitus, ipsilateral facial palsy, hearing loss, tinnitus, trigeminal sensory loss, and Horner's syndrome. Sensory loss or hemiparesis in the contralateral limbs may occur when lateral pons is involved.

Significance of Intracranial Atherosclerosis as a Cause of Cerebellar Infarction

Amarenco et al. [114] reviewed 88 pathologically proven cerebellar infarcts, and found that presumed causes include a cardiac embolism in 38 (43%) patients and atherosclerosis in the vertebrobasilar artery in 31 (35%) patients.

PICA infarction is caused by occlusion of the ICVA or PICA itself. According to previous studies, PICA occlusions are equally divided between in situ atherothrombosis and cardioembolism [114, 115]. Other less common causes include dissection (either VA or PICA).

Most SCA territory infarction is caused by embolism from atrial fibrillation, and less commonly from large artery atherosclerosis [106, 115, 116]. Atherosclerosis in the proximal part of the SCA as a cause of cerebellar infarction is uncommon. Dissection and fibromuscular dysphasia of the SCA are even less common [117–119].

For AICA territory infarction, atherothrombotic BA steno-occlusion seems to be the most common stroke mechanism [114, 120] (fig. 9). When BA atherostenosis is the cause invariably other areas of the posterior circulation are involved along with the AICA territory. Embolism is distinctly uncommon for isolated AICA territory infarction. According to Kumral et al. [121], large artery disease was the cause of stroke in 52%, cardiac embolism in 4% while 17% had both etiologies. Because AICA territory infarction is often associated with significant lower BA atherosclerosis, it should be kept in mind that this may herald massive BA thrombotic infarction [122]. In patients who showed deterioration of neurological function, early reperfusion therapy may have to be considered to prevent worsening of the symptoms (fig. 9).

Top of the Basilar Artery Syndrome

Infarction of the rostral brainstem and cerebral hemispherical regions fed by the distal BA causes a clinically recognizable syndrome characterized by visual, oculomotor, and behavioral abnormalities, often without significant motor dysfunction. Caplan [102] described this as 'the top of the basilar artery syndrome'. Typically there are bilateral multiple infarcts in the paramedian midbrain, medial thalamus, medial temporal areas and occipital lobes. However, the clinical features vary greatly depending on the damaged brain.

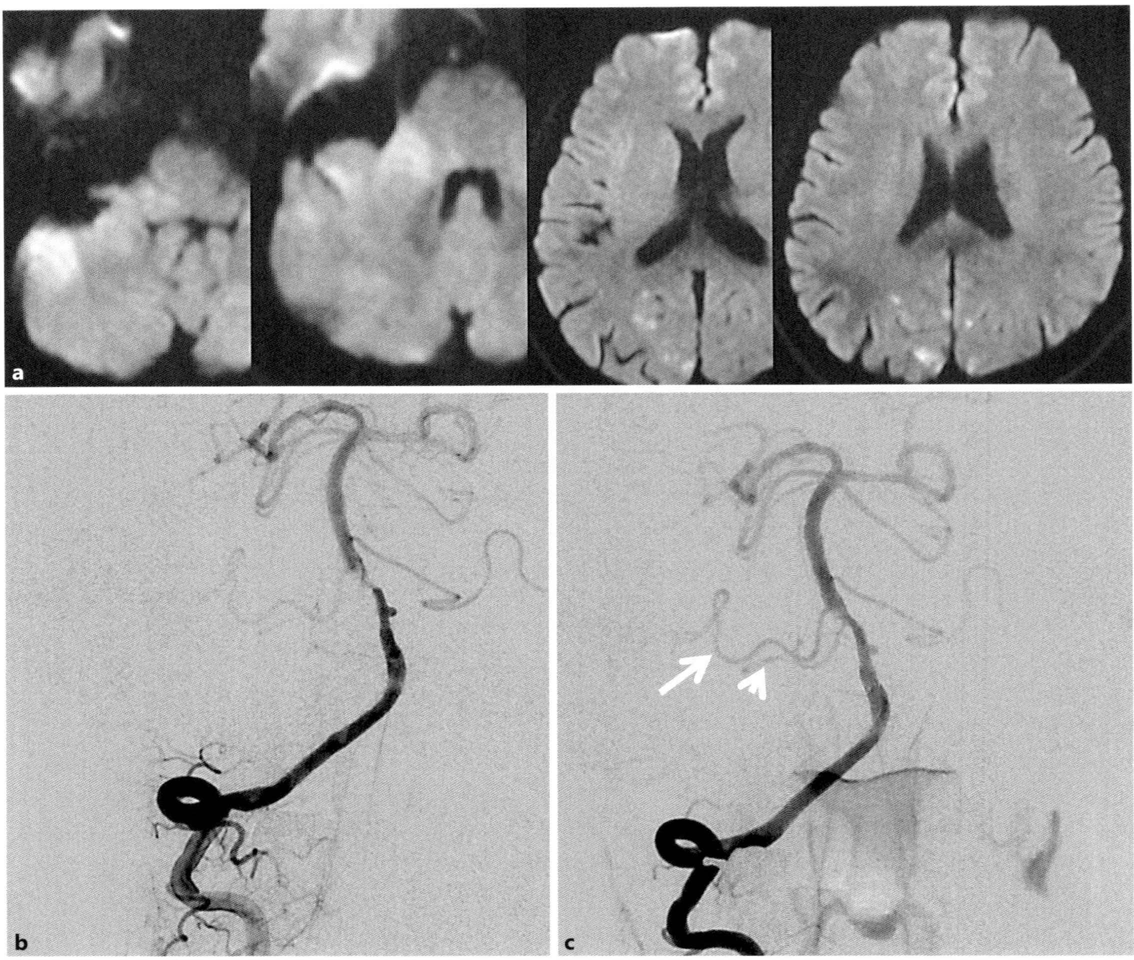

Fig. 9. A 55-year-old man with hypertension and diabetes developed dizziness. Examination showed right peripheral facial palsy, facial sensory loss, and hearing loss, and right- sided ataxia. Diffusion weighted MRI showed infarcts involving the left anterior inferior cerebellar artery (AICA) territory (lateral cerebellum and cerebellar peduncle) and bilateral occipital areas (**a**). Because his mentality fluctuated, catether angiography was performed, which revealed focal severe stenosis in the lower basilar artery (BA). Right AICA was poorly visualized as compared to the left one (**b**). Clot retrieval was tried using Solitaire device, but there remained segmental, severe BA stenosis. Balloon angioplasty and self expanding stent was performed. Final angiogram showed mild residual BA stenosis and well-visualization of two AICAs (**c**, long and short arrows). It seems that the patient had double AICAs.

BA Atherosclerosis as a Cause Top of Basilar Syndrome

Atherosclerosis is generally most severe in the proximal BA, and occlusions of the BA tip are usually embolic [102], more often from the diseased heart than proximal atherothrombosis. Although atherothrombosis occurring in the distal BA can also result in TOB [123], this is distinctly uncommon.

References

1 Kim JS, Nah HW, Park SM, Kim SK, Cho KH, Lee J, Lee YS, Kim J, Ha SW, Kim EG, Kim DE, Kang DW, Kwon SU, Yu KH, Lee BC: Risk factors and stroke mechanisms in atherosclerotic stroke: intracranial compared with extracranial and anterior compared with posterior circulation disease. Stroke 2012;43: 3313–3318.

2 Hong KS, Ko SB, Lee JS, Yu KH, Rha JH: Endovascular recanalization therapy in acute ischemic stroke: updated meta-analysis of randomized controlled trials. J Stroke 2015;17:268–281.

3 Lee JS, Hong JM, Lee KS, Suh HI, Demchuk AM, Hwang YH, Kim BM, Kim JS: Endovascular therapy of cerebral arterial occlusions: intracranial atherosclerosis versus embolism. J Stroke Cerebrovasc Dis 2015;24:2074–2080.

4 LHermitte F, Gautier JC, Derouesne C, Guiraud B: Ischemic accidents in the middle cerebral artery territory. A study of the causes in 122 cases. Arch Neurol 1968;19:248–256.

5 Lhermitte F, Gautier JC, Derouesne C: Nature of occlusions of the middle cerebral artery. Neurology 1970;20:82–88.

6 Gorelick PB, Caplan LR, Hier DB, Parker SL, Patel D: Racial differences in the distribution of anterior circulation occlusive disease. Neurology 1984;34:54–59.

7 Inzitari D, Hachinski VC, Taylor DW, Barnett HJ: Racial differences in the anterior circulation in cerebrovascular disease. How much can be explained by risk factors? Arch Neurol 1990;47:1080–1084.

8 Sacco RL, Kargman DE, Gu Q, Zamanillo MC: Race-ethnicity and determinants of intracranial atherosclerotic cerebral infarction. The northern Manhattan stroke study. Stroke 1995;26:14–20.

9 Min WK, Park KK, Kim YS, Park HC, Kim JY, Park SP, Suh CK: Atherothrombotic middle cerebral artery territory infarction: topographic diversity with common occurrence of concomitant small cortical and subcortical infarcts. Stroke 2000;31:2055–2061.

10 Lee DK, Kim JS, Kwon SU, Yoo SH, Kang DW: Lesion patterns and stroke mechanism in atherosclerotic middle cerebral artery disease: early diffusion-weighted imaging study. Stroke 2005;36: 2583–2588.

11 Caplan L, Babikian V, Helgason C, Hier DB, DeWitt D, Patel D, Stein R: Occlusive disease of the middle cerebral artery. Neurology 1985;35:975–982.

12 Bogousslavsky J, Barnett HJ, Fox AJ, Hachinski VC, Taylor W: Atherosclerotic disease of the middle cerebral artery. Stroke 1986;17:1112–1120.

13 Lyrer PA, Engelter S, Radu EW, Steck AJ: Cerebral infarcts related to isolated middle cerebral artery stenosis. Stroke 1997;28:1022–1027.

14 Yoo KM, Shin HK, Cahng HM, Caplan LR: Middle cerebral artery occlusive disease: the New England Medical Center Stroke Registry. J Stroke Cerebrovasc Dis 1998;7:344–351.

15 Lee PH, Oh SH, Bang OY, Joo IS, Huh K: Isolated middle cerebral artery disease: clinical and neuroradiological features depending on the pathogenesis. J Neurol Neurosurg Psychiatry 2004;75:727–732.

16 Bang OY, Heo JH, Kim JY, Park JH, Huh K: Middle cerebral artery stenosis is a major clinical determinant in striatocapsular small, deep infarction. Arch Neurol 2002;59:259–263.

17 Mok VC, Fan YH, Lam WW, Hui AC, Wong KS: Small subcortical infarct and intracranial large artery disease in chinese. J Neurol Sci 2003;216:55–59.

18 Cho AH, Kang DW, Kwon SU, Kim JS: Is 15 mm size criterion for lacunar infarction still valid? A study on strictly subcortical middle cerebral artery territory infarction using diffusion-weighted MRI. Cerebrovasc Dis 2007;23:14–19.

19 Nah HW, Kang DW, Kwon SU, Kim JS: Diversity of single small subcortical infarctions according to infarct location and parent artery disease: analysis of indicators for small vessel disease and atherosclerosis. Stroke 2010;41:2822–2827.

20 Gacs G, Fox AJ, Barnett HJM, Vinuela F: Occurrence and mechanisms of occlusion of the anterior cerebral-artery. Stroke 1983;14:952–959.

21 Bogousslavsky J, Regli F: Anterior cerebral-artery territory infarction in the lausanne stroke registry – clinical and etiologic patterns. Arch Neurol 1990;47: 144–150.

22 Kazui S, Sawada T, Naritomi H, Kuriyama Y, Yamaguchi T: Angiographic evaluation of brain infarction limited to the anterior cerebral-artery territory. Stroke 1993;24:549–553.

23 Kumral E, Bayulkem G, Evyapan D, Yunten N: Spectrum of anterior cerebral artery territory infarction: clinical and mri findings. Eur J Neurol 2002;9:615–624.

24 Sussman NM, Gur RC, Gur RE, Oconnor MJ: Mutism as a consequence of callosotomy. J Neurosurg 1983;59:514–519.

25 Ross MK, Reeves AG, Roberts DW: Post-commissurotomy mutism. Ann Neurol 1984;16:114–114.

26 Kang SY, Kim JS: Anterior cerebral artery infarction: stroke mechanism and clinical-imaging study in 100 patients. Neurology 2008;70:2386–2393.

27 Masdeu JC, Schoene WC, Funkenstein H: Aphasia following infarction of the left supplementary motor area: a clinicopathologic study. Neurology 1978;28: 1220–1223.

28 Alexander MP, Schmitt MA: The aphasia syndrome of stroke in the left anterior cerebral artery territory. Arch Neurol 1980;37:97–100.

29 Kim JS, Choi-Kwon S: Poststroke depression and emotional incontinence: Correlation with lesion location. Neurology 2000;54:1805–1810.

30 Kim JS: Involuntary movements after anterior cerebral artery territory infarction. Stroke 2001;32:258–261.

31 Klatka LA, Depper MH, Marini AM: Infarction in the territory of the anterior cerebral artery. Neurology 1998;51:620–622.

32 Nagamine Y, Fukuoka T, Hayashi T, Kato Y, Deguchi I, Maruyama H, Horiuchi Y, Sano H, Mizuno S, Tanahashi N: Research article: clinical characteristics of isolated anterior cerebral artery territory infarction due to arterial dissection. J Stroke Cerebrovasc Dis 2014;23:2907–2913.

33 Hass WK, Fields WS, North RR, Kircheff, II, Chase NE, Bauer RB: Joint study of extracranial arterial occlusion. Ii. Arteriography, techniques, sites, and complications. JAMA 1968;203:961–968.

34 Hutchinson EC, Yates PO: Carotico-vertebral stenosis. Lancet 1957;272:2–8.
35 Jorgensen L, Torvik A: Ischaemic cerebrovascular diseases in an autopsy series. I. Prevalence, location and predisposing factors in verified thrombo-embolic occlusions, and their significance in the pathogenesis of cerebral infarction. J Neurol Sci 1966;3:490–509.
36 Wechsler LR, Kistler JP, Davis KR, Kaminski MJ: The prognosis of carotid siphon stenosis. Stroke 1986;17:714–718.
37 Craig DR, Meguro K, Watridge C, Robertson JT, Barnett HJ, Fox AJ: Intracranial internal carotid artery stenosis. Stroke 1982;13:825–828.
38 Marzewski DJ, Furlan AJ, St Louis P, Little JR, Modic MT, Williams G: Intracranial internal carotid artery stenosis: longterm prognosis. Stroke 1982;13:821–824.
39 Sohn H, Kang DW, Kwon SU, Kim JS: Anterior choroidal artery territory infarction: lesions confined to versus beyond the internal capsule. Cerebrovasc Dis 2013;35:228–234.
40 Ueda K, Toole JF, McHenry LC Jr: Carotid and vertebrobasilar transient ischemic attacks: clinical and angiographic correlation. Neurology 1979;29:1094–1101.
41 Castaigne P, Lhermitte F, Gautier JC, Escourolle R, Derouesne C, Der Agopian P, Popa C: Arterial occlusions in the vertebro-basilar system. A study of 44 patients with post-mortem data. Brain 1973;96:133–154.
42 Cornhill JF, Akins D, Hutson M, Chandler AB: Localization of atherosclerotic lesions in the human basilar artery. Atherosclerosis 1980;35:77–86.
43 Kim JS: Pure lateral medullary infarction: clinical-radiological correlation of 130 acute, consecutive patients. Brain 2003;126:1864–1872.
44 Caplan LR: Posterior Circulation Disease: clinical Findings, Diagnosis, and Management. Boston, Blackwell Science, 1996.
45 Fisher CM, Karnes WE, Kubik CS: Lateral medullary infarction-the pattern of vascular occlusion. J Neuropathol Exp Neurol 1961;20:323–379.
46 Currier RDG, CL DeJong, RN: Some comments on Wallenberg's lateral medullary syndrome. Neurology 1961;1:778–792.
47 Kim JS, Lee JH, Suh DC, Lee MC: Spectrum of lateral medullary syndrome. Correlation between clinical findings and magnetic resonance imaging in 33 subjects. Stroke 1994;25:1405–1410.
48 Kim JS, Lee JH, Lee MC: Patterns of sensory dysfunction in lateral medullary infarction. Clinical-MRI correlation. Neurology 1997;49:1557–1563.
49 Kim JS: Sensory symptoms in ipsilateral limbs/body due to lateral medullary infarction. Neurology 2001;57:1230–1234.
50 Dejerine J: Semiologie des affections du système nerveux. Paris, Masson, 1914, pp 226–230.
51 Kim JS, Kim HG, Chung CS: Medial medullary syndrome. Report of 18 new patients and a review of the literature. Stroke 1995;26:1548–1552.
52 Park JY, Chun MH, Kang SH, Lee JA, Kim BR, Shin MJ: Functional outcome in poststroke patients with or without fatigue. Am J Phys Med Rehabil 2009;88:554–558.
53 Ropper AH, Fisher CM, Kleinman GM: Pyramidal infarction in the medulla: a cause of pure motor hemiplegia sparing the face. Neurology 1979;29:91–95.
54 Bassetti C, Bogousslavsky J, Mattle H, Bernasconi A: Medial medullary stroke: Report of seven patients and review of the literature. Neurology 1997;48:882–890.
55 Kim JS, Choi KD, Oh SY, Park SH, Han MK, Yoon BW, Roh JK: Medial medullary infarction: abnormal ocular motor findings. Neurology 2005;65:1294–1298.
56 Kim JS, Moon SY, Kim KY, Kim HC, Park SH, Yoon BW, Roh JK: Ocular contrapulsion in rostral medial medullary infarction. Neurology 2004;63:1325–1327.
57 Wallenberg A: Acute bulbar affection (embolie der art. Cerebellar post. Inf. Sinistra?) Arch Psychiatr Nervenkr 1895;27:504–540.
58 Sacco RL, Freddo L, Bello JA, Odel JG, Onesti ST, Mohr JP: Wallenberg's lateral medullary syndrome. Clinical-magnetic resonance imaging correlations. Arch Neurol 1993;50:609–614.
59 Vuilleumier P, Bogousslavsky J, Regli F: Infarction of the lower brainstem. Clinical, aetiological and mri-topographical correlations. Brain 1995;118:1013–1025.
60 Caplan LR: Occlusion of the vertebral or basilar artery. Follow-up analysis of some patients with benign outcome. Stroke 1979;10:277–282.
61 WG S: The symptom-complex of a lesion of the upper most portion of the anterior spinal and adjoining portion of the vertebral arteries. J Nerv Mednt Dis 1908;35:775–778.
62 Davison C: Syndrome of the anterior spinal artery of the medulla oblongata. Arch Neurol Psychiat 1937;37:91–107.
63 Fisher CM, Curry HB: Pure motor hemiplegia of vascular origin. Arch Neurol 1965;13:30–44.
64 Bassetti C, Bogousslavsky J, Barth A, Regli F: Isolated infarcts of the pons. Neurology 1996;46:165–175.
65 Kumral E, Bayulkem G, Evyapan D: Clinical spectrum of pontine infarction. Clinical-mri correlations. J Neurol 2002;249:1659–1670.
66 Erro ME, Gallego J, Herrera M, Bermejo B: Isolated pontine infarcts: etiopathogenic mechanisms. Eur J Neurol 2005;12:984–988.
67 Kataoka S, Hori A, Shirakawa T, Hirose G: Paramedian pontine infarction. Neurological/topographical correlation. Stroke 1997;28:809–815.
68 Fisher CM: Ataxic hemiparesis. A pathologic study. Arch Neurol 1978;35:126–128.
69 Fisher CM: A lacunar stroke. The dysarthria-clumsy hand syndrome. Neurology 1967;17:614–617.
70 Kim JS, Bae YH: Pure or predominant sensory stroke due to brain stem lesion. Stroke 1997;28:1761–1764.
71 Shintani S, Tsuruoka S, Shiigai T: Pure sensory stroke caused by a pontine infarct. Clinical, radiological, and physiological features in four patients. Stroke 1994;25:1512–1515.
72 Zee DS, Hain TC, Carl JR: Abduction nystagmus in internuclear ophthalmoplegia. Ann Neurol 1987;21:383–388.
73 Pierrot-Deseilligny C, Chain F, Serdaru M, Gray F, Lhermitte F: The 'one-and-a-half' syndrome. Electro-oculographic analyses of five cases with deductions about the physiological mechanisms of lateral gaze. Brain 1981;104:665–699.
74 Kubik CS, Adams RD: Occlusion of the basilar artery; a clinical and pathological study. Brain 1946;69:73–121.
75 Ferbert A, Bruckmann H, Drummen R: Clinical features of proven basilar artery occlusion. Stroke 1990;21:1135–1142.
76 Voetsch B, DeWitt LD, Pessin MS, Caplan LR: Basilar artery occlusive disease in the New England medical center posterior circulation registry. Arch Neurol 2004;61:496–504.

77 Fisher CM: The 'herald hemiparesis' of basilar artery occlusion. Arch Neurol 1988;45:1301–1303.
78 Biemond A: Thrombosis of the basilar artery and the vascularization of the brain stem. Brain 1951;74:300–317.
79 Kim JS, Cho KH, Kang DW, Kwon SU, Suh DC: Basilar artery atherosclerotic disease is related to subacute lesion volume increase in pontine base infarction. Acta Neurol Scand 2009;120:88–93.
80 Klein IF, Lavallee PC, Schouman-Claeys E, Amarenco P: High-resolution mri identifies basilar artery plaques in paramedian pontine infarct. Neurology 2005; 64:551–552.
81 Kim JS, Kim J: Pure midbrain infarction: Clinical, radiologic, and pathophysiologic findings. Neurology 2005;64:1227–1232.
82 Bogousslavsky J, Maeder P, Regli F, Meuli R: Pure midbrain infarction: clinical syndromes, mri, and etiologic patterns. Neurology 1994;44:2032–2040.
83 Schmahmann JD: Vascular syndromes of the thalamus. Stroke 2003;34:2264–2278.
84 Bogousslavsky J, Regli F, Uske A: Thalamic infarcts: clinical syndromes, etiology, and prognosis. Neurology 1988;38: 837–848.
85 Percheron G: The anatomy of the arterial supply of the human thalamus and its use for the interpretation of the thalamic vascular pathology. Z Neurol 1973;205:1–13.
86 Caplan LR, DeWitt LD, Pessin MS, Gorelick PB, Adelman LS: Lateral thalamic infarcts. Arch Neurol 1988;45: 959–964.
87 Kim JS: Pure sensory stroke. Clinical-radiological correlates of 21 cases. Stroke 1992;23:983–987.
88 Arboix A, Garcia-Plata C, Garcia-Eroles L, Massons J, Comes E, Oliveres M, Targa C: Clinical study of 99 patients with pure sensory stroke. J Neurol 2005;252: 156–162.
89 Fisher CM: Thalamic pure sensory stroke: a pathologic study. Neurology 1978;28:1141–1144.
90 Bogousslavsky J, Regli F, Assal G: The syndrome of unilateral tuberothalamic artery territory infarction. Stroke 1986; 17:434–441.
91 Ghika-Schmid F, Bogousslavsky J: The acute behavioral syndrome of anterior thalamic infarction: a prospective study of 12 cases. Ann Neurol 2000;48: 220–227.
92 Castaigne P, Lhermitte F, Buge A, Escourolle R, Hauw JJ, Lyon-Caen O: Paramedian thalamic and midbrain infarct: clinical and neuropathological study. Ann Neurol 1981;10:127–148.
93 Graff-Radford NR, Eslinger PJ, Damasio AR, Yamada T: Nonhemorrhagic infarction of the thalamus: behavioral, anatomic, and physiologic correlates. Neurology 1984;34:14–23.
94 Reilly M, Connolly S, Stack J, Martin EA, Hutchinson M: Bilateral paramedian thalamic infarction: a distinct but poorly recognized stroke syndrome. Q J Med 1992;82:63–70.
95 Wada K, Kimura K, Minematsu K, Yamaguchi T: Incongruous homonymous hemianopic scotoma. J Neurol Sci 1999;163:179–182.
96 Pessin MS, Lathi ES, Cohen MB, Kwan ES, Hedges TR, 3rd, Caplan LR: Clinical features and mechanism of occipital infarction. Ann Neurol 1987;21: 290–299.
97 Kumral E, Bayulkem G, Atac C, Alper Y: Spectrum of superficial posterior cerebral artery territory infarcts. Eur J Neurol 2004;11:237–246.
98 Cals N, Devuyst G, Afsar N, Karapanayiotides T, Bogousslavsky J: Pure superficial posterior cerebral artery territory infarction in the lausanne stroke registry. J Neurol 2002;249:855–861.
99 Steinke W, Mangold J, Schwartz A, Hennerici M: Mechanisms of infarction in the superficial posterior cerebral artery territory. J Neurol 1997;244: 571–578.
100 Yamamoto Y, Georgiadis AL, Chang HM, Caplan LR: Posterior cerebral artery territory infarcts in the new england medical center posterior circulation registry. Arch Neurol 1999;56: 824–832.
101 Lee E, Kang DW, Kwon SU, Kim JS: Posterior cerebral artery infarction: diffusion-weighted mri analysis of 205 patients. Cerebrovasc Dis 2009;28: 298–305.
102 Caplan LR: 'Top of the basilar' syndrome. Neurology 1980;30:72–79.
103 Kumral E, Bayulkem G, Akyol A, Yunten N, Sirin H, Sagduyu A: Mesencephalic and associated posterior circulation infarcts. Stroke 2002;33:2224–2231.
104 Wang X, Fan YH, Lam WW, Leung TW, Wong KS: Clinical features, topographic patterns on DWI and etiology of thalamic infarcts. J Neurol Sci 2008; 267:147–153.
105 Kwon JY, Kwon SU, Kang DW, Suh DC, Kim JS: Isolated lateral thalamic infarction: the role of posterior cerebral artery disease. Eur J Neurol 2012; 19:265–270.
106 Kase CS, Norrving B, Levine SR, Babikian VL, Chodosh EH, Wolf PA, Welch KM: Cerebellar infarction. Clinical and anatomic observations in 66 cases. Stroke 1993;24:76–83.
107 Tohgi H, Takahashi S, Chiba K, Hirata Y: Cerebellar infarction. Clinical and neuroimaging analysis in 293 patients. The tohoku cerebellar infarction study group. Stroke 1993;24:1697–1701.
108 Sypert GW, Alvord EC Jr.: Cerebellar infarction. A clinicopathological study. Arch Neurol 1975;32:357–363.
109 Amarenco P: The spectrum of cerebellar infarctions. Neurology 1991;41: 973–979.
110 Bogousslavsky J, Van Melle G, Regli F: The Lausanne stroke registry: Analysis of 1,000 consecutive patients with first stroke. Stroke 1988;19:1083–1092.
111 Barth A, Bogousslavsky J, Regli F: The clinical and topographic spectrum of cerebellar infarcts: a clinical-magnetic resonance imaging correlation study. Ann Neurol 1993;33:451–456.
112 Macdonell RA, Kalnins RM, Donnan GA: Cerebellar infarction: natural history, prognosis, and pathology. Stroke 1987;18:849–855.
113 Adams RD: Occlusion of the anterior infereior cereellar artery. Arch Neurol Psychiatry 1983;49:765.
114 Amarenco P, Hauw JJ, Gautier JC: Arterial pathology in cerebellar infarction. Stroke 1990;21:1299–1305.
115 Amarenco P, Hauw JJ: Cerebellar infarction in the territory of the superior cerebellar artery: a clinicopathologic study of 33 cases. Neurology 1990;40: 1383–1390.

116 Chaves CJ, Caplan LR, Chung CS, Tapia J, Amarenco P, Teal P, Wityk R, Estol C, Tettenborn B, Rosengart A, et al: Cerebellar infarcts in the New England medical center posterior circulation stroke registry. Neurology 1994;44:1385–1390.
117 Kalyan-Raman UP, Kowalski RV, Lee RH, Fierer JA: Dissecting aneurysm of superior cerebellar artery. Its association with fibromuscular dysplasia. Arch Neurol 1983;40:120–122.
118 Perez-Higueras A, Alvarez-Ruiz F, Martinez-Bermejo A, Frutos R, Villar O, Diez-Tejedor E: Cerebellar infarction from fibromuscular dysplasia and dissecting aneurysm of the vertebral artery. Report of a child. Stroke 1988; 19:521–524.
119 Caplan LR: Migraine and vertebrobasilar ischemia. Neurology 1991;41:55–61.
120 Amarenco P, Hauw JJ: Cerebellar infarction in the territory of the anterior and inferior cerebellar artery. A clinicopathological study of 20 cases. Brain 1990;113:139–155.
121 Kumral E, Kisabay A, Atac C: Lesion patterns and etiology of ischemia in the anterior inferior cerebellar artery territory involvement: a clinical – diffusion weighted – MRI study. Eur J Neurol 2006;13:395–401.
122 Amarenco P, Rosengart A, DeWitt LD, Pessin MS, Caplan LR: Anterior inferior cerebellar artery territory infarcts. Mechanisms and clinical features. Arch Neurol 1993;50:154–161.
123 Mehler MF: The rostral basilar artery syndrome: diagnosis, etiology, prognosis. Neurology 1989;39:9–16.

Jong S. Kim, MD, PhD
Department of Neurology, Asan Medical Center, University of Ulsan
Asanbyeongwon-gil 86, Songpa-gu
Seoul 138-736 (Korea)
E-Mail jongskim@amc.seoul.kr

Kim JS, Caplan LR, Wong KS (eds): Intracranial Atherosclerosis: Pathophysiology, Diagnosis and Treatment.
Front Neurol Neurosci. Basel, Karger, 2016, vol 40, pp 93–108 (DOI: 10.1159/000448304)

Biomarkers, Natural Course and Prognosis

Juan F. Arenillas[a] · Elena López-Cancio[b] · Ka Sing Wong[c]

[a]Department of Neurology, Hospital Clínico Universitario, University of Valladolid, Valladolid, and [b]Stroke Unit, Department of Neurosciences, Germans Trias i Pujol University Hospital, Badalona, Barcelona, Spain; [c]Department of Medicine and Therapeutics, The Chinese University of Hong Kong, Shatin, New Territory, HKSAR, Hong Kong, China

Abstract

Increasing our knowledge about intracranial atherosclerosis (ICAS) natural history and prognostic factors is essential to improve its preventive therapy and thus reduce the dramatic clinical consequences caused by this entity. ICAS is characterized by a chronic and progressive course until it becomes symptomatic, mostly through complication of an unstable intracranial atherosclerotic plaque. Population-based studies in healthy subjects have shown that the prevalence of asymptomatic ICAS is higher in Asian than in Caucasian populations. In both settings, asymptomatic ICAS is associated with classical vascular risk factors and with the metabolic syndrome, and it is burdened with an increasing risk of having incident stroke and cognitive impairment. When it reaches its symptomatic stage, ICAS is a dynamic and aggressive condition, and affected patients are at high risk of having recurrent stroke and other major vascular events. The Stenting versus Aggressive Medical Therapy for Intracranial Arterial Stenosis (SAMMPRIS) trial has recently shown a robust impact of intensive medical therapy reducing the risk of clinical recurrence of symptomatic ICAS. However, even under best medical therapy and degree of risk factor control, symptomatic ICAS-related recurrence risk continues to be the highest among all stroke etiologic subtypes. The second part of the chapter reviews the current understanding of prognostic factors that may help discriminate the high-risk ICAS patients, divided into local factors (vulnerable ICAS plaque) and systemic factors (vulnerable ICAS patient). Regarding research on local factors, high-resolution magnetic resonance imaging (HRMRI) is an emerging technique that allows in vivo evaluation of intracranial arterial wall, which is displacing our research focus from intracranial stenosis degree towards intracranial atherosclerotic plaque composition and activity. Characterization of the vulnerable ICAS patient may be improved with biomarker research. The latest contributions in this field help support the hypothesis that inflammation determines the risk of progression and complication of this disease, as it occurs in atherosclerosis affecting extracranial arterial beds.

Introduction

Intracranial atherosclerosis (ICAS) is characterized by the development, progression, and complication of atherosclerotic plaques affecting intracranial arteries [1]. ICAS represents the most common cause of ischemic stroke among Asian and African patients [2, 3], whereas it accounts for 8–10% of all ischemic strokes in Caucasians [4]. Thus, attending the distribution of the world's population, ICAS has been proposed to be the most common cause of stroke globally [5].

Atherosclerosis is a chronic inflammatory process of lipid-rich lesion growth in the vascular wall that can cause myocardial infarction and stroke [6]. The dynamics of atherosclerosis over time might be seen as a struggle between the processes of vascular injury and repair, where persistent inflammation leads to a predominance of aggressive mechanisms and to a derangement of vascular reparative capacity. Thus, the high-risk ICAS phenotype may also derive from an imbalance of basic mechanisms in favour of injury processes, which leads to progression, destabilization and complication of atherosclerotic plaques.

Although the process of atherogenesis may share common mechanisms across diverse arterial territories, there are important regional differences regarding the relative contribution of basic mechanisms to the progression of atherosclerotic plaques [7]. Atherosclerosis in intracranial arteries has unique characteristics related to the anatomical and hemodynamic peculiarities of the intracranial arterial system [8]. For instance, intracranial arteries are muscular-type arteries that contain only a few medial elastic fibers, a thick and dense internal elastic lamina, and a few adventitial vasa vasorum, and they lack an external elastic lamina [9]. Therefore, specific research may be needed to elucidate the molecular pathways that play a role in the natural history and prognosis of ICAS.

Our knowledge about ICAS natural history and prognosis has substantially improved during the past two decades. Our approach in this Chapter will try to integrate the main novelties that have emerged in the field lately. First, recently launched population-based prospective studies may allow a better understanding of ICAS development and prognostic impact from its asymptomatic stages in Asian and Caucasian populations [10, 11]. Second, the Stenting versus Aggressive Medical Therapy for Intracranial Arterial Stenosis (SAMMPRIS) study has opened a new era for symptomatic ICAS management, showing a striking impact of intensive medical therapy on disease's prognosis [12]. All the knowledge about ICAS natural history acquired during the pre-SAMMPRIS era needs to be reinterpreted in light of these major findings. Third, high-resolution magnetic resonance imaging (HRMRI) is an emerging technique that allows in vivo evaluation of intracranial arterial wall, which is displacing our research focus from intracranial stenosis degree to atherosclerotic plaque composition and activity [1]. And finally, biomarker research has provided us with relevant contributions, whose findings strongly support the hypothesis that inflammation determines the risk of progression and complication of ICAS [13].

Natural Course of Intracranial Atherosclerosis

The most feared clinical expression of ICAS is stroke followed by cognitive impairment and dementia [14]. Both entities are the cause of long-term disability and mortality. As atherosclerosis occurring elsewhere, atherosclerotic lesions in intracranial vessels develop silently over years before they give rise to clinical symptoms. However, the natural history of asymptomatic ICAS is still poorly understood. When it turns to symptomatic, ICAS becomes a dynamic and aggressive condition, even under aggressive medical management [12]. We will describe the main features that characterize the natural history of ICAS in both the asymptomatic and symptomatic stages.

Asymptomatic ICAS: Prevalence and Prognosis
Population-based studies aimed to determine the prevalence and risk factors of asymptomatic ICAS were firstly performed in Asian populations using transcranial Doppler [15–17]. Two similar

Table 1. Asymptomatic ICAS prevalence: population-based studies using transcranial ultrasonography

	n	Males, %	Age	Arteries explored	Prevalence, %	Associated vascular risk factors	Longitudinal study (prognosis)
Huang HW, China [15], 2007	1,068	34.6	64.4±9.6	MCA	5.9	DM, HT, age, male sex	No
Wong KS, China [16], 2007	3,057	40.8	55.8±11	MCA	12.6	DM, HT, age, DL	No
Bae HJ, Korea [17], 2007	1,228	40.1	58.1±11	All	24.5 (global)	DM, HT, age	No
APAC study, China [21], 2014	5,393	59.9	55.2±11	All	13.2	DM, HT, age, MetSynd	On-going
AsIA study, Spain [18, 20], 2012	933	64	66.3±8	MCA All	4.1 (MCA) 8.6 (global)	DM, HT, age, MetSynd	On-going

MCA = Middle cerebral artery; DM = diabetes mellitus; HT = hypertension; MetSynd = metabolic syndrome.

studies with a prospective design were developed in Caucasian and Asian populations: the Asymptomatic Intracranial Atherosclerosis (AsIA) study [11, 18] in Spain and the Asymptomatic Polyvascular Abnormalities Community study (APAC) in China [10, 11]. Table 1 summarizes the data on the prevalence of asymptomatic ICAS and associated vascular risk factors in the above mentioned studies. Although some methodological issues may preclude comparisons among studies, prevalence of asymptomatic ICAS was, as expected, higher in Asian populations. It is important to point out that Asian studies did not use contrast-agents in subjects with insufficient acoustic bone window, which may have led to underestimation of prevalence of ICAS. Interestingly, similar vascular risk factors were associated with asymptomatic ICAS across all populations that included age, diabetes, hypertension and metabolic syndrome. Both in Caucasian and Chinese populations, prevalence and severity of asymptomatic ICAS were higher with a higher vascular risk score (Framingham) [18, 19] and with increasing number of metabolic syndrome components [20, 21]. Thus, the different racial distribution of ICAS is poorly explained by classical vascular risk factors; genetic, molecular or environmental factors may play additional roles. Other European studies have reported the prevalence of asymptomatic ICAS among series of patients with TIA [22] and stroke [23, 24], which ranged from 5 to 15.5%. Although these are not population-based studies, they reinforced the importance of ICAS in Caucasian populations.

Regarding the prognostic impact of asymptomatic ICAS, current data is particularly scarce. In a Chinese prospective and hospital-based study including 2,144 type 2 diabetic subjects without history of stroke at baseline, presence of asymptomatic MCA stenosis (in 12.3% of the patients) was independently associated with incident stroke, acute coronary syndrome and vascular death after a median follow-up of 14 years [25]. In a stroke-free population of 2,924 subjects in Japan, ICAS conferred an annual stroke risk of 3.5% when combined with carotid plaques [26]. Recently, a subanalysis of the population-based Rotterdam study including 2,323 Caucasian stroke-free participants highlighted the importance of intracranial internal carotid artery calcification (ICAC) detected in simple CT as an independent risk factor of future stroke after 6 years of follow-up. ICAC predicted stroke better than vascular risk score assessment or calcification of other vessels such as carotid or aortic arch [27]. Although the direct association of intracranial carotid wall calcification on CT scans with an underlying atherosclerotic stenosis was not evaluated in this study, ICAC could be considered a marker of total ICASs. Ongoing prospective population-based studies will give us valuable information about the real prognostic impact and natural history of asymptomatic ICAS [10, 11]. These studies will also help us to identify clinical, molecular and genetic predictors of the conversion of subclinical ICAS to a more aggressive symptomatic stage. In a preliminary analysis of the longitudinal AsIA study, presence of asymptomatic intracranial stenosis emerged as a strong independent predictor not only for stroke but also for a composite of stroke, acute coronary syndrome and death, with higher hazard ratios that those conferred by carotid plaques or vascular risk score [28]. It has been proposed that ICAS may also play a role in cognitive impairment and dementia [29]. In this line, presence of intracranial stenosis in CT angiography was associated with a higher risk of progressing from mild cognitive impairment to dementia, independently of age and vascular risk factors, in a Chinese cohort of stroke-free individuals [30].

In conclusion, asymptomatic ICAS is a relatively frequent condition both in Asian and Caucasian populations. Prognostic impact of subclinical ICAS in incident stroke and incident cognitive impairment needs to be further investigated in longitudinal studies.

Symptomatic Intracranial Atherosclerosis: Risk of Stroke Recurrence and Risk of Other Vascular Events

Symptomatic ICAS is burdened with a high risk of stroke recurrence. Also, ICAS is associated with vascular events in other vascular beds and vascular death. The risk of having a recurrent ischemic stroke in the territory of a symptomatic stenosis varies depending on different local and systemic factors that will be discussed in the next part of the chapter.

Here we will summarize the natural history of symptomatic ICAS under medical treatment derived from the last prospective studies and randomized clinical trials. The most important finding is that stroke recurrence risk has been progressively lowered by aggressive management of vascular risk factors.

Wong et al. [31] followed-up 705 patients with ischemic stroke for a median of 42 months. The annual stroke recurrence was progressively higher among those with no vascular lesions (10.9%), those with ICAS only (17.1%) and those with extracranial carotid disease concurrent with ICAS (24.3%). The GESICA study investigators reported that during a median follow-up of 23.4 months, 38.2% of the 102 included patients had a stroke or a transient ischemic attack (TIA) in the same territory of the stenotic artery [32]. Recurrent cerebrovascular events were observed with a median time of 2 months after the initial episode. The WASID trial was the first randomized study that evaluated antithrombotic treatment in ICAS (warfarin versus aspirin) and included 569 patients with 50–99% symptomatic stenosis located in any intracerebral large-artery [33]. After a median follow-up of 1.8 years, the annual recurrence rate of a new ischemic stroke in the territory of the stenotic artery was 12% in the aspirin arm and 11% in the warfarin arm, and was up to 18% among those with a stenosis 70–99%. In the WASID trial, patients whose qualifying event for the trial occurred 17 days or fewer before enrolment had a significantly higher risk of recurrent stroke during follow-up than did patients whose qualifying event for the trial occurred more than 17 days (up to 90 days) before enrolment. The most important findings in the WASID trial were related to the importance of controlling risk factors to reduce major vascular events in ICAD patients. The results of WASID suggested that patients with poorly controlled systolic blood pressure (>140 mm Hg) and cholesterol (>5.20 mmol/l) during follow-up had the highest rates of major vascular events, including recurrent stroke [34]. Thus, in the following SAMMPRIS trial [35], aggressive risk factor management was performed, targeting LDL below 70 mg/dl, systolic blood pressure below 140 mm Hg, and a comprehensive lifestyle modification program. The SAMMPRIS study compared intensive medical therapy alone with intracranial stent placement combined with intensive medical therapy in patients with 70–99% intracranial stenosis who had had a TIA or stroke within 30 days before enrolment. Enrolment was discontinued early because of high rate of stroke and death in the stenting arm. The 1-year rate of the primary endpoint (any stroke or death within 30 days or ipsilateral stroke after 30 days) was significantly higher in the stent treatment group than in the medically managed group (20 vs. 12%).

Interestingly, patients in the aggressive medical management alone group of the SAMMPRIS trial had a much lower rate of stroke than expected (5.8% at 30 days and 12.2% at 1 year) compared with patients in the WASID trial who met the SAMMPRIS entry criteria and received aspirin or warfarin and usual management of vascular risk factors (10.7% at 30 days and 25% at 1 year). The fact that the lower risk in SAMMPRIS still persisted beyond 90 days after enrolment (when clopidogrel was stopped) suggests that intensive risk factor management had an important role beyond double antiplatelet treatment. Indeed, after adjustment for different baseline characteristics, stroke recurrence was still almost 2-fold higher in WASID patients that met inclusion criteria for SAMMPRIS [36]. In SAMMPRIS, within first 30 days, mean SBP decreased by over 5 mm Hg and mean LDL decreased by over 20 mg/dl, with both of these primary risk factor measures continuing to improve at 1 year. Improvements in secondary risk factor targets were also seen, with significantly better control of non-HDL cholesterol and HbA1c, weight loss, improved exercise, and smoking cessation compared to baseline [37]. This highlights the importance of aggressive control of risk factors. This is in line with the carotid intervention (endarterectomy) trials, which showed that in patients with asymptomatic carotid stenosis the stroke risk in the control group has lowered during the last 30 years with aggressive medical treatment including risk factor control [38].

Symptomatic ICAS patients are also exposed to an elevated risk of having coronary ischemic events and vascular death. In the WASID study, 30 (5.3%) patients had a major cardiac event (myocardial infarction or sudden death) during the study period [33]. The rate of fatal cardiac events has been shown to be extraordinarily high among patients with symptomatic intracranial ICA stenoses [39, 40]. Marzewski et al. [41] reported that 50% of the patients included in their series died during follow-up, 55% of them due to cardiac diseases. Thus, a significant proportion of patients with symptomatic ICAS may develop coronary artery disease within a few years after the initial event, often with fatal consequences. Therefore, coronary risk evaluation in patients with TIA and ischemic stroke caused by ICAS should be optimized.

Arenillas et al. [42] reported that up to 52% of patients with symptomatic ICAS who had no history of cardiac disease show abnormal myocardial perfusion SPECT studies suggesting the presence of occult coronary artery disease.

Prognosis

In the previous paragraph we have seen how patients affected by symptomatic ICAS are at a high risk of having recurrent ischemic stroke and other major vascular events. Intensive medical therapy is able to reduce this recurrence risk significantly, but even under the best possible conditions regarding medical treatment compliance and degree of vascular risk factor control, symptomatic ICAS- related recurrence risk continues to be the highest among all stroke main etiologic subtypes. Increasing our knowledge about the prognostic factors that help discriminate the high-risk ICAS patient seems a critical step in order to improve preventive therapy. In the near future, preventive treatment may need to be tailored according to an individual patient's risk, and those very high-risk patients who do not seem to respond sufficiently to conventional measures may benefit from additional or more aggressive therapies.

In this paragraph we will try to systematize ICAS prognostic factors according to the following schema (fig. 1). First, we will review the *local factors* and mechanisms that confer vulnerability to the culprit intracranial atherosclerotic plaque, which may be called *'vulnerable ICAS plaque'*. Second, we will describe the *systemic factors* that may promote the development of a more aggressive ICAS. These systemic factors can be evaluated globally at a patient's level and characterize the *'vulnerable ICAS patient'*, following the terminology used in the coronary literature [43, 44].

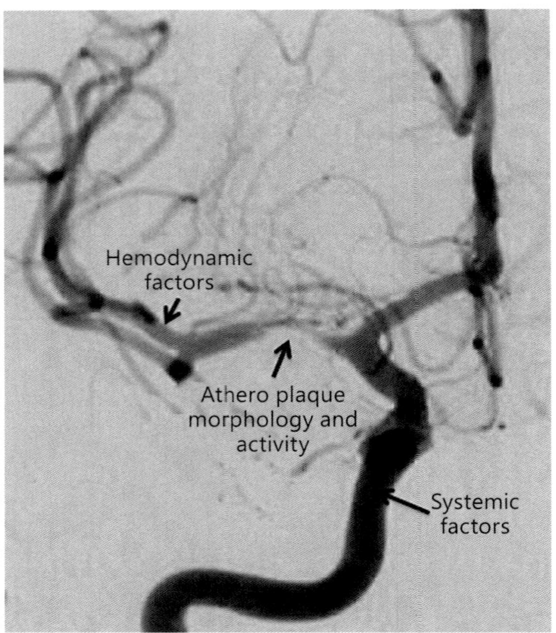

Fig. 1. Symptomatic intracranial atherosclerosis prognostic factor schema. The main prognostic factors in symptomatic intracranial atherosclerosis (ICAS) that we know thank to research done during the last decades could be summarized following this schema. These groups of factors interact amongst themselves in each ICAS patient and determine the risk of disease progression and clinical recurrence.

Local Factors (Vulnerable ICAS Plaque)

ICAS Plaque Morphology

Severity of the Symptomatic Intracranial Stenosis

In the WASID prospective study, the severity of the symptomatic ICAS was independently associated with a higher risk of subsequent stroke in the territory of the stenosed artery [45]. The risk of recurrent stroke in the territory of the symptomatic stenotic artery was the highest with stenosis ≥70% (hazard ratio 2.03; 95% confidence interval 1.29–3.22). The prognostic impact of stenosis severity had been previously shown for basilar artery stenosis in the WASID retrospective study, but not for other intracranial arteries [46]. Other investigators have found that the severity (>70%) of symptomatic ICAS is associated with early recurrent ischemic lesions on diffusion-weighted imaging [47]. Severe MCA stenoses often show a higher progression rate during TCD follow-up [48]. In the Chinese Intracranial Atherosclerosis (CICAS) Study, recurrence risk increased gradually with ICAS severity, being maximal in patients with complete intracranial atherothrombotic occlusions [49]. Finally, the medical arm of the SAMMPRIS study represents a unique opportunity to identify prognostic factors in patients with >70% symptomatic ICAS [50]. Among this very high-risk group, stenosis severity (>80%) was associated with a higher recurrence risk in the bivariate analysis. However, it was not an independent predictor when multivariate models were applied.

Location of the Symptomatic Intracranial Stenosis

No differences in recurrence risk were found according to the location of symptomatic ICAS in the WASID or SAMMPRIS studies, either considering each intracranial artery individually, or categorizing the involved vessels as the anterior or posterior circulation stenosis [45, 50]. In the CICAS study, posterior circulation stenoses were associated with a higher recurrence risk, only in the univariate analysis [49]. The presence of concomitant stenoses in the extracranial and intracranial portions of the same artery (tandem lesions) carries a higher recurrence risk [31].

Morphological Hallmarks of the Vulnerable ICAS Plaque

In extracranial arterial beds, it is accepted that plaque morphology provides information about its composition and vulnerability. Well recognized morphological hallmarks of plaque instability are: thin fibrous cap, irregular or ulcerated surface, presence of intraplaque hemorrhage, and rich lipid core, among others. However, how these concepts apply to ICAS remains still unclear, given the limited accessibility to the specimens of the diseased vessel.

The importance of vulnerable plaque may differ among different vascular trees; several histopathological studies have suggested that the relevance of the unstable atherosclerotic plaque might be greater in extracranial than in intracranial arteries [51, 52]. Nonetheless, plaques rich in inflammatory components have often been described in the intracranial vertebral and basilar arteries [53, 54], whereas they seem to occur less commonly in the MCA disease, where fibrous-stable plaques may predominate [55]. However, complicated plaques affecting the MCA showing rupture or intraplaque hemorrhage have also been reported [56].

In this context, HR-MRI may be a promising technique to examine characteristics of the intracranial atherosclerotic plaque that are associated with a higher recurrence risk [57, 58]. Some HR-MRI studies have already compared symptomatic versus asymptomatic MCA atherosclerotic plaques; symptomatic plaques seem to have a larger plaque area, positive remodeling, irregular surface and are more frequently located in the superior aspect of the arterial wall [59, 60]. However, it remains unclear whether these features predict the risk of recurrent strokes.

ICAS Plaque Activity

ICAS is a dynamic condition that often progresses over time. The risk of progression and clinical recurrence is determined by atherosclerotic plaque activity besides its morphology.

Indirect Evidence of ICAS Plaque Activity

Symptomatic vs. Asymptomatic Intracranial Stenosis. The risk of recurrent ischemic events appears to be much higher in patients with symptomatic than asymptomatic ICAS [26, 61, 62]. In patients with symptomatic ICAS, co-existent asymptomatic ICAS is frequently observed. The risk of future ischemic stroke caused by these asymptomatic lesions appears to be low [32]. Progression of stenosis in asymptomatic vessels is also much less frequent than that of symptomatic ones [63].

Old Infarct in the Territory of a Symptomatic Stenosis. This factor was identified as an independent predictor of the primary endpoint in the medical group in the SAMMPRIS trial [50]. The investigators interpret this finding as an indicator of unstable stenotic plaques or impaired collateral blood flow or both that put these patients at a high risk for further strokes in the territory.

Cortical Microinfarcts. The presence of cortical microinfarcts in 3T MRI was associated with ICAS in the CICAS cohort, and was significantly associated with a higher recurrence risk [64]. This novel prognostic factor may serve as an indirect marker of plaque instability and subsequent artery-to-artery microemboli.

Progression of Intracranial Stenosis. Two long-term follow-up studies using transcranial Doppler (TCD) showed that progression of symptomatic MCA stenosis was associated with a higher risk of further ischemic events, either related to the stenosed artery or not [65, 66]. Another longitudinal study showed a strong relationship between TCD-detected progression of ICAS and a higher risk of further brain ischemic events during follow-up [67].

Microembolic Signals (Transcranial Doppler). In patients with symptomatic MCA stenosis, detection of microembolic signals using TCD-monitoring within three days after onset of symptoms has been described as a predictor of future ischemic events in the stenotic MCA territory [68]. Moreover, a positive relationship has been found between the number of detected microembolic signals and the number of acute ischemic lesions visible on diffusion-weighted imaging [69]. These results suggest that microembolic signals detected during the acute phase of ischemic stroke might be considered an indirect sign of intracranial plaque instability. However, the presence of microembolic signals may imply a partial recanalization of an embolic occlusion rather than intrinsic atherosclerosis. Therefore thorough diagnostic work up may be required to rule out this possibility [70].

Direct Evidence of ICAS Plaque Activity

As mentioned above, there is a need to identify direct markers of ICAS plaque activity in vivo. Intracranial plaque post-contrast enhancement has been proposed as a marker of plaque activity [71], although the histopathological correlate of this HRMRI finding is still missing. Intracranial plaque enhancement has been recently shown to be associated with an increased stroke recurrence risk [72]. It remains to be elucidated whether the presence and intensity of plaque enhancement are really markers of plaque instability and degree of inflammatory activity.

Hemodynamic Factors

The hemodynamic impact caused by ICAS depends on the severity of lumen narrowing and on the capacity of collateral circulation to compensate distal blood flow reduction. Recent reports have consistently shown that poor collateral status as assessed by cerebral angiography determines ICAS prognosis [73]. From a clinical standpoint, patients with hemodynamic compromise affecting the territory of a stenosed artery characteristically report fluctuations in the intensity of the neurological deficits after changes in body position or with blood pressure drops. This clinical pattern may be present in around 15–20% of patients with symptomatic ICAS, who may have an extremely high risk of recurrent stroke [32].

Other ancillary examinations may allow noninvasive assessment of the hemodynamic impairment caused by a symptomatic ICAS. Fractional flow on MRA may identify hemodynamic compromise beyond the percent stenosis and has been reported to be associated with an increased stroke risk [74]. This parameter can be calculated using the distal/proximal signal intensity ratio, since the drop in signal intensity distal to the stenotic region is related to its hemodynamic impairment. Other methods include computational fluid dynamics models that can be reconstructed based on baseline computed tomographic angiography (CTA) source images. In patients with symptomatic 70–99% intracranial stenosis, the changes of shear strain rates and of velocities across the lesion were significantly related to recurrent territorial ischemic stroke within 1 year [75].

Systemic Factors (Vulnerable ICAS Patient)

Coexistent Vascular Disease

Extent and Severity of Cerebral Atherosclerosis

The number of diseased vessels within the cerebral arterial circulation has been shown to be associated with a higher risk of stroke recurrence and vascular death [31, 76]. Those patients with atherosclerotic stenoses affecting both extracranial and intracranial large arteries are exposed to a higher risk compared to patients with isolated ICAS. In the CICAS cohort, patients with stenosis affecting anterior and posterior circulation showed a higher recurrence risk. Nonetheless, other relevant studies failed to show an association between the number of ICAS and a higher risk of recurrent stroke [32]. Regarding disease progression, the number of ICAS is also associated with a higher risk of ICAS progression, as shown by TCD studies [67]. More recent studies have found an association between global cerebral atherosclerotic score (including extra and intracranial arteries) and the risk of MRA-defined progression of ICAS [77].

Coexistent Cerebral Small Vessel Disease

The prevalence of significant small vessel disease (defined by chronic lacunar infarctions and/or grade ≥2 white matter hyperintensities on MRI) in symptomatic ICAS patients was close to 50% in the SAMMPRIS study [78]. There are contradictory reports regarding the prognostic impact of coexistent small vessel disease in symptomatic ICAS. The Hong-Kong group identified the presence of small vessel disease as a predictor of stroke recurrence in patients with multiple ICAS [79], which, however, was not replicated in the study using SAMMPRIS cohort [78].

Intracranial Arterial Calcification

The degree of intracranial arterial calcification has been shown to predict stroke recurrence risk in stroke patients in general [80]. However, to our knowledge, the specific impact of intracranial arterial calcification on symptomatic ICAS prognosis has not been studied. Interestingly, the degree of intracranial arterial calcification on head CT has been shown to correlate with the severity of ICAS as defined by cerebral angiography [81].

Markers of Systemic Atherosclerosis: Low Ankle-Brachial Index

Ankle-brachial index (ABI) is considered a good indicator of the global extent of atherosclerosis. In the Vall d'Hebron cohort, ABI was systematically determined shortly after stroke in symptomatic ICAS patients, and 71% of them had pathologically low values, with severely low ABI (<0.8) being detected in 48% of the study patients. Patients with severely low ABI had a fourth fold increase in the risk of a recurrent major ischemic event [82].

Vascular Risk Factors

The role of vascular risk factors in the development of ICAS has been described in Chapter 4. Among the classical risk factors, diabetes mellitus and insulin resistance seem to play a preeminent role in ICAS. In European-Mediterranean patients, type 2 diabetes mellitus has been associated with a greater extent of ICAS, and consequently diabetic patients have a higher number of ICAS compared to non-diabetics [83]. Diabetes has also been found to be associated with a higher risk of recurrent stroke and vascular death among Asian symptomatic ICAS patients [31]. Post-hoc analysis of the WASID study identified poor risk factor control, in terms of elevated blood pressure and cholesterol levels, to be associated with an increased risk of stroke and other major vascular events in symptomatic ICAS patients [34]. In the SAMMPRIS study, intensive medical management may have succeeded in reducing stroke recurrence risk in part through improved vascular risk factor control. Regarding non-modifiable risk factors, age consistently appears as a predictor of recurrence risk [50].

Gender

Women with symptomatic ICAS appear to be at significantly greater risk for ischemic stroke and for the combined end point of stroke or vascular death in the WASID study [84]. The two-year rates of the primary end-point were 28.4 and

16.6% for women and men, respectively. In the medical arm of SAMMPRIS, female sex was also associated with a significantly higher risk for recurrent stroke, although this association was not apparent after multivariate adjustment [50].

Metabolic Syndrome
The relationship between the metabolic syndrome (MetS) and ICAS has been addressed [85]. Among ischemic stroke patients of Asian ancestry, the highest prevalence of MetS was observed in the subgroup of patients with ICAS (55%), even higher than the frequency of MetS observed in patients with extracranial carotid atherosclerosis (40%) [86]. Symptomatic ICAS patients with MetS had an excess risk of recurrent ischemic events in the WASID study [87] and in a study performed in China [88]. However, MetS was not predictive of stroke recurrence beyond its individual components. The relationship between insulin resistance and ICAS prognosis deserves further study.

Medical Treatment Prior to ICAS Related Ischemic Event
Failure of antithrombotic treatment (i.e. being on antiplatelets when an ICAS-related ischemic event occurs) was traditionally considered a poor prognostic factor [89]. However, prior antithrombotic therapy was not associated with an increased stroke recurrence risk in the medical arm of the WASID and SAMMPRIS studies [90, 91]. Regarding other treatments at study entry, absence of prior statin use emerged as an independent predictor of stroke recurrence in the SAMMPRIS medical arm.

Molecular Pathways
The following molecular pathways have been implicated in ICAS prognosis: inflammation, thrombosis & endogenous fibrinolysis, and angiogenesis. Given that blood biomarkers still represent our main methodological approach to assess ICAS pathophysiology non-invasively, the evidence about the role of these molecular pathways in determining ICAS progression and complication will be reviewed in the next paragraph (Biomarkers).

Genetic Factors
To our knowledge, research on genetics and ICAS has been mainly conducted in cross-sectional studies aiming to search for markers of ICAS vs. other stroke subtypes. The role of genetic polymorphisms on ICAS prognosis remains largely unknown.

Biomarkers and ICAS Prognosis

The ultimate aim of translational research is to provide applicable solutions to relevant clinical problems by means of a continuous crosstalk between clinical studies and basic research. In this context, blood biomarkers may have an increasing clinical applicability in the identification of high-risk ICAS patients and in monitoring the response to preventive therapies. Moreover, some of the biomarkers themselves could become therapeutic targets for preventive strategies. Finally, multimodal studies combining modern imaging methods and novel biomarker technology might be needed to clarify the role of the different molecular pathways in ICAS and its therapeutic potential.

Biomarkers in Asymptomatic ICAS
As reviewed previously, the presence of asymptomatic ICAS seems to confer a higher risk of developing stroke and other vascular events in Asian and Caucasian populations [25, 27, 28]. Therefore, subjects with asymptomatic ICAS may be considered in the future as a high-vascular risk population, similar to subjects with a high vascular risk score (Framingham), or to those with an increased intima-carotid thickness, presence of carotid plaque or high coronary calcium score. The Rotterdam study [27] raised the importance of calcification of intracranial carotid arteries in

the prediction of incident stroke. However, intracranial internal carotid artery calcification was identified in a large proportion (82%) of asymptomatic individuals, so it would not be a good screening tool to define a high-risk population. We do know that asymptomatic subjects with a large burden of vascular risk factors and a high number of metabolic syndrome components are at risk of having asymptomatic ICAS [18–21]. Similarly, in APAC study, those asymptomatic subjects that accomplished more ideal cardiovascular health metrics (nonsmoking, normal weight, physical activity at goal levels, and a healthy diet) were found to have less prevalence of ICAS [92]. Finally, evaluation of brachial-arm index has been proposed as a useful non-invasive tool in the screening of extra and intracranial large artery stenosis, especially in subjects at intermediate vascular risk [93].

Regarding circulating biomarkers involved in atherogenesis, some have been found to be associated with asymptomatic ICAS such as asymmetric-dimethylarginine (ADMA) [20], resistin [20] and Lipoprotein-associated phospholipase A2 (Lp-PLA2) [94]. Insulin resistance as measured by HOMA index has also been associated with the presence and severity of asymptomatic ICAS [20]. However, the role of these biomarkers in the progression and complication of asymptomatic ICAS has not yet been elucidated in order to be incorporated in the risk score of a single individual.

Biomarkers in Symptomatic ICAS

Inflammation

One of the crucial clinical problems that remains to be clarified is whether the inflammatory activity of the atherosclerotic plaque is a crucial contributor to the risk of clinical events in ICAS [13]. The relationship between inflammation and atherosclerosis might have to be considered from both local and systemic perspectives [95]. Locally, inflammatory infiltration within the atherosclerotic lesion renders the plaque more prone to rupture and to develop thrombotic complications. Systemically, persisting chronic inflammation is characterized by excessive circulating inflammatory cells and proinflammatory cytokines. Circulating monocytes can be recruited inside the evolving atherosclerotic lesion via adhesion molecules expressed on the dysfunctional endothelium, and then enter the plaque thereby kindling inflammatory reactions. Moreover, circulating inflammatory cytokines originating from different sources may exert their effects on the endothelium rendering it more proinflammatory and prothrombotic. In this context, inflammatory blood biomarkers may represent a valuable tool to assess the interplay between systemic and local inflammation. While the overexpression of some inflammatory mediators, such as interleukine-6 (IL-6) and C-reactive protein (CRP), may inform us about the existence of an ongoing chronic systemic inflammation [96], other inflammatory molecules, such as Lipoprotein associated phospholipase A2 (LpPLA2), are released to blood stream from the inflammatory cells that reside inside the atherosclerotic lesion, thus reflecting the plaque's intrinsic inflammatory activity [97].

Table 2 summarizes relevant studies examining the capacity of several inflammatory blood biomarkers to predict ICAS progression [67, 98] and the risk of recurrent stroke and other vascular events in symptomatic ICAS patients [99–102]. Baseline CRP [67] and IL-6 [98] level, in Caucasian and Asian symptomatic ICAS patients respectively, predicted ICAS progression in long-term follow-up studies. Regarding the risk of clinical recurrence, biomarkers of systemic inflammation, such as CRP and leukocyte count, were also found to predict further ischemic strokes and other major vascular events in symptomatic ICAS patients [99, 100, 102]. Taken together, these findings suggest that systemic inflammation may promote the progression and complication of ICAS. Besides these markers of systemic inflammation, other molecules that are

Table 2. Inflammatory biomarkers and ICAS prognosis

Reference	Study design	n	Main findings
Arenillas et al. [99], 2003	Single center, longitudinal, observational	71 consecutive symptomatic ICAS	High CRP as a predictor of further ICAS-related ischemic events and other vascular events
Ovbiagele et al. [100], 2007	Multicentric randomized clinical trial (WASID)	WASID sample symptomatic ICAS patients	Elevated WBC count at entry predicted increased risk of stroke and vascular death
Arenillas et al. [65], 2001	Single center, longitudinal, observational	75 consecutive symptomatic ICAS	CRP and PAI-1 as predictors of ICAS progression
Massot et al. [101], 2011	Single center, longitudinal, observational	75 consecutive symptomatic ICAS	LpPLA2 activity as a predictor of further vascular events Same series: CRP, E-selectin and PAI-1 as predictors of new ischemic stroke (unpublished)
Shimizu et al. [98], 2013	Single center, longitudinal, observational, MRA	48 AIS biomarkers <48 h onset	Baseline IL-6 level predicted MRA-assessed ICAS progression
Frankel et al. [102], 2014	Multicentric randomized clinical trial (SAMMPRIS) BIOSIS study	SAMMPRIS medical treatment arm; 227 symptomatic ICAS	LpPLA2 predictor of ICAS-related ischemic stroke, any ischemic stroke and stroke and vascular death E-Selectin and CRP predictors of any ischemic stroke and stroke and vascular death

CRP = C-reactive protein; ICAS = intracranial atherosclerosis; WBC = white blood cell; PAI-1 = plasminogen activator inhibitor-1; LpPLA2 = lipoprotein-associated phospholipase A2; IL-6 = interleukin-6; MRA = magnetic resonance angiography.

more informative about the local inflammatory activity within the atherosclerotic plaque, such as adhesion molecules and LpPLA2, have also been evaluated in these longitudinal studies [101, 102]. In this context, the most relevant findings derive from the BIOSIS study, a biomarker study affiliated with the SAMMPRIS clinical trial [102]. Interestingly, LpPLA2 level at study entry predicted further ischemic strokes within the symptomatic ICAS territory, as well as any major ischemic event during follow-up. This observation supports the hypothesis that local inflammation inside the ICAS plaque may determine its vulnerability.

Prothrombotic State and Impaired Endogenous Fibrinolysis

Thrombosis and defective endogenous fibrinolysis may also contribute to progression of atherosclerotic lesions systemically. Their potentially deleterious role on ICAS has been suggested by several biomarker studies. First, an elevated circulating level of Lp(a), an atherothrombogenic cholesterol rich lipoprotein that inhibits endothelial surface fibrinolysis by competing with plasminogen binding, was independently associated with a greater extent of ICAS [83]. Second, a positive correlation between homocysteine concentration and the number of ICAS has been reported. Homocysteine is known to exert prothrombotic effects on endothelial surface [103]. Third, a high level of plasminogen activator inhibitor-1 (PAI-1) emerged as a powerful predictor of the risk of ICAS progression [67] and stroke recurrence [82]. In this setting, an increased PAI-1 expression in atherosclerotic vessels may cause an impaired fibrinolytic response to mural thrombi, leading to a greater extent and persistence of thrombi in the arterial lumen. However, the BIOSIS study failed to demonstrate an association between PAI-1 level and the risk of recurrence ischemic stroke and vascular death [102].

Inhibited Endogenous Angiogenic Response
Angiogenesis is a complex and finely regulated process triggered by hypoxia that consists in the sprouting of new blood vessels from pre-existing vascular structures [104]. The endogenous angiogenic response to ischemia is the result of a complex balance between stimulants and inhibitors that interact in an orchestrated manner. A high circulating level of the angiogenesis inhibitor endostatin was independently associated with a higher recurrence risk and a higher progression rate of ICAS [105]. Endostatin impairs re-endothelization processes leading to plaque growth through excessive neointima formation. Researches are needed to evaluate whether the stimulation of angiogenesis may be a therapeutic alternative for patients with progressive ICAS.

References

1 Arenillas JF: Intracranial atherosclerosis: current concepts. Stroke 2011; 42(1 suppl):S20–S23.
2 Wong KS, Huang YN, Gao S, Lam WWM, Chan YL, Kay R: Intracranial stenosis in Chinese patients with acute stroke. Neurology 1998;50:812–813.
3 Kim JT, Yoo SH, Kwon JH, Kwon SU, Kim JS: Subtyping of ischemic stroke based on vascular imaging: analysis of 1167 acute, consecutive patients. J Clin Neurol 2006;2:225–230.
4 Sacco R, Kargman DE, Quiong Gu, Zamanillo MC: Race-ethnicity and determinants of intracranial atherosclerotic cerebral infarction: the Northern Manhattan Stroke Study. Stroke 1995;26:14–20.
5 Gorelick PB, Wong KS, Bae HJ, Pandey DK: Large artery intracranial occlusive disease: a large worldwide burden but a relatively neglected frontier. Stroke 2008;39:2396–2399.
6 Ross R: Atherosclerosis-an inflammatory disease. N Engl J Med 1999;340: 115–126.
7 Kiechl S, Willeit J: The natural course of atherosclerosis. Part I: incidence and progression. Arterioscler Thromb Vasc Biol 1999;19:1484–1490.
8 D'Armiento FP, Bianchi A, de Nigris F, et al: Age-related effects on atherogenesis and scavenger enzymes of intracranial and extracranial arteries in men without classic risk factors for atherosclerosis. Stroke 2001;32:2472–2479.
9 Ritz K, Denswil NP, Stam OC, van Lieshout JJ, Daemen MJ: Cause and mechanisms of intracranial atherosclerosis. Circulation 2014;130:1407–1414.
10 Wang A, Li Z, Luo Y, Liu X, Guo X, Wu S, Zhao X, Jonas JB: Asymptomatic Polyvascular Abnormalities in Community (APAC) Study in China: objectives, Design and Baseline Characteristics. PLoS One 2014;9:e113205.
11 Lopez-Cancio E, Dorado L, Millan M, Reverte S, Sunol A, Massuet A, et al: The population-based Barcelona-Asymptomatic Intracranial Atherosclerosis Study (ASIA): rationale and design. BMC Neurol 2011;11:22.
12 Chimowitz MI, Lynn MJ, Derdeyn CP, Turan TN, Fiorella D, Lane BF, Janis LS, Lutsep HL, Barnwell SL, Waters MF, Hoh BL, Hourihane JM, Levy EI, Alexandrov AV, Harrigan MR, Chiu D, Klucznik RP, Clark JM, McDougall CG, Johnson MD, Pride GL Jr, Torbey MT, Zaidat OO, Rumboldt Z, Cloft HJ; SAMMPRIS Trial Investigators. Stenting versus aggressive medical therapy for intracranial arterial stenosis. N Engl J Med 2011;365: 993–1003.
13 Arenillas JF: Intracranial atherosclerosis and in ammation: lessons from the East and the West. Brain Circ 2015;1:47–52.
14 Qureshi AI, Caplan LR: Intracranial atherosclerosis. Lancet 2014;383:984–998.
15 Huang HW, Guo MH, Lin RJ, et al: Prevalence and risk factors of middle cerebral artery stenosis in asymptomatic residents in Rongqi County, Guangdong. Cerebrovasc Dis 2007;24:111–115.
16 Wong KS, Ng PW, Tang A, Liu R, Yeung V, Tomlinson B: Prevalence of asymptomatic intracranial atherosclerosis in high-risk patients. Neurology 2007;68: 2035–2038.
17 Bae HJ, Lee J, Park JM, Kwon O, Koo JS, Kim BK, et al: Risk factors of intracranial cerebral atherosclerosis among asymptomatics. Cerebrovasc Dis 2007;24: 355–360.
18 Lopez-Cancio E, Dorado L, Millan M, Reverte S, Sunol A, Massuet A, et al: The Barcelona-Asymptomatic Intracranial Atherosclerosis (AsIA) study: prevalence and risk factors. Atherosclerosis 2012;221:221–225.
19 Zhang Y, Wu S, Jia Z, Zhou Y, Liu X, Wang W, Wang T, Wang L, Zhang S, Jin C, ZhaoX: The relationship of asymptomatic intracranial artery stenosis and Fr mingham stroke risk profile in a Northern Chinese industrial city. Neurol Res 2012;34:359–365.
20 López-Cancio E, Galán A, Dorado L, Jiménez M, Hernández M, Millán M, Reverté S, Suñol A, Barallat J, Massuet A, Alzamora MT, Dávalos A, Arenillas JF: Biological signatures of asymptomatic extra- and intracranial atherosclerosis: the Barcelona-AsIA (Asymptomatic Intracranial Atherosclerosis) study. Stroke 2012;43:2712–2719.
21 Wang A, Li Z, Luo Y, Liu X, Guo X, Wu S, Zhao X, Jonas JB: Asymptomatic intracranial arterial stenosis and metabolic syndrome: the APAC study. PLoS One 2014;9:e113205.
22 Meseguer E, Lavallee PC, Mazighi M, Labreuche J, Cabrejo L, Olivot JM, Abboud H, Slaoui T, Lapergue B, Guidoux C, Klein IF, Touboul PJ, Amarenco P: Yield of systematic transcranial Doppler in patients with transient ischemic attack. Ann Neurol 2010;68:9–17.

23 Homburg PJ, Plas GJ, Rozie S, van der Lugt A, Dippel DW: Prevalence and calcification of intracranial arterial stenotic lesions as assessed with multidetector computed tomography angiography. Stroke 2011;42:1244–1250.
24 Ovesen C, Abild A, Christensen AF, Rosenbaum S, Hansen CK, Havsteen I, Nielsen JK, Christensen H: Prevalence and long-term clinical significance of intracranial atherosclerosis after ischaemic stroke or transient ischaemic attack: a cohort study. BMJ Open 2013;3: e003724.
25 Duan JG, Chen XY, Lau A, Wong A, Thomas GN, Tomlinson B, Liu R, Chan JC, Leung TW, Mok V, Wong KS: Long-term risk of cardiovascular disease among type 2 diabetic patients with asymptomatic intracranial atherosclerosis: a prospective cohort study. PLoS One 2014;9:e10662.
26 Takahashi W, Ohnuki T, Ide M, Takagi S, Shinohara Y: Stroke risk of asymptomatic intra- and extracranial large-artery disease in apparently healthy adults. Cerebrovasc Dis 2006;22:263–270.
27 Bos D, van der Rijk MJ, Geeraedts TE, et al: Intracranial carotid artery atherosclerosis: prevalence and risk factors in the general population. Stroke 2012;43: 1878–1884.
28 Hennerici MG: ESC Abstract Awards: Highlights from the 23rd European Stroke Conference, Nice, May 6–9, 2014. Cerebrovasc Dis 2014;38:127–160.
29 Beach TG, Wilson JR, Sue LI, Newell A, Poston M, Cisneros R, Pandya Y, Esh C, Connor DJ, Sabbagh M, Walker DG, Roher AE: Circle of Willis atherosclerosis: association with Alzheimer's disease, neuritic plaques and neurofibrillary tangles. Acta Neuropathol 2007;113:13–21.
30 Zhu J, Wang Y, Li J, Deng J, Zhou H: Intracranial artery stenosis and progression from mild cognitive impairment to Alzheimer disease. Neurology 2014;82: 842–849.
31 Wong KS, Li H: Long-term mortality and recurrent stroke risk among Chinese stroke patients with predominant intracranial atherosclerosis. Stroke 2003;34:2361–2366.
32 Mazighi M, Tanasescu R, Ducrocq X, et al: Prospective study of symptomatic atherothrombotic intracranial stenoses: the GESICA study. Neurology 2006;66: 1187–1191.
33 Chimowitz MI, Lynn MJ, Howlett-Smith H, et al: Warfarin-Aspirin Symptomatic Intracranial Disease Trial Investigators. Comparison of warfarin and aspirin for symptomatic intracranial arterial stenosis. N Engl J Med 2005;352:1305–1316.
34 Chaturvedi S, Turan TN, Lynn MJ, et al; for WASID Study Group: Risk factor status and vascular events in patients with symptomatic intracranial stenosis. Neurology 2007;69:2063–2068.
35 Chimowitz MI, Lynn MJ, Derdeyn CP, et al: Stenting versus aggressive medical therapy for intracranial arterial stenosis. New Engl J Med 2011;365:993–1003.
36 Chaturvedi S, Turan TN, Lynn MJ, Derdeyn CP, Fiorella D, Janis LS, Chimowitz MI; SAMMPRIS Trial Investigators. Do patient characteristics explain the differences in outcome between medically treated patients in SAMMPRIS and WASID? Stroke 2015; 46:2562–2567.
37 Turan TN, Lynn MJ, Nizam A, Lane B, Egan BM, Le NA, Lopes-Virella MF, Hermayer KL, Benavente O, White CL, Brown WV, Caskey MF, Steiner MR, Vilardo N, Stufflebean A, Derdeyn CP, Fiorella D, Janis S, Chimowitz MI: Rationale, design, and implementation of aggressive risk factor management in the stenting and aggressive medical management for prevention of recurrent stroke in intracranial stenosis (SAMMPRIS) trial. Circulation Cardiovascular quality and outcomes. 2012;5:e51–e60.
38 Marquardt L, Geraghty OC, Mehta Z, Rothwell PM: Low risk of ipsilateral stroke in patients with asymptomatic carotid stenosis on best medical treatment: a prospective, population-based study. Stroke 2010;41:e11–e17.
39 Craig DR, Meguro K, Watridge C, Robertson JT, Barnett HJM, Fox AJ: Intracranial internal carotid artery stenosis. Stroke 1982;13:825–828.
40 Marzewski DJ, Furlan AJ, St. Louis P, Little JR, Modic MT, Williams G: Intracranial internal carotid artery stenosis: long term prognosis. Stroke 1982;13: 821–824.
41 Wechsler LR, Kistler JP, Davis KR, Kaminski MJ: The prognosis of carotid siphon stenosis. Stroke 1986;17:714–718.
42 Arenillas JF, Candell-Riera J, Romero-Farina G, et al: Silent myocardial ischemia in patients with symptomatic intracranial atherosclerosis: associated factors. Stroke 2005;36:1201–1206.
43 Naghavi M, Libby P, Falk E, et al: From vulnerable plaque to vulnerable patient: a call for new definitions and risk assessment strategies: Part I. Circulation 2003;108:1664–1672.
44 Naghavi M, Libby P, Falk E, et al: From vulnerable plaque to vulnerable patient: a call for new definitions and risk assessment strategies: Part II. Circulation 2003;108:1772–1778.
45 Kasner SE, Chimowitz MI, Lynn MJ, et al; Warfarin Aspirin Symptomatic Intracranial Disease Trial Investigators. Predictors of ischemic stroke in the territory of a symptomatic intracranial arterial stenosis. Circulation 2006;113: 555–563.
46 The Warfarin-Aspirin Symptomatic Intracranial Disease (WASID) Study Group. Prognosis of patients with symptomatic vertebral or basilar artery stenosis. Stroke 1998;29:1389–1392.
47 Kang DW, Kwon SU, Yoo SH, et al: Early recurrent ischemic lesions on diffusion-weighted imaging in symptomatic intracranial atherosclerosis. Arch Neurol 2007;64:50–54.
48 Jeon HW, Cha JK: Factors related to progression of middle cerebral artery stenosis determined using transcranial Doppler ultrasonograhy. J Thromb Thrombolysis 2008;25:265–269.
49 Wang Y, Zhao X, Liu L, Soo YO, Pu Y, Pan Y, Wang Y, Zou X, Leung TW, Cai Y, Bai Q, Wu Y, Wang C, Pan X, Luo B, Wong KS; CICAS Study Group. Prevalence and outcomes of symptomatic intracranial large artery stenoses and occlusions in China: the Chinese Intracranial Atherosclerosis (CICAS) Study. Stroke 2014;45:663–669.
50 Waters MF, Hoh BL, Lynn MJ, Kwon HM, Turan TN, Derdeyn CP, Fiorella D, Khanna A, Sheehan TO, Lane BF, Janis S, Montgomery J, Chimowitz MI; Stenting and Aggressive Medical Management for Preventing Recurrent Stroke in Intracranial Stenosis (SAMMPRIS) Trial Investigators. Factors Associated With Recurrent Ischemic Stroke in the Medical Group of the SAMMPRIS Trial. JAMA Neurol 2016:1–8. [Epub ahead of print].
51 Lammie GA, Sandercock PAG, Dennis MS. Recently occluded intracranial and extracranial carotid arteries. Relevance of the unstable atherosclerotic plaque. Stroke 1999;30:1319–1325.

52 Lhermitte F, Gautier JC, Derouesne C, Guiraud B: Ischemic accidents in the middle cerebral artery territory: a study of causes in 122 cases. Arch Neurol 1968;19:248–256.
53 Castaigne P, Lhermitte F, Gautier JC, et al: Arterial occlusions in the vertebro-basilar system. A study of 44 patients with post-mortem data. Brain 1973;96: 133–154.
54 Caplan L: Posterior circulation ischemia: then, now, and tomorrow. The Thomas Willis Lecture-2000. Stroke 2000;31: 2011–2023.
55 Schumacher HC, Tanji K, Mangla S, et al: Histopathological evaluation of middle cerebral artery after percutaneous intracranial transluminal angioplasty. Stroke 2003;34:170–173.
56 Ogata J, Masuda J, Yutani C, Yamaguchi T: Mechanisms of cerebral artery thrombosis: a histopathological analysis on eight necropsy cases. J Neurol Neurosurg Psychiatry 1994;57:17–21.
57 Bodle JD, Feldmann E, Swartz RH, Rumboldt Z, Brown T, Turan TN: High-resolution magnetic resonance imaging: an emerging tool for evaluating intracranial arterial disease. Stroke 2013;44: 287–292.
58 Turan TN, LeMatty T, Martin R, Chimowitz MI, Rumboldt Z, Spampinato MV, Stalcup S, Adams RJ, Brown T: Characterization of intracranial atherosclerotic stenosis using high-resolution MRI study – rationale and design. Brain Behav 2015;5:e00397.
59 Zhao DL, Deng G, Xie B, Ju S, Yang M, Chen XH, Teng GJ: High-resolution MRI of the vessel wall in patients with symptomatic atherosclerotic stenosis of the middle cerebral artery. J Clin Neurosci 2015;22:700–704.
60 Xu WH, Li ML, Gao S, Ni J, Zhou LX, Yao M, Peng B, Feng F, Jin ZY, Cui LY: In vivo high-resolution MR imaging of symptomatic and asymptomatic middle cerebral artery atherosclerotic stenosis. Atherosclerosis 2010;212:507–511.
61 Kern R, Steinke W, Daffertshofer M, Prager R, Hennerici M: Stroke recurrences in patients with symptomatic vs asymptomatic middle cerebral artery disease. Neurology 2005;65:859–864.
62 Kremer C, Schaettin T, Georgiadis D, Baumgartner RW: Prognosis of asymptomatic stenosis of the middle cerebral artery. J Neurol Neurosurg Psychiatry 2004;75:1300–1303.
63 Kwon SU, Cho YJ, Koo JS, et al: Cilostazol prevents the progression of the symptomatic intracranial arterial stenosis: the multicenter double-blind placebo-controlled trial of cilostazol in symptomatic intracranial arterial stenosis. Stroke 2005;36:782–786.
64 Fu R, Wang Y, Wang Y, Liu L, Zhao X, Wang DZ, Pan Y, Pu Y, Zhang C; Chinese IntraCranial AtheroSclerosis (CICAS) Study Group: The Development of Cortical Microinfarcts Is Associated with Intracranial Atherosclerosis: Data from the Chinese Intracranial Atherosclerosis Study. J Stroke Cerebrovasc Dis 2015;24:2447–2454.
65 Arenillas JF, Molina CA, Montaner J, Abilleira S, González-Sánchez MA, Álvarez-Sabín J: Progression and clinical recurrence of symptomatic middle cerebral artery stenosis. A long-term follow-up transcranial Doppler ultrasound study. Stroke 2001;32:2898–2904.
66 Wong KS, Li H, Lam WWM, Chan YL, Kay R: Progression of middle cerebral artery occlusive disease and its relationship with further vascular events after stroke. Stroke 2002;33:532–536.
67 Arenillas JF, Alvarez-Sabín J, Molina CA, Chacón P, Fernández-Cadenas I, Ribó M, Delgado P, Rubiera M, Penalba A, Rovira A, Montaner J: Progression of symptomatic intracranial large artery atherosclerosis is associated with a proinflammatory state and impaired fibrinolysis. Stroke 2008;39:1456–1463.
68 Gao S, Wong KS, Hansberg T, Lam WWM, Droste DW, Ringelstein EB: Microembolic signal predicts recurrent cerebral ischemic events in acute stroke patients with middle cerebral artery stenosis. Stroke 2004;35:2832–2836.
69 Wong KS, Gao S, Chan YL, et al: Mechanisms of acute cerebral infarctions in patients with middle cerebral artery stenosis: a diffusion-weighted imaging and microemboli monitoring study. Ann Neurol 2002;52:74–81.
70 Segura T, Serena J, Castellanos M, Teruel J, Vilar C, Dávalos A: Embolism in acute middle cerebral artery stenosis. Neurology 2001;56:497–501.
71 Vergouwen MD, Silver FL, Mandell DM, Mikulis DJ, Swartz RH: Eccentric narrowing and enhancement of symptomatic middle cerebral artery stenoses in patients with recent ischemic stroke. Arch Neurol 2011;68:338–342.
72 Kim JM, Jung KH, Sohn CH, Moon J, Shin JH, Park J, Lee SH, Hee Han M, Roh JK: Intracranial plaque enhancement from high resolution vessel wall magnetic resonance imaging predicts stroke recurrence. Int J Stroke 2016;11: 171–179.
73 Liebeskind DS, Cotsonis GA, Saver JL, Lynn MJ, Turan TN, Cloft HJ, Chimowitz MI; Warfarin-Aspirin Symptomatic Intracranial Disease (WASID) Investigators. Collaterals dramatically alter stroke risk in intracranial atherosclerosis. Ann Neurol 2011;69:963–974.
74 Liebeskind DS, Kosinski AS, Lynn MJ, Scalzo F, Fong AK, Fariborz P, Chimowitz MI, Feldmann E: Noninvasive fractional flow on MRA predicts stroke risk of intracranial stenosis. J Neuroimaging 2015;25:87–91.
75 Leng X, Scalzo F, Ip HL, Johnson M, Fong AK, Fan FS, Chen X, Soo YO, Miao Z, Liu L, Feldmann E, Leung TW, Liebeskind DS, Wong KS: Computational fluid dynamics modeling of symptomatic intracranial atherosclerosis may predict risk of stroke recurrence. PLoS One 2014;9:e97531.
76 Asil T, Balci K, Uzunca I, Kerimoglu M, Utku U: Six-month follow-up study in patients with symptomatic intracranial arterial stenosis. J Clin Neurosci 2006; 13:913–916.
77 Mizukami H, Shimizu T, Maki F, Shiraishi M, Hasegawa Y: Progression of intracranial major artery stenosis is associated with baseline carotid and intracranial atherosclerosis. J Atheroscler Thromb 2015;22:183–190.
78 Kwon HM, Lynn MJ, Turan TN, Derdeyn CP, Fiorella D, Lane BF, Montgomery J, Janis LS, Rumboldt Z, Chimowitz MI; SAMMPRIS Investigators. Frequency, Risk Factors, and Outcome of Coexistent Small Vessel Disease and Intracranial Arterial Stenosis: Results From the Stenting and Aggressive Medical Management for Preventing Recurrent Stroke in Intracranial Stenosis (SAMMPRIS) Trial. JAMA Neurol 2016; 73:36–42.
79 Fu JH, Chen YK, Chen XY, Mok V, Wong KS: Coexisting small vessel disease predicts poor long-term outcome in stroke patients with intracranial large artery atherosclerosis. Cerebrovasc Dis 2010;30:433–439.

80 Lee JG, Lee KB, Roh H, Ahn MY, Bae HJ, Lee JS, Woo HY, Hwang HW: Intracranial arterial calcification can predict early vascular events after acute ischemic stroke. J Stroke Cerebrovasc Dis 2014;23:e331–e337.
81 Kassab MY, Gupta R, Majid A, Farooq MU, Giles BP, Johnson MD, Graybeal DF, Rappard G: Extent of intra-arterial calcification on head CT is predictive of the degree of intracranial atherosclerosis on digital subtraction angiography. Cerebrovasc Dis 2009;28:45–48.
82 Massot A, Giralt D, Penalba A, Garcia-Berrocoso T, Navarro-Sobrino M, Arenillas JF, Ribó M, Molina CA, Alvarez-Sabín J, Montaner J, Delgado P: Predictive value of ankle-brachial index and PAI-1 in symptomatic intracranial atherosclerotic disease recurrence. Atherosclerosis 2014;233:186–189.
83 Arenillas JF, Molina CA, Chacón P, et al: High lipoprotein (a), diabetes and the extent of symptomatic intracranial atherosclerosis. Neurology 2004;63:27–32.
84 Williams JE, Chimowitz MI, Cotsonis GA, Lynn MJ, Waddy SP: Gender differences in outcomes among patients with symptomatic intracranial arterial stenosis. Stroke 2007;38:2055–2062.
85 Bang OY, Kim JW, Lee JH, et al: Association of the metabolic syndrome with intracranial atherosclerotic stroke. Neurology 2005;65:296–298.
86 Park JH, Kwon HM, Roh JK: Metabolic syndrome is more associated with intracranial atherosclerosis tran extracranial atherosclerosis. Eur J Neurol 2007;14: 379–386.
87 Obviagele B, Saver JL, Lynn MJ, Chimowitz M, for the WASID Study Group. Impact of metabolic syndrome on prognosis of symptomatic intracranial atherostenosis. Neurology 2006;66:1344–1349.
88 Mi D, Zhang L, Wang C, Liu L, Pu Y, Zhao X, Wang Y, Wang Y: Impact of metabolic syndrome on the prognosis of ischemic stroke secondary to symptomatic intracranial atherosclerosis in Chinese patients. PLoS One 2012; 7:e51421.
89 Thijs VN, Albers GW: Symptomatic intracranial atherosclerosis: outcome of patients who fail antithrombotic therapy. Neurology 2000;55:490–497.
90 Turan TN, Maidan L, Cotsonis G, Lynn MJ, Romano JG, Levine SR, et al; Warfarin-Aspirin Symptomatic Intracranial Disease Investigators. Failure of antithrombotic therapy and risk of stroke in patients with symptomatic intracranial stenosis. Stroke 2009;40:505–509.
91 Lutsep HL, Barnwell SL, Larsen DT, Lynn MJ, Hong M, Turan TN, Derdeyn CP, Fiorella D, Janis LS, Chimowitz MI, for the SAMMPRIS Investigators. Outcome in Patients Previously on Antithrombotic Therapy in the SAMMPRIS Trial. Stroke 2015;46:775–779.
92 Zhang Q , Zhang S, Wang C, Gao X, Zhou Y, Zhou H, Wang A, Wu J, Bian L, Wu S, Zhao X: Ideal cardiovascular health metrics on the prevalence of asymptomatic intracranial artery stenosis: a cross-sectional study. PLoS One 2013; 8:e58923.
93 Jiménez M, Dorado L, Hernández-Pérez M, Alzamora MT, Pera G , Torán P, Gomis M, Pérez de la Ossa N, Millán M, Escudero D, Dávalos A, Arenillas JF, López-Cancio E: Ankle-brachial index in screening for asymptomatic carotid and intracranial atherosclerosis. Atherosclerosis 2014;233:72–75.
94 Wang Y, Zhang J, Qian Y, Tang X, Ling H, Chen K, Gao P, Zhu D: Association of Lp-PLA2 Mass and Aysmptomatic Intracranial and Extracranial Arterial Stenosis in Hypertension Patients. PLoS One 2015;10:e0130473.
95 Libby P. Inflammation in atherosclerosis. Arterioscler Thromb Vasc Biol 2012; 32:2045–2051.
96 Ridker PM, Cannon CP, Morrow D, Rifai N, Rose LM, McCabe CH, Pfeffer MA, Braunwald E: C-reactive protein levels and outcomes after statin therapy. N Engl J Med 2005;352:20–28.
97 Virani SS, Nambi V: The role of lipoprotein-associated phospholipase A2 as a marker for atherosclerosis. Curr Atheroscler Rep 2007;9:97–103.
98 Shimizu K, Shimomura K, Tokuyama Y, Sakurai K, Isahaya K, Takaishi S, Kato B, Usuki N, Shimizu T, Yamada K, Hasegawa Y: Association between inflammatory biomarkers and progression of intracranial large artery stenosis after ischemic stroke. J Stroke Cerebrovasc Dis 2013;22:211–217.
99 Arenillas JF, Alvarez-Sabín J, Molina CA, Chacón P, Montaner J, Rovira A, Ibarra B, Quintana M: C-reactive protein predicts further ischemic events in first-ever transient ischemic attack or stroke patients with intracranial large-artery occlusive disease. Stroke 2003; 34:2463–2468.
100 Ovbiagele B, Lynn MJ, Saver JL, Chimowitz MI; WASID Study Group. Leukocyte count and vascular risk in symptomatic intracranial atherosclerosis. Cerebrovasc Dis 2007;24:283–288.
101 Massot A, Pelegri D, Penalba A, Arenillas J, Boada C, Giralt D, Ribó M, Molina CA, Rosell A, Alvarez-Sabín J, Chacón P, Rovira A, Delgado P, Montaner J: Lipoprotein-associated phospholipase A2 testing usefulness among patients with symptomatic intracranial atherosclerotic disease. Atherosclerosis 2011;218:181–187.
102 Frankel M, Quyyumi A, Zhao Y, Long Q, Ngoc-Anh L, Waller EK, Arenillas JF, Lane B, Chimowitz M, BIOSIS and SAMMPRIS investigators. Biomarkers of ischemic outcomes in symptomatic intracranial stenosis (BIOSIS) – preliminary results. Stroke 2014; 45:ATMP33.
103 Yoo JH, Chung CS, Kang SS: Relation of plasma homocyst(e)ine to cerebral infarction and cerebral atherosclerosis. Stroke 1998;29:2478–2483.
104 Marti H, Risau W: Angiogenesis in ischemic disease. Thromb Haemost 1999;82:44–52.
105 Arenillas JF, Álvarez-Sabín J, Montaner J, et al: Angiogenesis in symptomatic intracranial atherosclerosis: predominance of the inhibitor endostatin is related to a higher extent and risk of recurrence. Stroke 2005;36:92–97.

Juan F. Arenillas, MD, PhD
Department of Neurology, Hospital Clínico Universitario
University of Valladolid
Ramon y Cajal 3, 47003 Valladolid (Spain)
E-Mail jfarenillas@saludcastillayleon.es

Kim JS, Caplan LR, Wong KS (eds): Intracranial Atherosclerosis: Pathophysiology, Diagnosis and Treatment.
Front Neurol Neurosci. Basel, Karger, 2016, vol 40, pp 109–123 (DOI: 10.1159/000448308)

Vessel and Vessel Wall Imaging

Seung Chai Jung[a] · Dong-Wha Kang[b] · Tanya N. Turan[c]

[a]Department of Radiology and Research Institute of Radiology, and [b]Department of Neurology, University of Ulsan College of Medicine, Asan Medical Center, Seoul, Korea; [c]Department of Neurology, Medical University of South Carolina, Charleston, S.C., USA

Abstract

Angiography is a useful, important, common imaging method, with digital subtraction angiography (DSA) remaining the gold standard for luminal imaging. Computed tomography angiography (CTA) is minimally invasive and quite accurate in the evaluation of stenosis. Magnetic resonance angiography (MRA) is a good screening tool with the least invasiveness. Angiography mostly represents intracranial artery disease as luminal stenosis, which is often not sufficient to evaluate intracranial vascular pathology. The modalities provide indirect information about vascular pathology because luminal change, such as stenosis, results from the changes of vessel walls. Vessel wall imaging using high-resolution magnetic resonance imaging (HR-MRI) has been recently introduced for direct evaluation of vessel walls beyond just luminal information such as the severity of stenosis. HR-MRI for vessel walls can present the characteristic radiological findings for each intracranial artery disease such as atherosclerosis, dissection, moyamoya disease, and vasculitis. The radiological features are useful to differentiate among intracranial artery disease. This chapter discusses the role and radiological features of angiography and HR-MRI for vessel walls.

Luminal evaluation is the most common and traditional imaging method for intracranial artery diseases and focuses on the degree of stenosis. Digital subtraction angiography (DSA), computed tomography angiography (CTA), and magnetic resonance angiography (MRA) are representative modalities. DSA is the oldest modality [1] and serves as a reference standard, providing excellent resolution and hemodynamic information. DSA is limited by the radiation hazard, invasiveness, and the risk of stroke or fatal complications [2, 3]. CTA is a minimally invasive modality performed with the intravenous injection of iodinated contrast media. Benefits of CTA include short scan times and less imaging distortion and high diagnostic performance [4, 5], but CTA also involves radiation risks. MRA is a minimally invasive or noninvasive modality, depending on whether or not gadolinium-based contrast media is injected intravenously. MRA is widely used for screening for stenosis, but is vulnerable to imaging distortion [5]. All of these modalities provide indirect information about vascular pathology because luminal change, such as stenosis, results from the changes of vessel walls. Noninvasive and direct in vivo assessment of vessel walls via imaging may provide better information about vascular pathology. Vessel wall imaging using high-resolution magnetic resonance imaging (HR-MRI) can convey the morphology of the vessel wall and surrounding structure beyond just the luminal abnormalities. As such, vessel wall imaging was introduced as an emerging technique in cervical arteries and recently has been applied to intracranial artery diseases. HR-MRI enables us to observe vessel walls directly with high resolution and excellent soft tissue contrast without radiation hazard [6, 7]. This chapter discusses the role and radiological features of angiography and HR-MRI.

Angiography

Digital Subtraction Angiography (DSA)

Digital subtraction angiography (DSA) is still the gold standard for luminal imaging despite being the oldest technique, developed in 1927 [1]. Since the introduction of Seldinger's method of percutaneous catheterization in 1953 [8], the procedure gained wide acceptance and advanced technically in both subtraction and magnification. Modern DSA offers superb spatial resolution of less than 0.2 mm and superb contrast resolution, which are major reasons why DSA remains the gold standard. DSA is the most expensive and most invasive modality, available only at highly specialized centers [9, 10]. The invasiveness results in an increased risk of procedure-related complications, radiation hazard, and contrast media reactions. In a large retrospective study (n = 19,826), neurologic complications occurred in 2.63 % and permanent disability in 0.14% [2]. The risk of DSA in patients with transient ischemic attack (TIA) or stroke is even higher; with 3.0% had transient neurological deficits and 0.7% had permanent neurological deficit [10]. As a result of the complication rates and other factors mentioned, DSA is mostly used in patients with TIA or stroke when more detail is required to plan endovascular treatment or if small or medium sized arteries need to be examined. While there is a risk of neurological deficit with DSA, the risk is low and must be balanced against the risk of an incorrect diagnosis that may lead to a substantial risk of ischemic stroke [11, 12].

The degree of stenosis is currently the most important parameter to guide therapy in the evaluation of intracranial artery disease [11] and DSA has good interobserver and intraobserver agreement for measurement of stenosis [13]. The WASID formula is used to define the degree of stenosis as follows: percent stenosis = [(1 – (D(stenosis)/D(normal)))] ×100, where D(stenosis) = the diameter of the artery at the site of the most severe stenosis and D(normal) = the diameter of the proximal normal artery [13]. DSA also offers important hemodynamic information about the contribution of flow from the injected artery. Slow-flow vessels distal to a stenosis may be poorly filled with contrast media and therefore poorly visualized. In stenoocclusive disease with slow-flow, CTA may be better than DSA, because CTA can result in concentration of a larger volume of contrast media in distal vessels through a tight stenosis with a longer scan time [14]. With DSA, multiple artery injections with contrast media are required to show collateral flow and both vertebral arteries need to be injected to fully assess for posterior circulation stenosis.

Computed Tomography Angiography (CTA)

CT, developed by Sir Godfrey Hounsfield, generates cross-sectional imaging by using X rays and was first applied to brain imaging in 1972 [15]. Modern CT and CTA generate reconstructed 2D images in various viewing planes by continuous spiral acquisition of volume data from contiguous slices with short scan times using multi-row detectors. CTA can acquire complete images within the first pass of contrast media through an arterial system and display images using various post-processing techniques. First, multi-planar reformation (MPR) can display 2D images in various planes without any loss of information [16]. Second, maximum intensity projection (MIP) enhances high attenuation contrast tissues, such as blood vessels, wall calcification, and bone. Since dense calcifications or stents can interfere with the evaluation of the degree of stenosis, bone elimination is done during post-processing. The third post-processing technique is surface rendering, which provides a good 3D impression of the surface, but lacks accurate structural measurements.

CTA has similar or higher accuracy than MRA [5, 14, 17] and has a high sensitivity and specificity [4, 14, 18] in the evaluation of intracranial artery stenosis.

In a study of patients with acute stroke in the posterior circulation, CTA was reliable in evaluating basilar artery stenosis and more sensitive than DSA in showing retrograde flow in the distal basilar lesion. CTA was limited in the vertebral artery system because of artifacts from the skull base, which made it difficult to determine hypoplasia or stenosis [19]. CTA appears to be more accurate for identifying occlusion (sensitivity, 100%; specificity, 99.4–100%) than for measuring the degree of stenosis [4, 14, 18]. In a study comparing CTA and MRA using DSA as the gold standard, among arteries with stenosis ≥30%, CTA showed a sensitivity of 98% and specificity of 99% (positive predictive value, 93%; negative predictive value, 100%), which was higher than MRA [14]. For detection of stenoses ≥50%, CTA showed sensitivity of 99.6–97.1% and specificity of 99.4–99.5% (positive predictive value, 94.4–94.9%; negative predictive value, 99.6–99.8%) [4, 18], with a false positive rate of 2.4% at ≥30% stenosis, which is suggested as the screening cutoff point [18]. For measuring the degree of stenosis, agreement between CTA and DSA was 0.98 (95% confidence interval, 0.98–0.99) [18]. In the SONIA Study, the CTA cohort (n = 20) demonstrated less accuracy, with a positive predictive value of 46.7% (50–99% stenosis) and 13.3% (70–99% stenosis), and a negative predictive value of 73.0% (50–99% stenosis) and 83.8% (70–99% stenosis) [20, 21]. The diagnostic performance of CTA needs further evaluation, in particular with larger populations that have ≥70% stenosis that may require more aggressive and invasive therapy for stroke prevention.

Although CTA is known to reliably detect arterial size as small as 0.7 mm (DSA, 0.4 mm), accurate measurement is difficult in small arteries [22]. CTA does not appear to be as reliable as DSA for the determining the presence of stenosis in small arteries distal to the first 1 cm of the artery [22].

With the advent of the mechanical thrombectomy with stent-retriever, faster puncture time to endovascular therapy became the most important issue in acute ischemic stroke. Accordingly, CTA became a more important modality with short scan time and the evaluation of collaterals on multi-phase imaging, which can contribute to faster recanalization and better prognosis [23, 24].

Magnetic Resonance Angiography (MRA)

Since magnetic resonance angiography (MRA) was developed in the 1980s [25], it has been widely adopted as an imaging modality for evaluating intracranial artery disease. Time-of-flight (TOF) MRA and contrast-enhanced MRA (CE-MRA) are both used to evaluate intracranial artery flow. TOF-MRA uses flow-related enhancement phenomenon and saturation of background tissue without exogenous contrast media to generate angiographic images. TOF-MRA is vulnerable to flow-related artifact and imaging distortion, which may overestimate stenoocclusive lesions. CE-MRA usually covers the area from the intracranial to the neck vessels and so leads to poor spatial resolution of intracranial vessels, but compared to TOF-MRA, CE-MRA may lessen the overestimation of the length and degree of stenosis [26] and visualize small vessels better [27]. Modern TOF-MRA is generally acquired as a 3D sequence, using multiple overlapping thin slab acquisition (MOTSA) and tilted optimized non-saturation excitation (TONE) technique for the reduction of saturation effect. The saturation effect is caused by repeated excitation radiofrequency (RF) pulses and results in loss of signal leading to artifact and overestimation of stenosis [5, 28]. In a study of 28 patients, MRA had a sensitivity of 70% and specificity of 97% (positive predictive value, 65%; negative predictive value, 98%) using DSA as the gold standard for detecting ≥30% stenosis [14]. Choi et al. [29] reported a sensitivity of 78–85% and specificity of 95% (positive predictive value, 75–79%; negative predictive value, 95–97%) for detecting ≥30% stenosis in 39 patients. For detecting arterial occlusion, MRA has a sensitivity and specificity of 87–100% and 98–100%, respectively [14, 29, 30]. The studies described above are limited by retrospective design, single institute studies, and small sample size.

The SONIA trial (n = 407) reported that 3D TOF-MRA had a positive predictive value of 59% (95 % confidence interval, 54–65) and negative predictive value of 91% (95 % confidence interval, 89–93) for detecting a stenosis ≥50–99% [20]. In other words, TOF-MRA is a reliable test to exclude intracranial arterial disease with high negative predictive value, but the positive predictive value is low and so TOF-MRA is not sufficient for accurately quantifying intracranial artery stenosis. Since the positive predictive value relies on the prevalence of the disease [31], the relatively low prevalence of intracranial atherosclerosis in Caucasians may have impacted the positive predictive value in the SONIA study.

TOF-MRA may have a higher positive predictive value in an Asian population where there is a higher prevalence of intracranial atherosclerosis [32].

MRA is the least invasive modality for evaluating intracranial artery disease, almost free from procedure-related complications, radiation hazard, and does not require exogenous contrast media (in TOF-MRA), but MRA tends to overestimate the severity of stenosis and is vulnerable to artifacts from metallic devices [5]. MRA has been widely used as a first and/or screening imaging modality for intracranial artery evaluation.

HR-MRI for Vessel Wall Imaging

Techniques

HR-MRI requires good resolution for depicting vessel walls, an imaging plane perpendicular to the arterial course, and an adequate image contrast to characterize vessel walls [7, 33]. Given the small diameter of intracranial arteries (anterior cerebral artery, 2–3 mm; middle cerebral artery, 3–5 mm; vertebral artery, 3–4 mm), high-resolution imaging is required to see the vessel wall [34–36]. HR-MRI with resolution of less than 1 mm has been clinically used by 1.5 tesla or 3 tesla machines [7]. Higher resolution has recently been studied with 7 tesla machines, but its use is not widespread.

Positioning of the imaging plane perpendicular to the long axis of the artery enables the most accurate characterization of the vessel wall (e.g. eccentricity, wall thickness). It is sometimes difficult to differentiate true pathology from pseudo-vessel wall components or pseudo-enhancement because intracranial arteries are bordered by dura and meninges and normal meninges or veins can be enhanced [37]. Other imaging planes are also useful, which has resulted in the preference of 3D HR-MRI. Black-blood techniques and multi-contrast imaging, including contrast-enhanced imaging, contribute to better image contrast [38]. HR-MRI generally consists of T1-weighted imaging, T2-weighted imaging, proton density imaging, and contrast-enhanced T1-weighted imaging. T1-weighted and T2-weighted imaging generally show basic characteristics of vessel walls, such as the morphology and signal intensity. Proton density imaging is useful to demarcate outer arterial walls, but not as good for characterization of components within vessel walls. Contrast-enhanced T1-weighted imaging shows the most notable contrast and wall enhancement, which may be an indicator of disease activity. It is acquired by using gadolinium based contrast media, but the optimal dose, time interval from injection to scan, and injection method of contrast media are not standardized.

Susceptibility-weighted imaging is also useful to evaluate the components of vessel walls. It can be defined as 3D fully flow compensated high-resolution gradient echo imaging with phase information. Susceptibility-weighted imaging is known to present higher sensitivity than traditional T2* gradient-echo imaging [39] for detecting intracranial vessel wall hemorrhage [39, 40]. Black-blood techniques improve the contrast of vessel walls by suppressing signals of luminal blood and surrounding cerebrospinal fluid [7, 33]. Black-blood techniques include double inversion recovery, motion-sensitized driven equilibrium (MSDE) or improved motion-sensitized driven equilibrium (iMSDE) and delay alternating with nutation for tailored excitation (DANTE). Double inversion recovery consists of an initial nonselective inversion recovery pulse to invert the magnetization of the whole body and then a second selective inversion recovery pulse to re-invert the imaging section. This leads to inverting the magnetization of blood from outside the imaging section, whereas the magnetization within the imaging section is unchanged with a zero-sum of inversion [6]. Double inversion recovery generally applies to two-dimensional (2D) imaging because of the sequential slice acquisition, which results in a limited spatial resolution, a long scan time, and partial volume effects [33]. MSDE or iMSDE which uses preparation radiofrequency pulses of flip angles of 90° and 180° before acquiring imaging has the advantages of a shorter preparation time and larger coverage than double inversion recovery. However, this can cause signal loss during the preparation time and incomplete suppression of blood or cerebrospinal fluid signals, and is susceptible to field inhomogeneity [7, 33, 41]. DANTE has been recently introduced in intracranial vessel wall imaging to improve black-blood techniques, which induces the attenuation of static tissue signal less than MSDE [42]. DANTE uses a series of low flip angle nonselective pulses interleaved with gradient pulses with short repetition times, which lead to static tissue signals being preserved and flowing tissue signals being attenuated. The suppression is insensitive to flow rates above 0.1 cm/s [43].

Intracranial Atherosclerosis

Intracranial atherosclerosis is the most common intracranial artery pathology causing ischemic stroke [44]. Dissection, moyamoya disease, and vasculitis are also important causes of intracranial vascular pathology that are sometimes confused with atherosclerosis. HR-MRI is expected to aid in the diagnosis and understanding of intracranial atherosclerosis and other intracranial artery diseases.

Lipid, fibrous tissue, intraplaque hemorrhage, and calcium are the major components of atherosclerotic plaques. In extracranial carotid arteries, vulnerable plaques can be differentiated from stable plaques based on plaque components using HR-MRI [6, 45]. Intracranial plaques are more difficult to characterize in detail because of smaller arterial size and limited resolution.

Imaging characteristics consistent with intraplaque hemorrhage on T1-weighted imaging and plaque enhancement on contrast-enhanced T1-weighted imaging may be most important for characterization of intracranial atherosclerosis. Intracranial intraplaque hemorrhage appears as a bright high-signal intensity and is usually defined as signal intensity of >1.5 times that of adjacent muscles on T1-weighted imaging [46, 47]. This definition was based on a few histopathological and radiological reports and data from the cervical carotid artery representing recent or fresh hemorrhage [6, 46, 48, 49]. This definition may not always apply to intraplaque hemorrhage. Intraplaque hemorrhage in the cervical carotid artery shows iso- or high signal intensities (contrast ratios to adjacent muscles, 1.01–2.57) according to different techniques of T1-weighted sequences [50]. Intramural hematoma in intracranial artery dissection has also been shown to have similar signal intensities [51]. Therefore, Intraplaque hemorrhage may be more accurately interpreted based on multi-contrast imaging, such as T2-weighted imaging or susceptibility weighted imaging. Nevertheless, intracranial intraplaque hemorrhage is one of the important components to determine plaque vulnerability. Intraplaque hemorrhage was detected in more plaques associated with infarctions than plaques not associated with infarction (30.4 vs. 15.4%) in a postmortem study [52], and was significantly associated with ipsilateral stroke [46]. Because intracranial arteries have a relative paucity of vaso-vasorum that is the source of neovascularization and ultimate intraplaque hemorrhage in other extracranial arteries, intraplaque hemorrhage may not be as prevalent in intracranial vulnerable plaque as in other vascular beds [53, 54].

Although the intracranial plaque components of lipid core, fibrous cap, and calcification cannot be definitely differentiated on HR-MRI, the components may have signal intensities consistent with those seen in the cervical carotid artery [55]. In a case report of intracranial atherosclerosis plaque features seen on HR-MRI and correlated with pathology, lipid core was isointense on T1-weighted imaging and hypo- to isointense on T2-weighted imaging; fibrous component was isointense on T1- and T2-weighted imaging; and calcification was dark signal intensity on T1- and T2-weighted imaging [55].

Wall or plaque enhancement is one of the most reliable and notable features in intracranial artery disease. Stronger plaque enhancement has been shown to be related to more recent ischemic stroke and more severe inflammatory activity [56–58]. Contrast enhancement was detected more frequently in symptomatic plaques than asymptomatic plaques (70 vs. 8%) and the degree of enhancement was higher in symptomatic plaques (1.63 vs. 1.23) [58]. The degree of enhancement in symptomatic plaques has also been shown to decrease over time [57]. Plaques resulting in ischemic stroke may be identified according to the degree of enhancement [56]. Plaque enhancement has also been shown to indicate neovascularization or increased permeability of the endothelium [59, 60]. This finding is not specific to atherosclerosis, as vessel wall enhancement is also seen in generalized inflammatory diseases, such as vasculitis, and even moyamoya disease [7].

Plaque morphology is useful for determining vascular pathology. Asymmetric irregular wall thickening, so-called eccentricity, is the classic finding of atherosclerotic plaques, whereas vasculitis tends to show smooth concentric wall thickening [61]. The distribution of the plaque is also important. Both asymptomatic and symptomatic atherosclerotic plaques in the middle cerebral artery usually tend to form on the opposite side (ventral and inferior wall) to the orifices of perforators (superior wall). Symptomatic plaques in the middle cerebral artery tend to be located at the superior walls, which may mean that superiorly located plaques are more likely to cause perforator infarction [62–64].

Quantitative and qualitative methods may be useful for determining vascular pathology and vulnerability in intracranial plaques. Intracranial arterial lumen and wall measurements showed excellent reproducibility (interclass correlation coefficients, 0.87–0.97) [65] and were sufficient to determine other characteristics, such as positive remodeling vs negative remodeling, and plaque volume or area [66]. Positive and negative remodeling, as described in coronary artery atherosclerosis, is also seen in intracranial plaques [66]. The remodeling index formula is as follows: maximum outer wall area / ([proximal normal arterial area + distal normal arterial area] / 2). If the index is ≥1.0, the area is defined as positive remodeling; otherwise, the area is defined as negative remodeling [66]. Positive remodeling tends to be associated with symptomatic plaques [67–69]. More plaque burden and less luminal area were associated with plaque vulnerability [70]. The morphology and distribution of plaque in vessel walls may indicate vulnerability and the stroke mechanism, as well as distinguish among vascular pathologies (fig. 1).

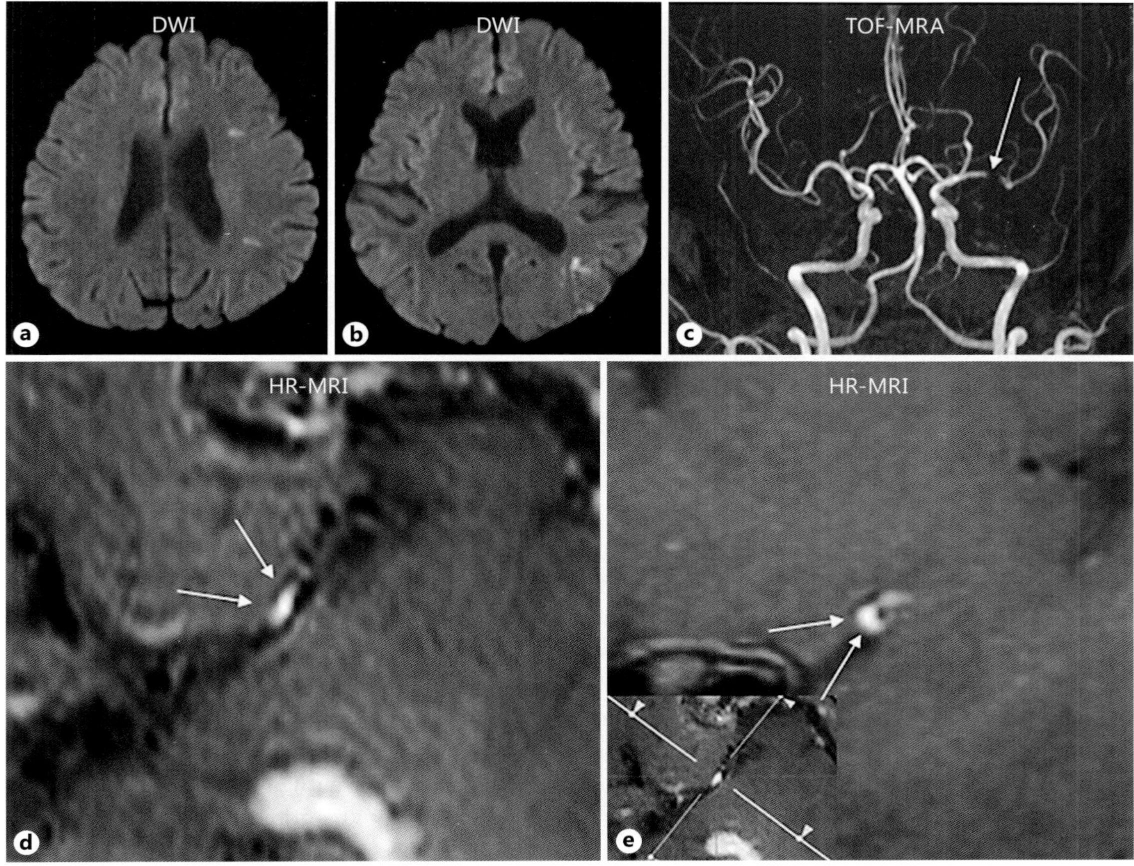

Fig. 1. A 52-year-old man developed right sided limb weakness. DWI showed multiple embolic infarctions in the left cerebral hemisphere (**a**, **b**). TOF-MRA showed a focal severe stenosis of the left middle cerebral artery (arrow) (**c**). A HR-MR transverse T1-weighted image showed a contrast-enhanced plaque in the middle cerebral artery (arrows) (**d**). A HR-MR T1-weighted image with the perpendicular plane to the arterial long axis (small figure) showed an eccentric plaque with strong enhancement (arrows) (**e**).

Intracranial Artery Dissection

Intracranial artery dissection is an important cause of ischemic stroke in young adults [71]. Ischemic symptoms are present in 52% of patients with intracranial artery dissections, followed by subarachnoid hemorrhage in 28% of patients [72].

In young patients with minimal risk atherosclerotic factors, middle cerebral artery stenoocclusive disease may be due to moyamoya disease, vasculitis, or dissection, rather than atherosclerosis, and HR-MRI may be useful to differentiate among these pathologies [73].

The conventional radiological findings of arterial dissection include the presence of intimal flap, double lumen, intramural hematoma, aneurysmal dilatation, tapered stenosis, occlusion, and sting-of-pearls sign, established mainly by using angiography [72]. A clear geometric change on follow-up luminal imaging is also characteristic [74]. In intracranial artery dissection, the findings of intimal flap, double lumen and intramural hematoma were more commonly detected on HR-MRI than angiography [40, 51, 75].

Vessel wall enhancement on HR-MRI has been seen with intracranial artery dissection. Although the pathology is not fully understood, wall enhancement may be caused by inflammation [76], slow blood flow in the false lumen, or enhancement of the vasa vasorum [77]. Pathological (18F)-fluorodeoxyyglucose uptake in positron emission tomography (PET)-CT was observed at the location of the enhancement in vessel walls with dissection and the enhancement resolved within weeks, which may indicate a generalized transient inflammatory arteriopathy [76].

Intramural hematoma is one of the most common dissection findings on HR-MRI. If intramural hematoma is seen without intimal flap or double lumen, intracranial artery dissection should be considered first in the differential diagnosis. The possibility of intraplaque hemorrhage also has to be considered in an ambiguous clinical setting. For example, in the middle cerebral artery (one of the most common locations of atherosclerosis) ischemic symptoms are more common than typical symptoms of dissection such as headache [40, 71], making dissection and atherosclerosis difficult to differentiate. Intramural hematoma with no connection between the true and false lumen is also reported in dissection and may be the result of rupture of the vasa vasorum or new vessels [78]. Intramural hematoma can also show signal intensities similar to intraplaque hemorrhage (hyper-intensity, 73.9%; iso-intensity, 8.7%; hypo-intensity, 13% on T1-weighted imaging) [51]. Distinguishing intramural hematoma from intraplaque hemorrhage is sometimes challenging and may rely on clinical findings and other radiologic features, such as a clear geometric change on follow-up vascular imaging.

In contrast to atherosclerosis, arterial dissection results in subsequent geometric change, with rapid and spontaneous normalization [74]. Among patients with unruptured intracranial artery dissections, geometric changes were seen within 2 weeks to 2 months in 83.9%, and, among these, 61.5% and 18.3% showed radiological improvement and complete normalization, respectively [74]. In unruptured intracranial vertebral artery dissections, 37.4–75% showed spontaneous improvement [79, 80]. The normalization rate for intracranial artery dissection is higher than that (<30%) of intracranial atherosclerosis when intensive stroke prevention medication is administered [81, 82]. Since HR-MRI findings can change over time, subsequent geometric changes are useful in differentiation between pathologies (fig. 2).

Moyamoya Disease

Moyamoya disease is described as abnormal vascular networks, and spontaneous and progressive stenosis or occlusion at the terminal internal carotid artery [83]. Moyamoya disease is traditionally defined on DSA as pathognomonic findings of bilateral steno-occlusive lesions at terminal internal carotid arteries, the proximal anterior cerebral arteries, or middle cerebral arteries. Unilateral involvement suggestive of probable moyamoya disease may eventually progress into bilateral lesions in up to 40% of patients [83]. The angiographic features can be unclear and the pathognomonic findings can only be observed during the intermediate stage. Distinguishing moyamoya disease from atherosclerosis is challenging in some cases, especially in East Asian populations that have high prevalence of both moyamoya disease and intracranial atherosclerosis, and in patients with ambiguous clinical and radiological features [84].

HR-MRI has attempted to identify radiological differences between moyamoya disease and atherosclerosis. Smaller outer vessel wall diameter, along with concentric and weaker wall enhancement, are the most important findings that differentiate moyamoya disease from atherosclerosis [85, 86]. Intimal hyperplasia and medial thinning are well-known pathological features of moyamoya disease. Intimal hyperplasia results from the proliferation of smooth muscle cells and luminal

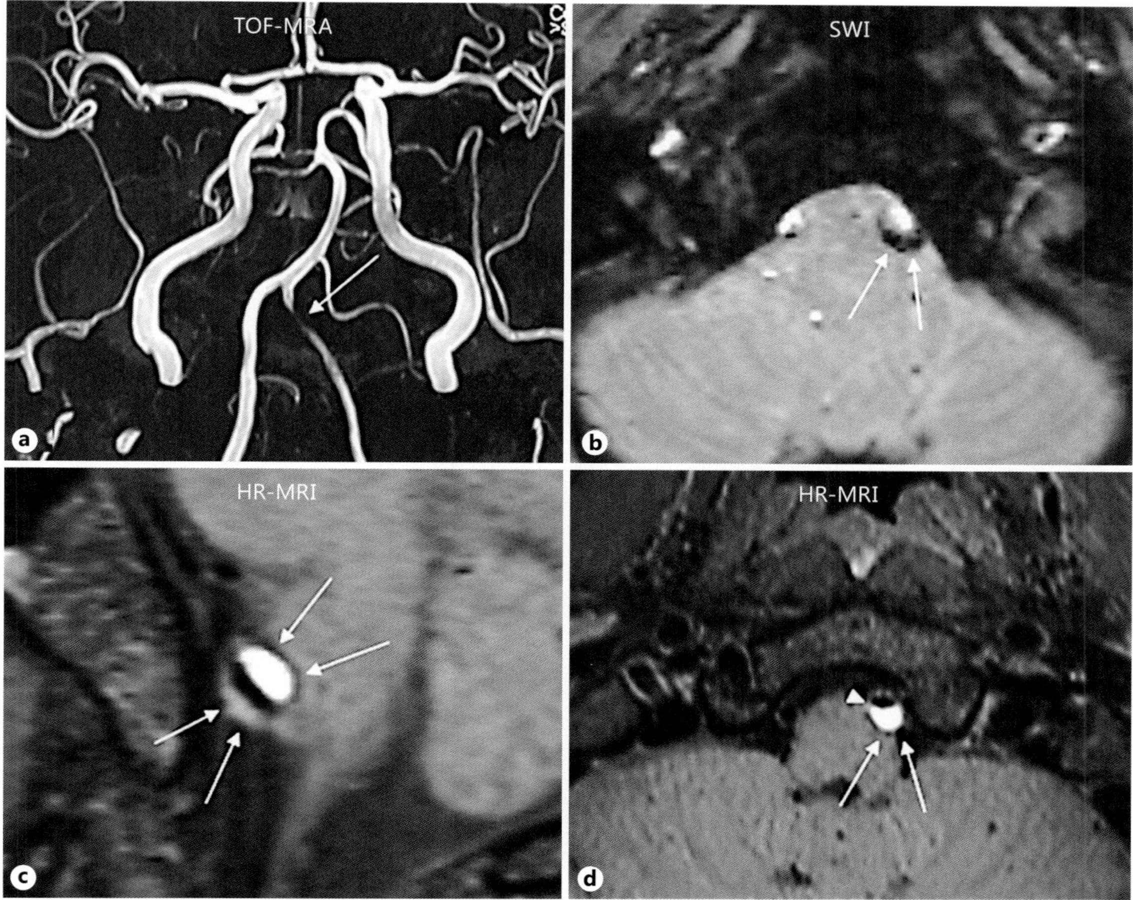

Fig. 2. A 50-year-old woman had a sudden occipital headache. TOF-MRA showed a focal severe stenosis in the left distal vertebral artery (arrow) (**a**). Susceptibility-weighted imaging showed an intramural hematoma with blooming artifact (arrows) (**b**). A HR-MR sagittal T1-weighted image showed an aneurysmal dilatation and intramural hematoma (arrows) (**c**). A HR-MR T1-weighted transverse image showed an intramural hematoma (arrows) and intimal flap (arrowhead) (**d**).

thrombosis leads to steno-occlusive lesions. Thinning of the media is caused by degradation of smooth muscle cells. Caspase-dependent apoptosis and overproduction of matrix metalloproteinase are known to be the mechanisms of the arterial pathology of moyamoya disease [87]. The degradation of vessel walls is associated with media thinness, which seems to contribute to smaller outer diameter on HR-MRI. Intimal hyperplasia may result in diffuse concentric enhancement [85, 86]. On HR-MRI, measurement of the minimal outer diameters was significantly different between moyamoya and atherosclerosis (1.61–2.01 vs. 3.03–3.31 mm, respectively) [84, 85]. The HR-MRI remodeling index and wall area also showed significant differences (mean remodeling index: 0.19 vs. 1.00; mean wall area: 0.32–0.39 vs. 1.64–6.00 mm^2) [84, 86]. The proportion of concentric enhancement is higher, whereas the degree of enhancement is lower in moyamoya disease compared to

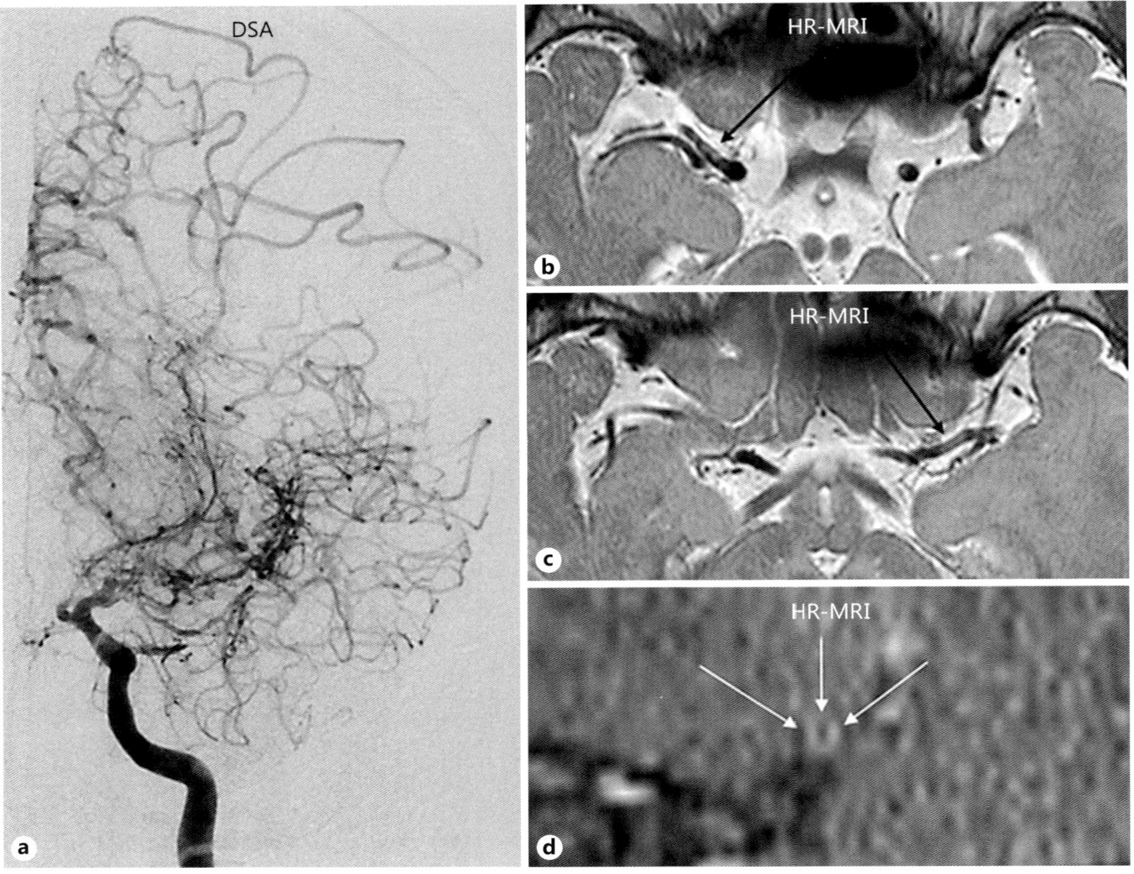

Fig. 3. A 44-year-old male patient presented became abulic. A DSA showed severe stenosis of the left terminal internal carotid artery and middle cerebral artery with basal collaterals (**a**). A HR-MR transverse proton-density image showed that the outer diameters of both middle cerebral arteries were decreased (black arrows) (**b**, **c**). A HR-MR contrast-enhanced T1-weighted image with perpendicular plane to the arterial long axis showed mild and concentric wall enhancement (arrows) (**d**).

atherosclerosis. Bilateral lesions occurred more commonly in moyamoya disease [85, 86]. Moyamoya disease is the typical pathology seen with small outer artery wall diameter, but congenital agenesis, chronic localized arteritis, and dissection are considered in the differential diagnosis [88, 89]. Moyamoya vessel walls on T1-weighted and T2-weighted imaging appeared to have more homogeneous signal intensity than atherosclerosis [84, 85]. As moyamoya disease progresses, the outer diameter seems to decrease [84] (fig. 3).

Vasculitis

Central nervous system (CNS) vasculitis is a rare cerebrovascular disease including a broad spectrum of conditions that present with various inflammatory and destructive characteristics. The average annual rate is 2.4 cases per 1 million person-years [90]. Primary CNS vasculitis indicates primary angiitis and secondary CNS vasculitis results from systemic inflammatory or infectious conditions [91]. The diagnosis of primary CNS angiitis was made as follows: (1) the presence of

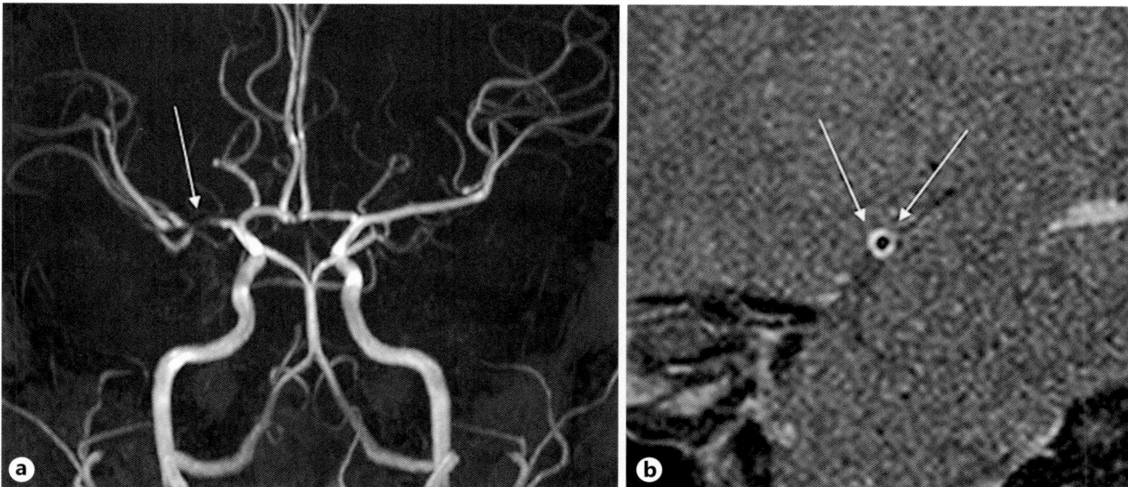

Fig. 4. A 19-year-old male patient had transient left side weakness. A TOF-MRA image showed a focal severe stenosis of the right middle cerebral artery (arrow) (**a**). A HR-MR contrast-enhanced T1-weighted image with perpendicular plane to the arterial long axis showed strong and concentric wall enhancement (arrows) (**b**). This patient's condition is considered to be vasculitis.

an acquired or otherwise unexplainable neurological or psychiatric deficit, (2) the presence of classic angiographic or histopathological features, and (3) no evidence of secondary vasculitis [91]. One of the major differential diagnoses is premature atherosclerosis.

Patients with atherosclerosis usually present with vascular risk factors and a normal cerebrospinal fluid study [91]. Atherosclerosis can involve any arteries, whereas the classic primary CNS vasculitis tends to involve medium to small sized vessels, and single lesions in multiple arteries are more common than multiple lesions in a single artery. The medium size is defined as arteries distal to the bifurcation of the middle cerebral artery and anterior- and posterior communicating artery. Small size can be beyond the resolution of DSA [92, 93]. Diffuse, bilateral, and alternating lesions of stenosis and dilatation are classic angiographic feature in primary CNS vasculitis. These features are not specific [91, 92]. On HR-MRI, eccentric and irregular plaques are the characteristic finding of atherosclerosis, whereas vasculitis tends to show luminal narrowing with smooth wall thickening. The degree of enhancement decreases with favorable treatment responses, and so may be a marker for disease activity in vasculitis [94, 95]. Ischemic infarctions in vasculitis may involve both white and gray matter and present different ages and occur in different vascular territories [91] (fig. 4).

References

1 Moniz E: L'encephalographie arterielle, son impartance dans la localisaton des tumeurs cerebrales. Revue Neurologique 1927;2:72–90.

2 Kaufmann TJ, Huston J 3rd, Mandrekar JN, Schleck CD, Thielen KR, Kallmes DF: Complications of diagnostic cerebral angiography: evaluation of 19,826 consecutive patients. Radiology 2007;243:812–819.

3 Leng X, Wong KS, Liebeskind DS: Evaluating intracranial atherosclerosis rather than intracranial stenosis. Stroke 2014;45:645–651.

4 Duffis EJ, Jethwa P, Gupta G, Bonello K, Gandhi CD, Prestigiacomo CJ: Accuracy of computed tomographic angiography compared to digital subtraction angiography in the diagnosis of intracranial stenosis and its impact on clinical decision-making. J Stroke Cerebrovasc Dis 2013;22:1013–1017.

5 Carvalho M, Oliveira A, Azevedo E, Bastos-Leite AJ: Intracranial arterial stenosis. J Stroke Cerebrovasc Dis 2014;23:599–609.

6 Oppenheim C, Naggara O, Touze E, Lacour JC, Schmitt E, Bonneville F, Crozier S, Guegan-Massardier E, Gerardin E, Leclerc X, Neau JP, Sirol M, Toussaint JF, Mas JL, Meder JF: High-resolution mr imaging of the cervical arterial wall: what the radiologist needs to know. Radiographics 2009;29:1413–1431.

7 Dieleman N, van der Kolk AG, Zwanenburg JJ, Harteveld AA, Biessels GJ, Luijten PR, Hendrikse J: Imaging intracranial vessel wall pathology with magnetic resonance imaging: current prospects and future directions. Circulation 2014;130:192–201.

8 Seldinger SI: Catheter replacement of the needle in percutaneous arteriography; a new technique. Acta Radiol 1953;39:368–376.

9 Theodotou BC, Whaley R, Mahaley MS: Complications following transfemoral cerebral angiography for cerebral ischemia. Report of 159 angiograms and correlation with surgical risk. Surg Neurol 1987;28:90–92.

10 Cloft HJ, Joseph GJ, Dion JE: Risk of cerebral angiography in patients with subarachnoid hemorrhage, cerebral aneurysm, and arteriovenous malformation: a meta-analysis. Stroke 1999;30:317–320.

11 Chimowitz MI, Lynn MJ, Howlett-Smith H, Stern BJ, Hertzberg VS, Frankel MR, Levine SR, Chaturvedi S, Kasner SE, Benesch CG, Sila CA, Jovin TG, Romano JG: Comparison of warfarin and aspirin for symptomatic intracranial arterial stenosis. NEJM 2005;352:1305–1316.

12 Warfarin-Aspirin Symptomatic Intracranial Disease Trial I: Design, progress and challenges of a double-blind trial of warfarin versus aspirin for symptomatic intracranial arterial stenosis. Neuroepidemiology 2003;22:106–117.

13 Samuels OB, Joseph GJ, Lynn MJ, Smith HA, Chimowitz MI: A standardized method for measuring intracranial arterial stenosis. AJNR Am J Neuroradiol 2000;21:643–646.

14 Bash S, Villablanca JP, Jahan R, Duckwiler G, Tillis M, Kidwell C, Saver J, Sayre J: Intracranial vascular stenosis and occlusive disease: evaluation with CT angiography, MR angiography, and digital subtraction angiography. AJNR Am J Neuroradiol 2005;26:1012–1021.

15 Buzug TM: Computed tomography: from photon statistics to modern cone-beam CT. Berlin, Springer, 2008.

16 Lell MM, Anders K, Uder M, Klotz E, Ditt H, Vega-Higuera F, Boskamp T, Bautz WA, Tomandl BF: New techniques in CT angiography. Radiographics 2006;26:S45–S62.

17 Skutta B, Furst G, Eilers J, Ferbert A, Kuhn FP: Intracranial stenoocclusive disease: double-detector helical ct angiography versus digital subtraction angiography. AJNR Am J Neuroradiol 1999;20:791–799.

18 Nguyen-Huynh MN, Wintermark M, English J, Lam J, Vittinghoff E, Smith WS, Johnston SC: How accurate is ct angiography in evaluating intracranial atherosclerotic disease? Stroke 2008;39:1184–1188.

19 Graf J, Skutta B, Kuhn FP, Ferbert A: Computed tomographic angiography findings in 103 patients following vascular events in the posterior circulation: potential and clinical relevance. J Neurol 2000;247:760–766.

20 Feldmann E, Wilterdink JL, Kosinski A, Lynn M, Chimowitz MI, Sarafin J, Smith HH, Nichols F, Rogg J, Cloft HJ, Wechsler L, Saver J, Levine SR, Tegeler C, Adams R, Sloan M, Stroke O, Neuroimaging of Intracranial Atherosclerosis Trial Investigated; The stroke outcomes and neuroimaging of intracranial atherosclerosis (sonia) trial. Neurology 2007;68:2099–2106.

21 Liebeskind DS, Kosinski AS, Saver JL, Feldmann E, Investigators S: Computed tomography angiography in the stroke outcomes and neuroimaging of intracranial atherosclerosis (sonia) study. Interv Neurol 2014;2:153–159.

22 Villablanca JP, Rodriguez FJ, Stockman T, Dahliwal S, Omura M, Hazany S, Sayre J: Mdct angiography for detection and quantification of small intracranial arteries: comparison with conventional catheter angiography. AJR Am J Roentgenol 2007;188:593–602.

23 Campbell BC, Mitchell PJ, Kleinig TJ, Dewey HM, Churilov L, Yassi N, Yan B, Dowling RJ, Parsons MW, Oxley TJ, Wu TY, Brooks M, Simpson MA, Miteff F, Levi CR, Krause M, Harrington TJ, Faulder KC, Steinfort BS, Priglinger M, Ang T, Scroop R, Barber PA, McGuinness B, Wijeratne T, Phan TG, Chong W, Chandra RV, Bladin CF, Badve M, Rice H, de Villiers L, Ma H, Desmond PM, Donnan GA, Davis SM, Investigators E-I: Endovascular therapy for ischemic stroke with perfusion-imaging selection. N Engl J Med 2015;372:1009–1018.

24 Goyal M, Demchuk AM, Menon BK, Eesa M, Rempel JL, Thornton J, Roy D, Jovin TG, Willinsky RA, Sapkota BL, Dowlatshahi D, Frei DF, Kamal NR, Montanera WJ, Poppe AY, Ryckborst KJ, Silver FL, Shuaib A, Tampieri D, Williams D, Bang OY, Baxter BW, Burns PA, Choe H, Heo JH, Holmstedt CA, Jankowitz B, Kelly M, Linares G, Mandzia JL, Shankar J, Sohn SI, Swartz RH, Barber PA, Coutts SB, Smith EE, Morrish WF, Weill A, Subramaniam S, Mitha AP, Wong JH, Lowerison MW, Sajobi TT, Hill MD, Investigators ET: Randomized assessment of rapid endovascular treatment of ischemic stroke. N Engl J Med 2015;372:1019–1030.

25 Pipe JG: Limits of time-of-flight magnetic resonance angiography. Topics in Magn Reson Imaging 2001;12:163–174.

26 Jung H, et al: Contrast-enhanced mr angiography for the diagnosis of intracranial vascular disease: optimal dose of gadopentetate dimeglumine. Am J Roentgenol 1995;165:1251–1255.

27 Yang JJ, et al: Comparison of pre- and postcontrast 3d time-of-flight mr angiography for the evaluation of distal intracranial branch occlusions in acute ischemic stroke. Am J Radiol 2002;23:557–567.

28 Carr JC, Carroll TJ: Magnetic resonance angiography: principles and applications. New York, Springer, 2012.

29 Choi CG, Lee DH, Lee JH, Pyun HW, Kang DW, Kwon SU, Kim JK, Kim SJ, Suh DC: Detection of intracranial atherosclerotic steno-occlusive disease with 3d time-of-flight magnetic resonance angiography with sensitivity encoding at 3t. AJNR Am J Neuroradiol 2007;28: 439–446.
30 Sadikin C, Teng MM, Chen TY, Luo CB, Chang FC, Lirng JF, Sun YC: The current role of 1.5t non-contrast 3d time-of-flight magnetic resonance angiography to detect intracranial steno-occlusive disease. J Formos Med Assoc 2007;106:691–699.
31 Altman DF, Bland JM: Diagnostic tests 2: Predictive values. BMJ 1994;309:102.
32 Feldmann E, Daneault N, Kwan E, Ho KJ, Pessin MS, Langenberg P, Caplan LR: Chinese-white differences in the distribution of occlusive cerebrovascular disease. Neurology 1990;40:1541–1545.
33 Choi YJ, Jung SC, Lee DH: Vessel wall imaging of the intracranial and cervical carotid arteries. J Stroke 2015;17:238–255.
34 Jain KK: Some observations on the anatomy of the middle cerebral artery. Can J Surg 1964;7:134–139.
35 Kamath S: Observations on the length and diameter of vessels forming the circle of willis. J Anat 1981;133:419–423.
36 Akgun V, Battal B, Bozkurt Y, Oz O, Hamcan S, Sari S, Akgun H: Normal anatomical features and variations of the vertebrobasilar circulation and its branches: an analysis with 64-detector row ct and 3t mr angiographies. ScientificWorldJournal 2013;2013:620162.
37 Mineyko A, Kirton A, Ng D, Wei XC: Normal intracranial periarterial enhancement on pediatric brain mr imaging. Neuroradiology 2013;55:1161–1169.
38 Mossa-Basha M, Hwang WD, De Havenon A, Hippe D, Balu N, Becker KJ, Tirschwell DT, Hatsukami T, Anzai Y, Yuan C: Multicontrast high-resolution vessel wall magnetic resonance imaging and its value in differentiating intracranial vasculopathic processes. Stroke 2015;46:1567–1573.
39 Kim TW, Choi HS, Koo J, Jung SL, Ahn KJ, Kim BS, Shin YS, Lee KS: Intramural hematoma detection by susceptibility-weighted imaging in intracranial vertebral artery dissection. Cerebrovasc Dis 2013;36:292–298.
40 Gao PH, Yang L, Wang G, Guo L, Liu X, Zhao B: Symptomatic unruptured isolated middle cerebral artery dissection: Clinical and magnetic resonance imaging features. Clin Neuroradiol 2016;26: 81–91.
41 Zhu C, Graves MJ, Yuan J, Sadat U, Gillard JH, Patterson AJ: Optimization of improved motion-sensitized driven-equilibrium (imsde) blood suppression for carotid artery wall imaging. J Cardiovasc Magn Reson 2014;16:61.
42 Li L, Chai JT, Biasiolli L, Robson MD, Choudhury RP, Handa AI, Near J, Jezzard P: Black-blood multicontrast imaging of carotid arteries with dante-prepared 2d and 3d mr imaging. Radiology 2014;273:560–569.
43 Xie Y, Yang Q, Xie G, Pang J, Fan Z, Li D: Improved black-blood imaging using dante-space for simultaneous carotid and intracranial vessel wall evaluation. Magn Reson Med 2016;75:2286–2294.
44 Arenillas JF: Intracranial atherosclerosis: current concepts. Stroke 2011;42:S20–S23.
45 Fleg JL, Stone GW, Fayad ZA, Granada JF, Hatsukami TS, Kolodgie FD, Ohayon J, Pettigrew R, Sabatine MS, Tearney GJ, Waxman S, Domanski MJ, Srinivas PR, Narula J: Detection of high-risk atherosclerotic plaque: report of the nhlbi working group on current status and future directions. JACC Cardiovasc Imaging 2012;5:941–955.
46 Xu WH, Li ML, Gao S, Ni J, Yao M, Zhou LX, Peng B, Feng F, Jin ZY, Cui LY: Middle cerebral artery intraplaque hemorrhage: prevalence and clinical relevance. Ann Neurol 2012;71:195–198.
47 Turan TN, Bonilha L, Morgan PS, Adams RJ, Chimowitz MI: Intraplaque hemorrhage in symptomatic intracranial atherosclerotic disease. J Neuroimaging 2011;21:e159–e161.
48 Altaf N, MacSweeney ST, Gladman J, Auer DP: Carotid intraplaque hemorrhage predicts recurrent symptoms in patients with high-grade carotid stenosis. Stroke 2007;38:1633–1635.
49 Chen XY, Wong KS, Lam WW, Ng HK: High signal on t1 sequence of magnetic resonance imaging confirmed to be intraplaque haemorrhage by histology in middle cerebral artery. Int J Stroke 2014; 9:E19.
50 Saito A, Sasaki M, Ogasawara K, Kobayashi M, Hitomi J, Narumi S, Ohba H, Yamaguchi M, Kudo K, Terayama Y: Carotid plaque signal differences among four kinds of t1-weighted magnetic resonance imaging techniques: a histopathological correlation study. Neuroradiology 2012;54:1187–1194.
51 Wang Y, Lou X, Li Y, Sui B, Sun S, Li C, Jiang P, Siddiqui A, Yang X: Imaging investigation of intracranial arterial dissecting aneurysms by using 3 t high-resolution mri and dsa: from the interventional neuroradiologists' view. Acta Neurochir 2014;156:515–525.
52 Chen XY, Wong KS, Lam WW, Zhao HL, Ng HK: Middle cerebral artery atherosclerosis: histological comparison between plaques associated with and not associated with infarct in a postmortem study. Cerebrovasc Dis 2008;25:74–80.
53 Aydin F: Do human intracranial arteries lack vasa vasorum? A comparative immunohistochemical study of intracranial and systemic arteries. Acta Neuropathol 1998;96:22–28.
54 Virmani R, Kolodgie FD, Burke AP, Finn AV, Gold HK, Tulenko TN, Wrenn SP, Narula J: Atherosclerotic plaque progression and vulnerability to rupture: angiogenesis as a source of intraplaque hemorrhage. Arterioscler Thromb Vasc Biol 2005;25:2054–2061.
55 Turan TN, Rumboldt Z, Granholm AC, Columbo L, Welsh CT, Lopes-Virella MF, Spampinato MV, Brown TR: Intracranial atherosclerosis: Correlation between in-vivo 3t high resolution mri and pathology. Atherosclerosis 2014;237: 460–463.
56 Qiao Y, Zeiler SR, Mirbagheri S, Leigh R, Urrutia V, Wityk R, Wasserman BA: Intracranial plaque enhancement in patients with cerebrovascular events on high-spatial-resolution mr images. Radiology 2014;271:534–542.
57 Skarpathiotakis M, Mandell DM, Swartz RH, Tomlinson G, Mikulis DJ: Intracranial atherosclerotic plaque enhancement in patients with ischemic stroke. AJNR Am J Neuroradiol 2013;34:299–304.
58 Vakil P, Vranic J, Hurley MC, Bernstein RA, Korutz AW, Habib A, Shaibani A, Dehkordi FH, Carroll TJ, Ansari SA: T1 gadolinium enhancement of intracranial atherosclerotic plaques associated with symptomatic ischemic presentations. AJNR Am J Neuroradiol 2013;34:2252–2258.

59 Sluimer JC, Kolodgie FD, Bijnens AP, Maxfield K, Pacheco E, Kutys B, Duimel H, Frederik PM, van Hinsbergh VW, Virmani R, Daemen MJ: Thin-walled microvessels in human coronary atherosclerotic plaques show incomplete endothelial junctions relevance of compromised structural integrity for intraplaque microvascular leakage. J Am Coll Cardiol 2009;53:1517–1527.
60 Qiao Y, Etesami M, Astor BC, Zeiler SR, Trout HH 3rd, Wasserman BA: Carotid plaque neovascularization and hemorrhage detected by mr imaging are associated with recent cerebrovascular ischemic events. AJNR Am J Neuroradiol 2012;33:755–760.
61 Swartz RH, Bhuta SS, Farb RI, Agid R, Willinsky RA, Terbrugge KG, Butany J, Wasserman BA, Johnstone DM, Silver FL, Mikulis DJ: Intracranial arterial wall imaging using high-resolution 3-tesla contrast-enhanced mri. Neurology 2009; 72:627–634.
62 Zhao DL, Deng G, Xie B, Gao B, Peng CY, Nie F, Yang M, Ju S, Teng GJ: Wall characteristics and mechanisms of ischaemic stroke in patients with atherosclerotic middle cerebral artery stenosis: a high-resolution mri study. Neurol Res 2015;1743132815Y0000000088.
63 Xu WH, Li ML, Gao S, Ni J, Zhou LX, Yao M, Peng B, Feng F, Jin ZY, Cui LY: Plaque distribution of stenotic middle cerebral artery and its clinical relevance. Stroke 2011;42:2957–2959.
64 Sui B, Gao P, Lin Y, Jing L, Qin H: Distribution and features of middle cerebral artery atherosclerotic plaques in symptomatic patients: a 3.0 t high-resolution mri study. Neurol Res 2015;37:391–396.
65 Yang WQ, Huang B, Liu XT, Liu HJ, Li PJ, Zhu WZ: Reproducibility of high-resolution mri for the middle cerebral artery plaque at 3t. Eur J Radiol 2014; 83:e49–e55.
66 Zhu XJ, Du B, Lou X, Hui FK, Ma L, Zheng BW, Jin M, Wang CX, Jiang WJ: Morphologic characteristics of atherosclerotic middle cerebral arteries on 3t high-resolution mri. AJNR Am J Neuroradiol 2013; 34:1717–1722.
67 Xu WH, Li ML, Gao S, Ni J, Zhou LX, Yao M, Peng B, Feng F, Jin ZY, Cui LY: In vivo high-resolution mr imaging of symptomatic and asymptomatic middle cerebral artery atherosclerotic stenosis. Atherosclerosis 2010;212:507–511.
68 Lee WJ, Choi HS, Jang J, Sung J, Kim TW, Koo J, Shin YS, Jung SL, Ahn KJ, Kim BS: Non-stenotic intracranial arteries have atherosclerotic changes in acute ischemic stroke patients: a 3t mri study. Neuroradiology 2015;57:1007–1013.
69 Zhao DL, Deng G, Xie B, Ju S, Yang M, Chen XH, Teng GJ: High-resolution mri of the vessel wall in patients with symptomatic atherosclerotic stenosis of the middle cerebral artery. J Clin Neurosci 2015;22:700–704.
70 Teng Z, Peng W, Zhan Q, Zhang X, Liu Q, Chen S, Tian X, Chen L, Brown AJ, Graves MJ, Gillard JH, Lu J: An assessment on the incremental value of high-resolution magnetic resonance imaging to identify culprit plaques in atherosclerotic disease of the middle cerebral artery. Eur Radiol 2016;26:2206–2214.
71 Sikkema T, Uyttenboogaart M, Eshghi O, De Keyser J, Brouns R, van Dijk JM, Luijckx GJ: Intracranial artery dissection. Eur J Neurol 2014;21:820–826.
72 Tsukahara T, Minematsu K: Overview of spontaneous cervicocephalic arterial dissection in japan. Acta Neurochir Suppl 2010;107:35–40.
73 Ahn SH, Lee J, Kim YJ, Kwon SU, Lee D, Jung SC, Kang DW, Kim JS: Isolated mca disease in patients without significant atherosclerotic risk factors: a high-resolution magnetic resonance imaging study. Stroke 2015;46:697–703.
74 Mizutani T: Natural course of intracranial arterial dissections. J Neurosurg 2011;114:1037–1044.
75 Han M, Rim NJ, Lee JS, Kim SY, Choi JW: Feasibility of high-resolution mr imaging for the diagnosis of intracranial vertebrobasilar artery dissection. Eur Radiol 2014;24:3017–3024.
76 Pfefferkorn T, Saam T, Rominger A, Habs M, Gerdes LA, Schmidt C, Cyran C, Straube A, Linn J, Nikolaou K, Bartenstein P, Reiser M, Hacker M, Dichgans M: Vessel wall inflammation in spontaneous cervical artery dissection: a prospective, observational positron emission tomography, computed tomography, and magnetic resonance imaging study. Stroke 2011;42:1563–1568.
77 Sakurai K, Miura T, Sagisaka T, Hattori M, Matsukawa N, Mase M, Kasai H, Arai N, Kawai T, Shimohira M, Yamawaki T, Shibamoto Y: Evaluation of luminal and vessel wall abnormalities in subacute and other stages of intracranial vertebrobasilar artery dissections using the volume isotropic turbo-spin-echo acquisition (VISTA) sequence: a preliminary study. J Neuroradiol 2013;40:19–28.
78 Yoon W, Seo JJ, Kim TS, Do HM, Jayaraman MV, Marks MP: Dissection of the v4 segment of the vertebral artery: clinicoradiologic manifestations and endovascular treatment. Eur Radiol 2007;17: 983–993.
79 Kim BM, Kim SH, Kim DI, Shin YS, Suh SH, Kim DJ, Park SI, Park KY, Ahn SS: Outcomes and prognostic factors of intracranial unruptured vertebrobasilar artery dissection. Neurology 2011;76: 1735–1741.
80 Arauz A, Marquez JM, Artigas C, Balderrama J, Orrego H: Recanalization of vertebral artery dissection. Stroke 2010;41:717–721.
81 Tan TY, Kuo YL, Lin WC, Chen TY: Effect of lipid-lowering therapy on the progression of intracranial arterial stenosis. J Neurol 2009;256:187–193.
82 Kwon SU, Cho YJ, Koo JS, Bae HJ, Lee YS, Hong KS, Lee JH, Kim JS: Cilostazol prevents the progression of the symptomatic intracranial arterial stenosis: The multicenter double-blind placebo-controlled trial of cilostazol in symptomatic intracranial arterial stenosis. Stroke 2005;36:782–786.
83 Scott RM, Smith ER: Moyamoya disease and moyamoya syndrome. N Engl J Med 2009;360:1226–1237.
84 Yuan M, Liu ZQ, Wang ZQ, Li B, Xu LJ, Xiao XL: High-resolution mr imaging of the arterial wall in moyamoya disease. Neurosci Lett 2015;584:77–82.
85 Kim YJ, Lee DH, Kwon JY, Kang DW, Suh DC, Kim JS, Kwon SU: High resolution mri difference between moyamoya disease and intracranial atherosclerosis. Eur J Neurol 2013;20:1311–1318.
86 Ryoo S, Cha J, Kim SJ, Choi JW, Ki CS, Kim KH, Jeon P, Kim JS, Hong SC, Bang OY: High-resolution magnetic resonance wall imaging findings of moyamoya disease. Stroke 2014;45:2457–2460.

87 Achrol AS, Guzman R, Lee M, Steinberg GK: Pathophysiology and genetic factors in moyamoya disease. Neurosurg Focus 2009;26:E4.

88 Hui FK, Zhu X, Jones SE, Uchino K, Bullen JA, Hussain MS, Lou X, Jiang WJ: Early experience in high-resolution mri for large vessel occlusions. J Neurointerv Surg 2015;7:509–516.

89 Kim SM, Ryu CW, Jahng GH, Kim EJ, Choi WS: Two different morphologies of chronic unilateral middle cerebral artery occlusion: evaluation using high-resolution mri. J Neuroimaging 2014;24:460–466.

90 Salvarani C, Brown RD, Jr., Calamia KT, Christianson TJ, Weigand SD, Miller DV, Giannini C, Meschia JF, Huston J 3rd, Hunder GG: Primary central nervous system vasculitis: analysis of 101 patients. Ann Neurol 2007;62:442–451.

91 Hajj-Ali RA, Calabrese LH: Diagnosis and classification of central nervous system vasculitis. J Autoimmu 2014; 48–49:149–152.

92 Gomes LJ: The role of imaging in the diagnosis of central nervous system vasculitis. Curr Allergy Asthma Rep 2010; 10:163–170.

93 Obusez EC, Hui F, Hajj-Ali RA, Cerejo R, Calabrese LH, Hammad T, Jones SE: High-resolution mri vessel wall imaging: spatial and temporal patterns of reversible cerebral vasoconstriction syndrome and central nervous system vasculitis. AJNR Am J Neuroradiol 2014;35:1527–1532.

94 Kuker W, Gaertner S, Nagele T, Dopfer C, Schoning M, Fiehler J, Rothwell PM, Herrlinger U: Vessel wall contrast enhancement: a diagnostic sign of cerebral vasculitis. Cerebrovasc Dis 2008;26:23–29.

95 Saam T, Habs M, Pollatos O, Cyran C, Pfefferkorn T, Dichgans M, Dietrich O, Glaser C, Reiser MF, Nikolaou K: High-resolution black-blood contrast-enhanced t1 weighted images for the diagnosis and follow-up of intracranial arteritis. Br J Radiol 2010;83:e182–e184.

Seung Chai Jung, MD, PhD
Department of Radiology and Research Institute of Radiology
University of Ulsan College of Medicine, Asan Medical Center
86 Asanbyeongwon-Gil, Songpa-Gu
Seoul 138-736 (Republic of Korea)
E-Mail dynamics79@gmail.com

Kim JS, Caplan LR, Wong KS (eds): Intracranial Atherosclerosis: Pathophysiology, Diagnosis and Treatment.
Front Neurol Neurosci. Basel, Karger, 2016, vol 40, pp 124–140 (DOI: 10.1159/000448309)

Transcranial Doppler

Vijay K. Sharma[a] • Ka Sing Wong[b] • Andrei V. Alexandrov[c]

[a]Yong Loo Lin School of Medicine, National University of Singapore and National University Hospital, Singapore, Singapore; [b]Department of Medicine and Therapeutics, The Chinese University of Hong Kong, Shatin, New Territory, HKSAR, Hong Kong, China; [c]Department of Neurology, The University of Tennessee Health Science Center, Memphis, Tenn., USA

Abstract

Transcranial Doppler ultrasonography (TCD) is the only diagnostic modality that provides a reliable evaluation of intracranial blood flow patterns in real-time. The physiological information obtained from TCD is complementary to the anatomical details obtained from other neuroimaging modalities. TCD is relatively cheap, can be performed bedside, and allows monitoring in acute emergency settings. TCD criteria for intracranial stenosis have been validated against various forms of angiographic studies and serve as reliable tools for screening, diagnostic as well as follow up purposes. TCD findings of intracranial stenosis have acceptable accuracy parameters for anterior as well as posterior circulation. Extended applications of TCD, especially emboli monitoring and assessment of vasomotor reactivity, provide important information about the pathophysiology of cerebrovascular ischemia and risk stratification. Therefore, TCD has become an integral component of the armamentarium of stroke neurologists for understanding stroke etiopathogenesis, planning and monitoring definitive treatment and determining the prognosis. We present the basic principles of TCD, techniques of test performance, diagnostic methods as well as some of the advanced applications of TCD in patients with intracranial stenosis.

Transcranial Doppler

Among a variety of neuroimaging techniques that investigate intracranial arteries for the presence of an atherosclerotic stenosis, Transcranial Doppler (TCD) is the most convenient, cheapest, and noninvasive test [1]. TCD is portable test that can be performed bedside. It provides information about cerebral hemodynamics and various pathological alterations in real-time. In the past several decades, TCD has been brought to acute stroke units, emergency rooms, operating rooms, outpatient clinics and even to the community for screening, to reveal stenosis of large arteries, assess the hemodynamic effects and monitor progression of atherosclerotic lesions. This novel technique is very helpful in understanding the mechanism of the cerebrovascular disease and aids in optimizing various treatment strategies [2–10]. While sickle cell anemia and vasospasm monitoring in patients after subarachnoid hemorrhage remain the established or effective indications, TCD plays an important role in the evaluation of intracranial steno-occlusive disease, emboli monitoring, vasomotor reactivity testing, brain death as well as monitoring during carotid endarterectomy, coronary artery bypass graft operations and thrombolysis for acute ischemic stroke [11].

For patients with intracranial atherosclerotic disease, TCD serves as an initial and reliable screening tool. Unlike the magnetic resonance angiography (MRA), computerized tomographic angiography (CTA) and digital subtraction angiography (DSA), TCD examination is considered operator-dependent. In order to improve its accuracy for the diagnosis of an intracranial stenosis in a neurovascular laboratory, employing a consistent standard scanning protocol and validation of the findings against CTA, DSA or even MRA are the two most important tools. Other relevant factors that influence the reliability of TCD include Sonographers' knowledge of intracranial arteries and changes in flow spectra in various physiological and pathological states. Frequent validations of TCD findings and feedback from referring physicians also play important role in improving and maintaining the quality of TCD results. Neurosonologists or Neurologists responsible for the interpretation of TCD findings are advised to take various certification examinations (administered by the American Society of Neuroimaging and World Federation of Neurology). Similarly, the neurovascular laboratories are advised to get accreditation from various recognized bodies (like Intersocietal Accreditation Commission (IAC) for vascular laboratorios).

Since TCD deploys a 2-MHz pulsed wave transducer, it able to detect transient high intensity signals, it is also used to detect microembolic signals (MES) caused by large artery stenosis or monitor MES intra-operatively during carotid interventions and cardiac surgery [12–15]. Continuous TCD monitoring may also enhance recanalization during thrombolytic therapy for acute ischemic stroke. This is a newly developed therapeutic application of this technology [16].

The Physics and Principles of Transcranial Doppler

Physical Principles

Ultrasound

A normal human ear is capable of hearing the sounds within a frequency range of 20–20,000 Hertz (Hz). A sound wave with the vibration frequency above 20,000 Hz is called ultrasound. The diagnostic frequency of ultrasound in most of thes commercial diagnostic equipments varies between 2–20 MHz. However, the newer diagnostic systems have started providing transducer with higher frequency, especially when the equipment is used for imaging superficial structures. On the other hand, currently available TCD machines employ a fixed frequency transducer that emits 2-MHz ultrasound waves. Current commercial ultrasound systems have no adverse biological effects since the emitted spatial peak and temporal average intensity below 700 mW/cm^2.

Doppler Effects

Ultrasound, including TCD, is based on the Doppler effect, which was named after the famous mathematician, Christian Doppler, who in 1842 explained the color shift of moving galaxies. Doppler effect explains the phenomenon by which an observer can appreciate the direction and speed of a moving object that produces sound continuously. Accordingly, the sound wave from a moving source is perceived as having a higher pitch (due to increased frequency) when the source is approaching the listener and a lower pitch (due to decreased frequency) when the source is moving away. If the sound source is stationary and the reflector is moving, the frequency of reflected sound will still change. This relative difference in the observed frequency (from the emitted frequency) is called Doppler shift. Therefore, the faster velocities of a moving object would produce a greater change in the observed frequency. If the change in frequency is known, the velocity and the direction of the reflector movement can be calculated. However, measurement of the frequency shift will be most accurate if the reflector moves in a direction parallel to the emission ultrasound. In TCD, the reflectors of the ultrasound are tiny red blood cells and it is assumed that these reflectors or the vessels, in which they are moving, are intercepted at an angle of zero or 180 degrees. Since the cosine values of 0 and 180 degree angle are +1 and –1, respectively, the obtained flow velocities are considered real. Furthermore, the assumed 0 or 180 degree angle on TCD never allows overestimation of the velocities.

Continuous Wave Mode and Pulse Wave Mode

Ultrasound is emitted and received by the transducer which utilizes the piezoelectric effect to convert electrical energy into mechanical ultrasound energy and vice versa. The initial ultrasound systems employed two transducers. While one of them continuously produced (speaker or moth-piece of the system) ultrasound waves, the other transducer served the function of a receiver (the ear-piece). Such systems were called as continuous wave (CW) Doppler equipments. Since the time elapsed between produced and perceived sound waves remains unknown in CW Doppler systems, they cannot identify the distance from the reflector to the transducer. Therefore, CW Doppler systems are labeled as 'range ambiguous'.

The current ultrasound systems employ only a single piezoelectric crystal. This crystal emits a bundle of ultrasound waves (pulse) and then waits for the signals returning from various tissue layers or moving red blood cells. Such systems are employ 'pulsed wave' (PW) mode technology. Since the time elapsed between the emitted pulse and returning signal is known, PW ultrasound can identify the distance between the reflector and the transducer. All currently available commercial ultrasound used for medical diagnostics use the PW Doppler technology.

Transcranial Power Motion Mode

Mark Moehring first introduced transcranial power motion mode (PMD or M-mode) in 2002 and this technology has become an integral part of most of the TCD equipments [17]. It can facilitate window location and alignment of the US beam to view blood flow from multiple vessels simultaneously. Since the PMD equipment displays flow from a moving particle at any depth along the ultrasound beam, it helps an inexperienced person to find the acoustic window. Furthermore, the major intracranial arteries are arranged in a fixed fashion (with some variations among individuals), the direction of flow in an arterial segment and, its relationship to the flow spectra in an adjacent artery provides an immense help in easy identification of various branches of the circle of Willis. PMD technology helps in simultaneous monitoring of multiple vessels as well multi-depth emboli tracking. While the red and blue color flow in the duplex systems is determined by the technical settings on the machine, these colors are fixed on TCD and represent the direction of blood flow. Accordingly, red color on PMD indicates blood flow towards the probe and blue color represents blood flow away from the probe (fig. 1).

Transcranial Color-Coded Duplex Sonography

Although spectral Doppler velocity measurement remains the mainstay of vascular ultrasound examinations, the transcranial color-coded duplex sonography (TCCD) has also been developed to help guide Doppler examinations with structural brightness-modulated (B-mode) and functional

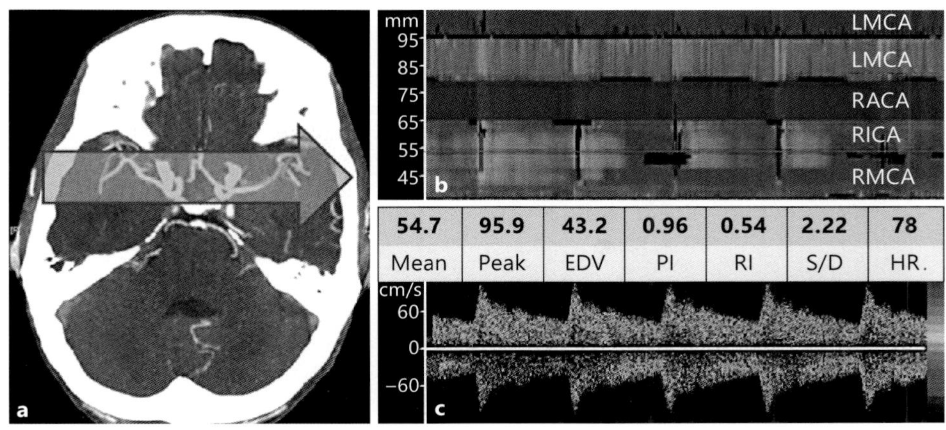

Fig. 1. Transcranial insonation of anterior circulation. Power-mode multigated Trancranial Doppler (TCD) employs 2-MHz ultrasound that penetrates the entire diameter of the skull (**a**). In an average adult skull, midline is believed to be at 75 mm. Thus, the flow signals obtained from beyond 75mm are from contralateral arteries. Panel **b** shows the Power Motion-mode signatures from various intracranial arteries when TCD insonation is performed via right temporal acoustic window red color denoted flow 'towards' the transducer while blue represents flow 'away' from the ultrasound transducer. The arteries are represented according to their depths-right middle cerebral artery (RMCA), right terminal internal carotid artery (RICA), right anterior cerebral artery (RACA), left anterior cerebral artery (LACA) and left middle cerebral artery (LMCA). Panel **c** shows the flow characteristics and velocities obtained from a depth of 54 mm.

color flow imaging of the brain and proximal vasculature. TCCD can identify arteries more accurately since branches of the circle of Willis are recognized more easily with imaging [18]. Previous studies showed that the velocities measured with angle correction on TCCD were significantly greater than those attained with TCD in all vessels [19, 20]. Due to the differences in transducers and emitting crystals, TCCD generally tends to fail more often than TCD to detect acoustic windows. Many centers use commercially available ultrasound contrast agents to overcome the problem of suboptimal temporal acoustic windows. TCCD requires technical skills since the intracranial arteries are quite small (less than 5 mm) in their diameter.

Hemodynamic Principles [21]

Flow Resistance

Similar to the electric current, the blood flow rate (Q) in a vessel is determined by the pressure difference between the beginning and the end of the vessel (ΔP) and the resistance (R):

$$Q = \frac{\Delta P}{R}.$$

Under ideal conditions of laminar flow and constant viscosity in a rigid cylindrical tube, The Hagen-Poiseuille law describes further flow dependence on the following:

$$Q = \frac{\Delta P r^4 \pi}{8 \eta l}.$$

The flow rate is dependent on the viscosity (η), length (l) and radius of the tube (r). If equations A and B are combined, the flow resistance will be:

$$R = \frac{8 \eta l}{\pi r^4}.$$

Thus, increased viscosity and decreased vessel radius will lead to high resistance.

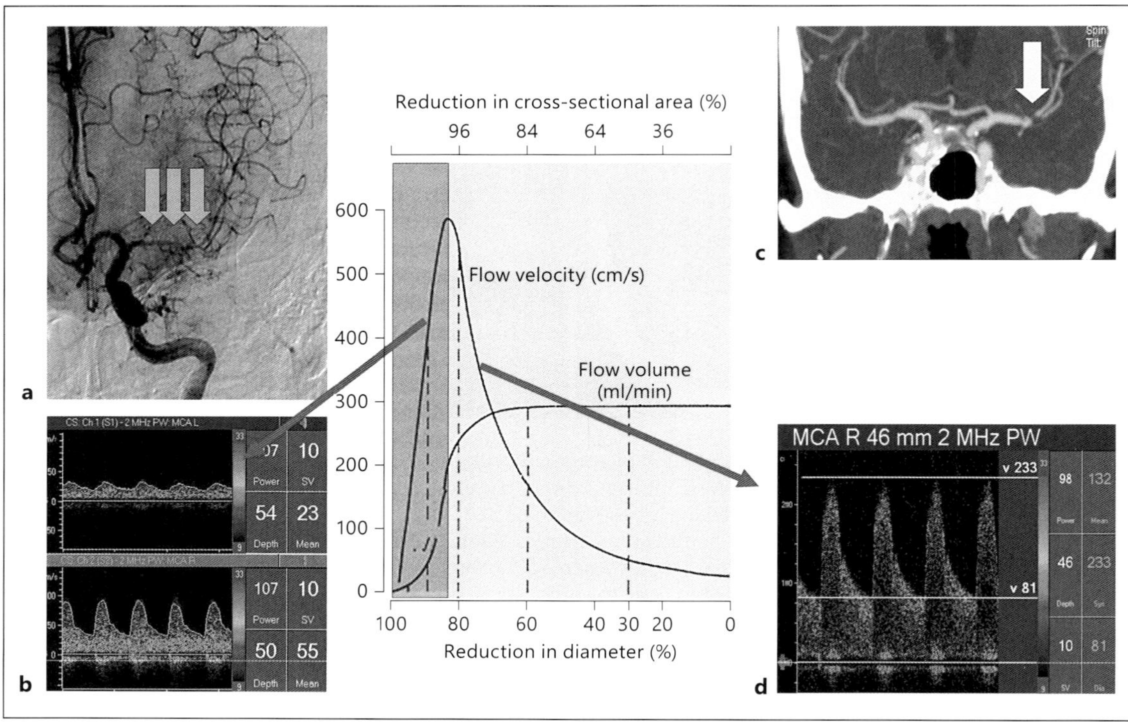

Fig. 2. The Spencer's curve of cerebral hemodynamics. The relationship between decrease in arterial luminal diameter and cross-sectional area with the changes in flow volume and flow velocities is represented in the center. A severe and long (diffuse) segment of middle cerebral artery (MCA) stenosis seen on angiography (**a**) results in 'blunted' spectral waveforms on transcranial Doppler (**b**) from left MCA (compare normal waveforms obtained simultaneously from the right MCA). This relationship is depicted on the shaded pink area on the Spencer's curve (central panel) as rapid decrease in flow velocities and flow volume in the presence of a severe stenosis. In comparison a moderate and 'focal' MCA stenosis on CT angiography (**c**) results in the expected marked elevation of flow velocity on transcranial Doppler (**d**), representing the 'upslope' of the Spencer's curve.

Flow Velocity

The arterial flow velocity (V) is proportional to the flow rate (Q) and inversely proportional to the vessel cross-sectional area (πr^2):

$$V = \frac{Q}{\pi r^2}.$$

Accordingly, reduction of the vessel radius to its half would quadruple the velocity. The relationship between residual arterial luminal diameter, flow velocity and flow volume is represented in the Spencer's curve of cerebral hemodynamics. This curve explains that a reduction in the arterial luminal diameter would lead to increased flow velocity. However, until a critical reduction in the lumen, the flow volume remains almost constant and any further reduction in the former would lead to paradoxical reduction in the flow velocities (fig. 2).

Turbulent Flow

In normal human large arteries, blood flows in various layers (laminar flow), where the flow velocities are fastest in the center and gradually reduces in the peripheral layers (parabolic). However, this arrangement may be disturbed in the

Table 1. Various acoustic windows, arteries insonated through them and their flow characteristics

Artery	Acoustic window	Insonation depth, cm	Frequency shift	Pulsatility
MCA	Temporal	30–65	Positive	Low (<1.2)
ACA	Temporal	60–75	Negative	Low
PCA	Temporal	55–75	P1: Positive; P2: Negative	Low
TICA	Temporal	60–70	Positive	Low
OA	Orbital	40–50	Positive	High
Siphon ICA	Orbital	60–75	Positive or Negative	Low
VA	Occipital	40–75	Negative	Low
BA	Occipital	75–120	Negative	Low

arterial segments with significant stenosis. The Reynolds number summarizes the effect of various physical factors that will lead to a turbulent flow: flow velocity (v), vessel diameter (r), and density of the blood (ρ):

$$Re = 2rv\,\frac{\eta}{\rho}.$$

With smooth vessel walls, turbulent flow will appear if the Reynolds number exceeds 2000. It is important for the sonographers that turbulent flow may also be observed in tortuous arteries, patients with hyperdynamic circulatory states and with wrong scale (pulse repetition frequency) settings on the ultrasound system. Turbulence occurs in high-grade stenosis, due to the chaotic motion of blood in the segment with post-stenotic dilation. Since TCD examination is usually performed with a large sample volume (gate) that covers both stenotic and post-stenotic segments, the turbulence can be heard along with maximal velocities at the site of exit of the stenosis.

There are several findings that indicate the presence of turbulence in intracranial vessels:

(1) Low frequency turbulence appears as high intensity – low frequency signals above and below the baseline; usually seen in systolic and may be accompanied by an audible bruit (fig. 2d).

(2) High frequency turbulence appears as spindle-like clusters near the baseline which may be accompanied by a more pronounced audible component.

(3) Musical murmurs appear as short arch-like signals aligned above and below the baseline symmetrically and accompanied by sounds that resemble musical tones (fig. 2).

These turbulent signals are often recognized by sonographers. However, their presence may not be employed in reliable grading of the severity of an arterial stenosis.

Examination Techniques for Intracranial Arteries

In TCD examination, an artery can be identified by the following criteria (table 1) [21, 22]. First, determine the position and the angle of the probe; second, the insonation depth and third, the direction of the flow. The power, sample volume, gain, scale, zero line and envelope should be adjusted properly to display the spectrum clearly.

Since TCD is operator dependent, it is important for sonographers to obtain sufficient training and follow a standard insonation protocol [21–24].

Middle Cerebral Artery (Figure 2)

(1) Position and the Angle of the Probe. Put the probe at the preauricular temporal window, which is above the zygomatic arch and anterior

to the tragus of the ear. The probe should be aimed slightly upward and anterior to intercept M1 and M2 segments of the MCA. In our experience, following the course of ipsilateral eyebrow of the patient often helps to locate his MCA.

(2) Insonation Depth: The origin of MCA is located at 60–70 mm while the distal segment can be as shallow as 30 mm. It is better to start from the stem of M1 MCA, which will be at the depth of 50–60 mm, and then follow the signal to the distal M1 and M2 at the depth of 30–50 mm, then MCA-ACA bifurcation at depths of 60–65 mm, and to the terminal ICA at depth of 65–70 mm. Since M1 MCA is the continuation of the terminal ICA, it is difficult to differentiate these two clearly. A general rule for a reliable performance is to 'go with the flow'.

(3) Flow Direction. Positive M1 MCA signal (flow spectra above the baseline) means that the blood flow moves toward the probe. A negative signal with the depth less than 50 mm may suggests M2 segment or transcortical collateral flow the in the presence of ipsilateral ICA severe stenosis or occlusion.

Anterior Cerebral Artery (Figure 1)

(1) Position and the Angle of the Probe. Continue temporal window examination and visualize bi-directional signals with increasing depth of insonation.

(2) Insonation Depth. A1 ACA can be detected from depth of 60–75 mm.

(3) Flow Direction. The signal is negative. However, in the presence of severe ipsilateral ICA severe stenosis or occlusion, the A1 ACA flow can reverse due to anterior cross-filling from the contralateral ICA through the anterior communicating Artery (AcomA). Under this condition, the positive signal can be traced from the depth of the MCA to 80 mm. Negative signals can also be present if retrograde filling of the ICA siphon occurs from the same collateral flow.

Posterior Cerebral Artery (PCA)

(1) Position and the Angle of the Probe. Continue with the temporal window insonation and turn the transducer posteriorly and slightly downward if necessary away from the MCA-ACA bifurcation signal.

(2) Insonation Depth. P1 and P2 PCA can be detected from depth of 55–75 mm. P1 PCA will be detected at a deeper depth than P2 PCA.

(3) Flow Direction. The signal is positive for P1 PCA and proximal P2, negative for more distal aspect of P2. In the presence of posterior circulation stenosis, the posterior communicating artery (PcomA) is negative because the collateral flow is established from the anterior circulation, and vice versa. It also can be bi-directional due to tortuosity of PcomA and adjacent vessels.

Ophthalmic Artery and Internal Carotid Artery Siphon (Figure 3)

(1) Position and the Angle of the Probe. Put the probe gently over the closed eyelid on a more lateral aspect and aim slightly towards the inner corner of the orbit.

(2) Insonation Depth. OA can be detected from depth of 40–60 mm while the ICA siphon flow signals are obtained from a depth of 60–75 mm.

(3) Flow Direction. The signal is positive for OA, positive for cavernous segment of the siphon and negative for its supraclinoid segment. A reversed OA flow with low pulsatility is a sensitive sign for severe stenosis or occlusion in the ipsilateral ICA [25]. However, a considerable proportion of patients with ICA occlusion do not have reversed OA due to competency of the intracranial collaterals of the circle of Willis.

Vertebral Artery (VA) and Basilar Artery (BA) (Figure 4)

(1) Position and the Angle of the Probe. Have the patient sit or lie laterally with the head slightly tilted forward, put the probe slightly to the right or the left of the midline.

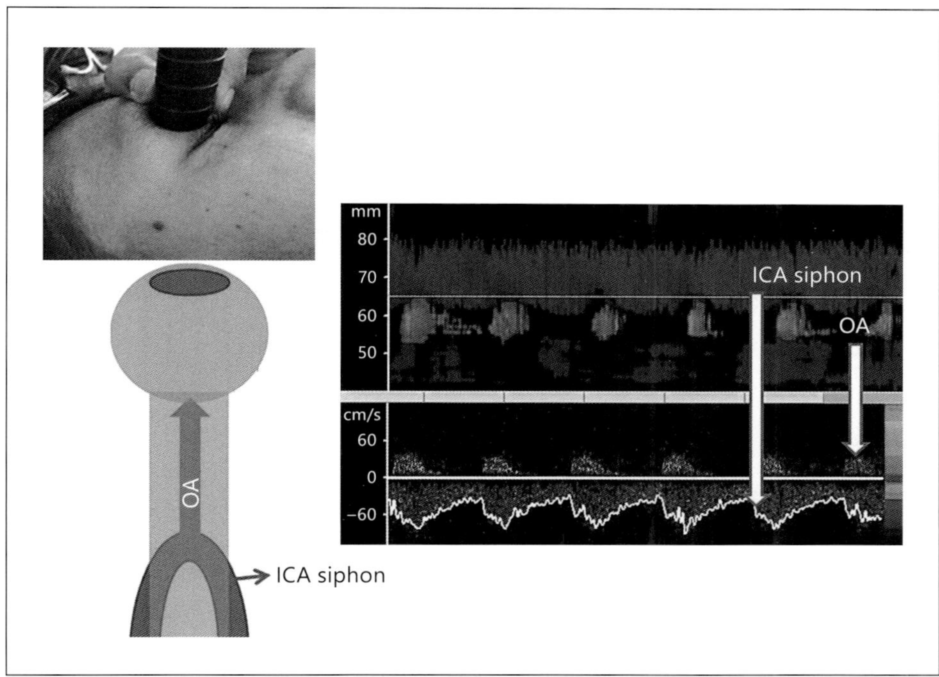

Fig. 3. Transorbital insonation of ophthalmic artery and internal carotid artery siphón. With closed eyed, the transducer is gently kept on the eye, slightly lateral to the mid-point, pointed upwards and medially. Between the depth of 45–60 mm, high resistance flow signals towards the transducer represent flow in the ophthalmic artery. Flow signals between 60 to 75 mm originate from the internal carotid artery siphón. The direction of flow in the sipón can be towards or away from the transducer, depending upon which limb is being insonated.

(2) Insonation Depth. VA can be detected from depths of 40–75 mm, and BA from 75–110 mm. In our neurovascular laboratories, any flow signal at or beyond 100 mm is considered to represent distal BA.

(3) Flow Direction. The signal is negative for VA and BA. Positive signals can originate from the posterior inferior (PICA), anterior inferior (AICA), and superior (SCA) cerebellar arteries. In the presence of a severe stenosis or occlusion in the ipsilateral proximal subclavian artery, VA flow can reverse completely or in systoli showing an alternating signal with high pulsatility towards the probe since the VA supplies the arm also. If the collateral flow comes from the anterior circulation through BA, the flow of BA will also reverse. Flow reversal (complete or only during systole) in the VA or BA represents subclavian steal syndrome.

Diagnosis for Intracranial Large Artery Stenosis

Numerous studies have explored the accuracy and best criteria for the diagnosis of intracranial large artery stenosis [26–36]. TCD has higher accuracy for detection of stenoses in the MCA and BA than in other vessels, largely due to the tortuosity in the latter. Current diagnostic criteria focus mainly on the MCA stenosis of >50% and are mostly based on velocity alone (peak velocity or mean velocity). In

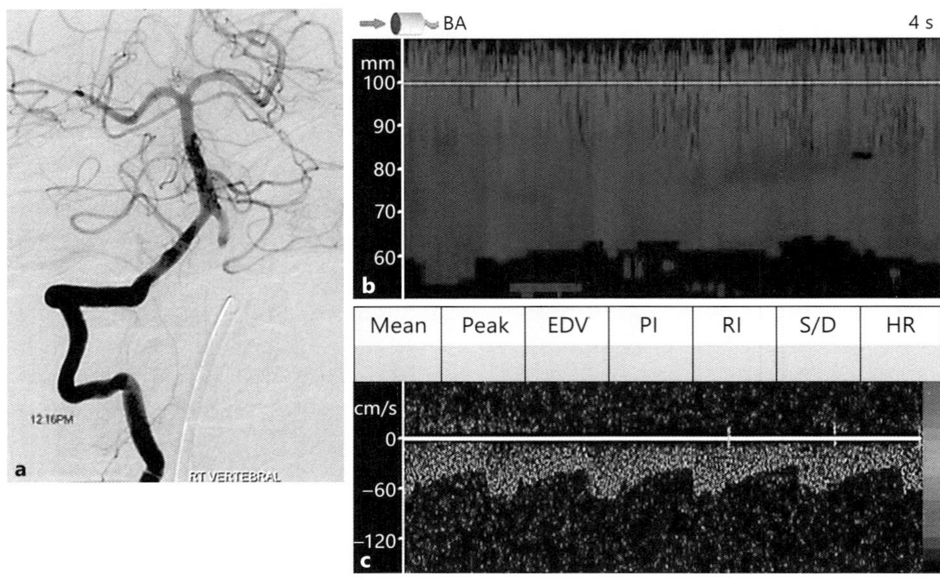

Fig. 4. Sub-occipital insonation of the vertebrobasilar circulation. Flow signals in the vertebral and basilar artery are away from the transducer (**a**, **b**). The transducer is kept just below the insertion of sternocleidomastoid muscle at the mastoid process. Vertebral artery flow is obtained from a depth of 45–85 mm while basilar artery flow signals may be obtained up to a depth of 110 mm (**c**).

clinical practice, interpretation of TCD findings should take multiple parameters into account and be individualized, i.e. not only the velocity values, but also spectrum, waveform patterns, flow pulsatility, presence of collateral flows, conditions of extracranial vessels, systemic conditions, etc. Generally, all these parameters can be divided into direct changes detected at the stenosis, and the indirect changes seen in other vessels. We have recently published these extended criteria for better grading and quantifying the severity of stenosis [37].

Diagnostic Criteria for MCA Stenosis

Navarro et al. [38] systematically reviewed the accuracy of TCD, when compared with digital subtraction angiography (DSA) for the diagnosis of ≥50% MCA stenosis. In this review, mean flow velocities (MFV) of 80 cm/s and MFV of 100 cm/s were frequently used as the cutoff value. In addition, one study also adopted segmental increase in systolic peak frequency of more than 20% [26]; another study used a prestenotic to stenotic MCA velocity ratio of 1: ≥2 in addition to the MFV threshold [32]. This review also showed the overall accuracy of MFV = 100 cm/s was more balanced with sensitivity = 91.8%, specificity = 92.2%, PPV = 88.8%, NPV = 98.4%. Due to differences in patient populations, scanning protocols and analyzed parameters, these published data can be used as a guide for development and validation of local diagnostic criteria to be used by a particular laboratory.

In addition to the focal velocity increase, the velocity decrease should also be considered seriously. In patients with severe stenosis or occlusion, the velocity cannot continue to increase beyond a certain point and start to fall paradoxically, to the ‘other side of the Spencer’s curve’ [39, 40]. Diffuse intracranial stenosis can also produce a decrease in velocity with high pulsatility [35]. To identify these abnormally decreased velocities, it is important to examine the differences between homologous arteries, the differences between anterior and posterior circulation, the waveform pattern and Pulsatility index (PI) values.

To diagnose MCA stenosis, the following parameters should be considered [24]:

(1) Focal velocity increase: MFV ≥100 cm/s or PSV >140 cm/s or follow locally validated velocity criteria; if velocity increase appears to be global, i.e. in ACA, PCA and VA-BA, check systemic hemodynamics (for example, anemia can produce these findings). Velocity decrease: MFV <30 cm/s with MCA < ACA or any other intracranial artery: suspicious of MCA subtotal stenosis or near occlusion. Note that diffuse intracranial disease can produce low velocity and PI ≥1.2 in multiple vessels.

(2) The difference between bilateral MCAs, MCA and ACA, MCA and PCA: a difference >30% should be considered abnormal for high velocity findings.

(3) The spectrum pattern: presence of low frequency turbulence, high frequency turbulence, contour oscillation, musical murmurs suggest significant stenosis (fig. 5e).

(4) The waveform pattern: blunted waveform with low pulsatility usually suggests stenosis proximal to the site of insonation; dampened waveform with high pulsatility usually suggest distal obstructions (fig. 5c).

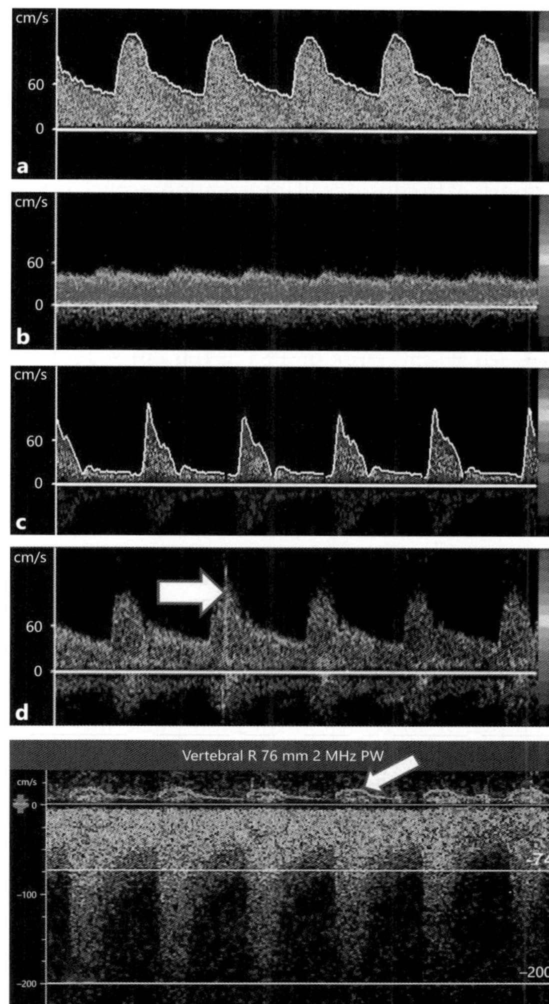

Fig. 5. Various forms of Doppler spectra on transcranial Doppler. A normal flow spectra (**a**) is composed of a rapid upstroke and considerable diastolic flow (between 1/3rd to 1/2 of the peak systolic flow). Panel **b** demonstrates the 'blunted' waveform with delayed upstroke, obtained from arteries distal to the severe stenosis. Arterial segment proximal to the severe stenosis demonstrate 'dampened' flow spectra (**c**), characterised by high resistance flow. Spontaneous microembolic signals (**d**) may be noted during continuous monitoring. In arteries with severe stenosis, the bruit due to turbulent flow may aquire a musical character (**e**), represented by a sinusoidal line.

Diagnostic Criteria for Other Arteries [24]

There are few reports about the diagnostic criteria for the ACA, PCA, siphon and terminal ICA and the VA-BA complex. One study used MFV ≥100 cm/s as abnormal for ACA, MFV ≥50 cm/s for PCA, VA and BA [35] while another study uses PSV ≥120 cm/s for ACA and ICA siphon, PSV ≥100 cm/s for PCA, VA and BA [6]. The multi-center SONIA study showed when diagnosing >50% stenosis with a single velocity threshold, the accuracy is not as reliable (PPV = 55%, NPV = 83%) when using cutoff value of MFV = 90 cm/s for intracranial ICA, 80 cm/s for VA and BA [41]. Besides simplification of diagnostic criteria, these results may be due to tortuosity of these vessels which will compromise the accuracy because of the increased insonation angle. Another reason is that anatomical variations are common in ACA and VA which may further contribute to velocity asymmetry. Therefore, it is important to consider all information, especially related to various hemodynamica adjustments in severe stenosis. Generally, criteria include [24]:

(1) Focal velocity increase [6, 35, 41]: ACA, MFV ≥100 cm/s or PSV ≥120 cm/s; PCA, VA and BA, MFV ≥50 cm/s or PSV ≥100 cm/s; ICA siphon, MFV ≥90 cm/s or PSV ≥120 cm/s.

(2) The normal hierarchy of flow velocity is disrupted: MCA ≥ ACA ≥ ICA ≥ PCA ≥ BA ≥ VA.

(3) Spectral analysis: the presence of low frequency turbulence, high frequency turbulence, contour oscillation, and musical murmurs suggest significant stenosis.

(4) Waveform patterns: blunted waveform with low pulsatility usually suggests a steno-occlusive lesion proximal to the site of insonation; dampened waveform with high pulsatility usually suggests a distal obstruction. Especially for the A2, distal P2, distal BA, and cervical VA which are difficult to insonate, these indirect findings could be quite useful yet need to be cautiously applied due to suboptimal angle of insonation or hypoplasia that are common with these vessels.

Other Applications in Intracranial Atherosclerosis

Microembolic Signal Detection

The detection of arterial emboli using TCD is a well-established technique, which has been commonly used in interventional procedures such as cerebral and coronary angiography, carotid angioplasty, carotid endarterectomy and coronary angiography and in patients with carotid and intracranial large artery atherosclerotic stenosis [14]. Increasing number of studies have shown that microemboli detection is useful in risk stratification, evaluating the effectiveness of novel therapies and in perioperative monitoring [14].

Characteristics of Microembolic Signals

Wide difference between the acoustic impedance of air, thrombus, platelet aggregates, or atheroma and red blood cells causes a significantly increased ultrasound intensity of reflected echoes relative to the blood flow background [12, 14, 43]. In general, characteristics of microembolic signals include: high-intensity (usually above 3–9 dB or higher), transient (duration, 10–100 ms), unidirectional within the flow spectra and accompanied by a characteristic chirp sound [12, 14, 42] (fig. 5d).

Werner et al. reported four kinds of artifacts: changes of TCD settings, probe movement, low flow artifact and electrocautery [44]. Elimination of artifact can be achieved by standard practices and proper parameter settings. To differentiate true emboli and artifact, it is necessary not only to apply automated artifact rejection software but also review possible MES. In contrary to true emboli, artifacts are usually bidirectional and maximal at low frequencies, appearing simultaneously at two depths [42]. True emboli signals may also produce bidirectional signals, yet will have a time delay between two depths of insonation and characteristic chirping sounds. Multi-depths monitoring and synchronous audio recording are encouraged when performing MES detection.

Regarding the nature of the emboli, there are no definite criteria for differentiating the solid and gas emboli [44, 45]. In patients with TCD-detected emboli, determining the source of emboli is important. Accordingly, appearances of an embolic signal in the distal MCA might represent an atherosclerotic plaque in the ipsilateral MCA or the carotid artery. On the contrary, detection of embolic signals in multiple arteries, especially when bilateral, represents the origin to be in the arch of aorta or heart [46]. Gao and Wong [15] reported 3 types of emboli according to the fre-

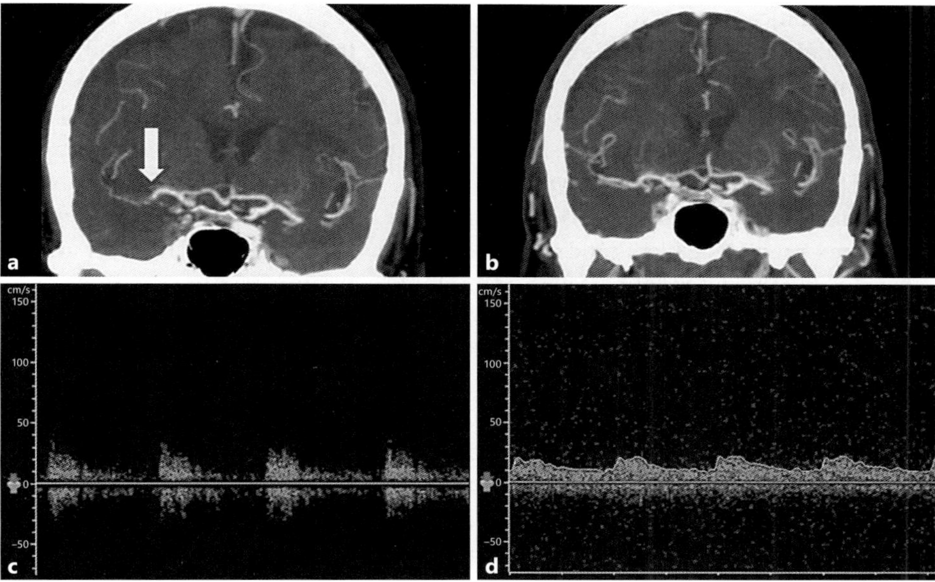

Fig. 6. Transcranial Doppler monitoring during intravenous thrombolysis for acute ischemic stroke. Computed tomographic angiography (CTA) performed before thrombolysis (**a**) demonstrates an occlusion of the right middle cerebral artery (MCA), which recanalised completely (**b**), accompanied by clinical recovery. Transcranial Doppler (TCD) can monitor the offending intracranial artery during thrombolysis. Pre-thrombolysis TCD from the proximal MCA shows high-resistance flow spectra (**c**), suggestive of distal occlusion. At 26 min after thrombolytic bolus injection, rapid recanalization of the right MCA (**d**) was noted, with normalization of the flow spectra and accompanied by clinical recovery.

quencies of these signals displayed on post-FFT (fast Fourier transform- the current method of displaying flow spectra) spectrum: focused-frequency signals (FFSs), bottom-frequency signals (BFSs), and multifrequency signals (MFSs). MES from MCA atherosclerotic lesions may possess special characteristics of multiple frequency on both post-FFT spectra and pre-FFT time domain signals (fig. 5d).

Regarding the time course, most emboli can be detected several days after the ischemic event, and the prevalence will decrease over time, but still are present even 2 weeks after the onset of symptoms [46–49]. Note, that artery-to-artery MES in the MCA can change flow velocity implying that some of these emboli have sizes sufficient to alter cerebral blood flow.

Techniques for Microembolic Signal Detection

In 1998, the International Consensus Group on Microembolus (MES) Detection published criteria for MES detection. According to the consensus statement [14], parameters affect detectability of MES and should be reported in a research paper: ultrasound device, transducer type and size, insonated artery, insonation depth, algorithms for signal intensity measurement, scale settings, detection threshold, axial extension of sample volume, fast Fourier transform size, FFT lengths (time), FFT overlap, transmitted ultrasound frequency, high pass filter settings and recording time. Recently, Droste et al. [50] suggested that the use of 1 MHz instead of 2 MHz may be useful when evaluating the recordings off-line by an experienced blinded observer.

Clinical Significance of MES

Early studies showed that MES are quite common during interventional procedures and in patients with carotid stenosis, carotid dissection, aortic arch atherosclerosis and cardiac disorders [51–57]. MES are more prevalent in symptomatic patients with severe carotid stenosis [52], and these emboli can predict the likelihood of stroke recurrence [58, 59]. Even for patients with asymptomatic significant (≥60%) carotid stenosis, MES can predict the stroke event at 1 year follow-up. If MES are detected from asymptomatic lesions, these patients might also benefit from carotid endarterectomy or stenting [60]. A large ongoing multi-centre prospective study, Asymptomatic Carotid Emboli Study (ACES), will reveal more about the relationship between of MES and carotid stenosis.

For intracranial atherosclerosis, Nabavi and Wong reported MES in acute stroke patients with MCA stenosis [61, 62]. During the last decade, numerous studies have described the association between MES and severity of the MCA stenosis, extension of the ischemic lesions on DWI, recurrent ischemic events, and the effects of therapeutic measures [47, 48, 63–69].

Postert et al. reported MES to be common in large artery stenosis compared with other subtype groups (TOAST stroke classification) [57, 64, 65] and even more common in patients with severe stenoses. In one study, all the patients with peak velocity ≥210 cm/s had MES despite anticoagulation [65, 70]; in another study, 48% patients with severe stenosis on MRA had MES [65, 70]. The number of MES can predict the number of acute infarcts on Diffusion-weighted (DWI) MRI; artery to artery emboli tend to cause multiple small cerebral infarct along the border zone region because of impaired clearance [63, 69, 71].

MES can also predict the recurrence of ischemic events. In a 13.8 months follow up, the presence of MES was the only predictor of a further ischemic stroke/TIA by Cox regression (adjusted odds ratio, 8.45; 95% CI, 1.69–42.22; p = 0.01) [65]. Iguchi found that MES detected at 48 hours of stroke onset were associated with recurrent ischemic lesions on DWI on day 7 [47]; in addition, MES presence after day 7 but not within 24 hours of stroke onset could be a predictor of stroke recurrence at 3 months [47].

Finally, the number of MES is affected by treatment. One study reported more frequent MES in anticoagulated patients than in patients receiving antiplatelet treatment [64]. The relationship between antiplatelet therapy and MES frequency has been investigated in several studies [67, 68, 72], which showed that the number of MES may serve as a marker for assessing the therapeutic efficacy in preventing TIA and stroke recurrence. However the quality control of TCD monitoring remains an important issue.

Intra-Intervention Monitoring

TCD monitoring during the cardiac and vascular interventions can help to guide management strategies and change techniques to avoid complications [73, 74]. Several studies report lower complication rate with monitoring compared to historic controls [74–76]. Numerous microemboli can be detected during intravascular procedures despite the uniform use of distal protection devices, but most of them are asymptomatic [73, 77–80]. Some studies report that early postoperative appearances of MES can predict the perioperative stroke and most of MES are detected within 30 minutes after procedures [13, 81]. However multi-center trial with large sample is required to confirm these findings. De Borst et al. [82] also performed postoperative MES monitoring in addition to intra-intervention monitoring to compare the influence of antiplatelet therapy, which showed no significant difference between the number of postoperative MES among the three groups (Asasantin, Asasantin plus clopidogrel, Asasantin plus Rheomacrodex).

Application of Ultrasound in Stroke Therapy
During systemic thrombolysis for acute ischemic stroke, TCD shows hemodynamic changes with timing, speed and degree of arterial recanalization and reocclusion (fig. 6) [83–86]. Furthermore, 2 MHz TCD also has a safe therapeutic effect of enhancement of enzymatic thrombolysis with tissue plasminogen activator (TPA) [16, 87]. The CLOTBUST trial (Combined Lysis Of Thrombus in Brain ischemia using transcranial Ultrasound and Systemic TPA) showed a higher recanalization rate in patients who received continuous TCD insonation [88]. Microspheres-potentiated ultrasound-enhanced thrombolysis also can promote the ability of sonolysis to induce early arterial recanalization [89]. However, a confirmatory phase 3 study is awaited to establish the role of sonothrombolysis in improving outcome in acute ischemic stroke.

In conclusion, TCD provides important information as a rapid and reliable screening tool for intracranial large artery atherosclerotic stenosis, assess its severity and evaluate various hemodynamic adjustments and collaterals. Detection of microembolic signals, in arterial segments distal to stenosis, aids further in risk stratification. Emboli monitoring by TCD may also help in optimization of anti-thrombotic therapy. Furthermore, continuous monitoring of the occluded intracranial artery in acute stroke during intravenous thrombolysis may help in enhancing the rates of recanalization.

References

1 Alexandrov AV, Babikian VL, Adams RJ, Tegeler CH, Caplan LR, Spencer MP: The evolving role of transcranial doppler in stroke prevention and treatment. J Stroke Cerebrovasc Dis 1998;7:101–104.

2 Budingen HJ, von Reutern GM, Freund HJ: Diagnosis of cerebro-vascular lesions by ultrasonic methods. Int J Neurol 1977;11:206–218.

3 Aaslid R, Markwalder TM, Nornes H: Noninvasive transcranial Doppler ultrasound recording of flow velocity in basal cerebral arteries. J Neurosurg 1982;57: 769–774.

4 Bogdahn U, Becker G, Schlief R, Reddig J, Hassel W: Contrast-enhanced transcranial color-coded real-time sonography. Results of a phase-two study. Stroke 1993;24:676–684.

5 Alexandrov AV, Demchuk AM, Wein TH, Grotta JC: Yield of transcranial Doppler in acute cerebral ischemia. Stroke 1999;30:1604–1609.

6 Wong KS, Li H, Chan YL, et al: Use of transcranial Doppler ultrasound to predict outcome in patients with intracranial large-artery occlusive disease. Stroke 2000;31:2641–2647.

7 Huang HW, Guo MH, Lin RJ, et al: Prevalence and risk factors of middle cerebral artery stenosis in asymptomatic residents in Rongqi County, Guangdong. Cerebrovasc Dis 2007;24:111–115.

8 Arenillas JF, Molina CA, Montaner J, Abilleira S, Gonzalez-Sanchez MA, Alvarez-Sabin J: Progression and clinical recurrence of symptomatic middle cerebral artery stenosis: a long-term follow-up transcranial Doppler ultrasound study. Stroke 2001;32:2898–2904.

9 Purroy F, Montaner J, Delgado P, et al: [Usefulness of urgent combined carotid/transcranial ultrasound testing in early prognosis of TIA patients]. Med Clin (Barc) 2006;126:647–650.

10 Imray CH, Tiivas CA: Are some strokes preventable? The potential role of transcranial doppler in transient ischaemic attacks of carotid origin. Lancet Neurol 2005;4:580–586.

11 Sloan MA, Alexandrov AV, Tegeler CH, et al: Assessment: transcranial Doppler ultrasonography: report of the Therapeutics and Technology Assessment Subcommittee of the American Academy of Neurology. Neurology 2004;62: 1468–1481.

12 Markus HS, Tegeler CH: Experimental aspects of high-intensity transient signals in the detection of emboli. J Clin Ultrasound 1995;23:81–87.

13 Levi CR, O'Malley HM, Fell G, et al: Transcranial Doppler detected cerebral microembolism following carotid endarterectomy. High microembolic signal loads predict postoperative cerebral ischaemia. Brain 1997;120:621–629.

14 Markus H: Monitoring embolism in real time. Circulation 2000;102:826–828.

15 Gao S, Wong KS: Characteristics of microembolic signals detected near their origins in middle cerebral artery stenoses. J Neuroimaging 2003;13:124–132.

16 Molina CA, Alexandrov AV: Transcranial ultrasound in acute stroke: from diagnosis to therapy. Cerebrovasc Dis 2007;24(suppl 1):1–6.

17 Moehring MA, Spencer MP: Power M-mode Doppler (PMD) for observing cerebral blood flow and tracking emboli. Ultrasound Med Biol 2002;28:49–57.

18 Bartels E, Flugel KA: Quantitative measurements of blood flow velocity in basal cerebral arteries with transcranial duplex color-flow imaging. A comparative study with conventional transcranial Doppler sonography. J Neuroimaging 1994;4:77–81.

19 Martin PJ, Evans DH, Naylor AR: Measurement of blood flow velocity in the basal cerebral circulation: advantages of transcranial color-coded sonography over conventional transcranial Doppler. J Clin Ultrasound 1995;23:21–26.
20 Schoning M, Buchholz R, Walter J: Comparative study of transcranial color duplex sonography and transcranial Doppler sonography in adults. J Neurosurg 1993;78:776–784.
21 Reutern GM, Budingen HJ, Ultrasound Diagnosis of Cerebrovascular Disease. Thieme Medical Publishers, 1993.
22 Alexandrov AV, Sloan MA, Wong LK, et al: Practice standards for transcranial Doppler ultrasound: part I – test performance. J Neuroimaging 2007;17:11–18.
23 Bartels E: Color-Coded Duplex Ultrasonography of the Cerebral vessels. Schattauer, Germany, 1999.
24 Alexandrov AV: Cerebrovascular Ultrasound in Stroke Prevention and Treatment. Blackwell Publishing, 2004.
25 Christou I, Felberg RA, Demchuk AM, et al: A broad diagnostic battery for bedside transcranial Doppler to detect flow changes with internal carotid artery stenosis or occlusion. J Neuroimaging 2001;11:236–242.
26 de Bray JM, Joseph PA, Jeanvoine H, Maugin D, Dauzat M, Plassard F: Transcranial Doppler evaluation of middle cerebral artery stenosis. J Ultrasound Med 1988;7:611–616.
27 Zanette EM, Fieschi C, Bozzao L, et al: Comparison of cerebral angiography and transcranial Doppler sonography in acute stroke. Stroke 1989;20:899–903.
28 Ley-Pozo J, Ringelstein EB: Noninvasive detection of occlusive disease of the carotid siphon and middle cerebral artery. Ann Neurol 1990;28:640–647.
29 Rorick MB, Nichols FT, Adams RJ: Transcranial Doppler correlation with angiography in detection of intracranial stenosis. Stroke 1994;25:1931–1934.
30 Demchuk AM, Christou I, Wein TH, et al: Accuracy and criteria for localizing arterial occlusion with transcranial Doppler. J Neuroimaging 2000;10:1–12.
31 Gao S, Lam WW, Chan YL, Liu JY, Wong KS: Optimal values of flow velocity on transcranial Doppler in grading middle cerebral artery stenosis in comparison with magnetic resonance angiography. J Neuroimaging 2002;12:213–218.
32 Felberg RA, Christou I, Demchuk AM, Malkoff M, Alexandrov AV: Screening for intracranial stenosis with transcranial Doppler: the accuracy of mean flow velocity thresholds. J Neuroimaging 2002;12:9–14.
33 Suwanwela NC, Phanthumchinda K, Suwanwela N: Transcranial Doppler sonography and CT angiography in patients with atherothrombotic middle cerebral artery stroke. AJNR Am J Neuroradiol 2002;23:1352–1355.
34 Bang OY, Cho JH, Han BI, Joo IS, Kim DI, Huh K: Transcranial Doppler findings in middle cerebral arterial occlusive disease in relation to degree of stenosis and presence of concomitant stenoses. J Clin Ultrasound 2003;31:142–151.
35 Sharma VK, Tsivgoulis G, Lao AY, Malkoff MD, Alexandrov AV: Noninvasive detection of diffuse intracranial disease. Stroke 2007;38:3175–3181.
36 Tsivgoulis G, Sharma VK, Lao AY, Malkoff MD, Alexandrov AV: Validation of transcranial Doppler with computed tomography angiography in acute cerebral ischemia. Stroke 2007;38:1245–1249.
37 Hao Q, Gao S, Leung TW, Guo MH, You Y, Wong KS: Pilot study of new diagnostic criteria for middle cerebral artery stenosis by transcranial Doppler. J Neuroimaging 2010;20:122–129.
38 Navarro JC, Lao AY, Sharma VK, Tsivgoulis G, Alexandrov AV: The accuracy of transcranial Doppler in the diagnosis of middle cerebral artery stenosis. Cerebrovasc Dis 2007;23:325–330.
39 Spencer MP, Reid JM: Quantitation of carotid stenosis with continuous-wave (C-W) Doppler ultrasound. Stroke 1979;10:326–330.
40 Alexandrov AV: The Spencer's Curve: clinical implications of a classic hemodynamic model. J Neuroimaging 2007;17:6–10.
41 Feldmann E, Wilterdink JL, Kosinski A, et al: The Stroke Outcomes and Neuroimaging of Intracranial Atherosclerosis (SONIA) trial. Neurology 2007;68:2099–2106.
42 Ringelstein EB, Droste DW, Babikian VL, et al: Consensus on microembolus detection by TCD. International Consensus Group on Microembolus Detection. Stroke 1998;29:725–729.
43 Mess WH, Titulaer BM, Ackerstaff RG: A new algorithm for off-line automated emboli detection based on the pseudowigner power distribution and the dual gate TCD technique. Ultrasound Med Biol 2000;26:413–418.
44 Thoennissen NH, Allroggen A, Dittrich R, et al: Can Doppler time domain analysis of microembolic signals discriminate between gaseous and solid microemboli in patients with left ventricular assist device? Neurol Res 2005;27:780–784.
45 Darbellay GA, Duff R, Vesin JM, et al: Solid or gaseous circulating brain emboli: are they separable by transcranial ultrasound? J Cereb Blood Flow Metab 2004;24:860–868.
46 Sliwka U, Lingnau A, Stohlmann WD, et al: Prevalence and time course of microembolic signals in patients with acute stroke. A prospective study. Stroke 1997;28:358–363.
47 Iguchi Y, Kimura K, Kobayashi K, Ueno Y, Shibazaki K, Inoue T: Microembolic signals at 48 hours after stroke onset contribute to new ischaemia within a week. J Neurol Neurosurg Psychiatry 2008;79:253–259.
48 Iguchi Y, Kimura K, Kobayashi K, Yamashita S, Shibazaki K, Inoue T: Microembolic signals after 7 days but not within 24 hours of stroke onset should be predictor of stroke recurrence. J Neurol Sci 2007;263:54–58.
49 Segura T, Serena J, Castellanos M, Teruel J, Vilar C, Davalos A: Embolism in acute middle cerebral artery stenosis. Neurology 2001;56:497–501.
50 Droste DW, Lerner T, Dittrich R, Ritter M, Ringelstein EB: Comparison of a 1-MHz and a 2-MHz probe for microembolus detection using transcranial Doppler ultrasound. Neurol Res 2005;27:471–476.
51 Hellings WE, Ackerstaff RG, Pasterkamp G, De Vries JP, Moll FL: The carotid atherosclerotic plaque and microembolisation during carotid stenting. J Cardiovasc Surg (Torino) 2006;47:115–126.
52 Droste DW, Dittrich R, Kemeny V, Schulte-Altedorneburg G, Ringelstein EB: Prevalence and frequency of microembolic signals in 105 patients with extracranial carotid artery occlusive disease. J Neurol Neurosurg Psychiatry 1999;67:525–528.

53 Koennecke HC, Mast H, Trocio SH Jr, et al: Frequency and determinants of microembolic signals on transcranial Doppler in unselected patients with acute carotid territory ischemia. A prospective study. Cerebrovasc Dis 1998;8:107–112.
54 Markus HS, Droste DW, Brown MM: Detection of asymptomatic cerebral embolic signals with Doppler ultrasound. Lancet 1994;343:1011–1012.
55 Grosset DG, Georgiadis D, Abdullah I, Bone I, Lees KR: Doppler emboli signals vary according to stroke subtype. Stroke 1994;25:382–384.
56 Orlandi G, Fanucchi S, Gallerini S, et al: Impaired clearance of microemboli and cerebrovascular symptoms during carotid stenting procedures. Arch Neurol 2005;62:1208–1211.
57 Azarpazhooh MR, Chambers BR: Clinical application of transcranial Doppler monitoring for embolic signals. J Clin Neurosci 2006;13:799–810.
58 Valton L, Larrue V, Pavy Le Traon A, Geraud G: Cerebral microembolism in patients with stroke or transient ischaemic attack as a risk factor for early recurrence. J Neurol Neurosurg Psychiatry 1997;63:784–787.
59 Markus HS, MacKinnon A: Asymptomatic embolization detected by Doppler ultrasound predicts stroke risk in symptomatic carotid artery stenosis. Stroke 2005;36:971–975.
60 Spence JD, Tamayo A, Lownie SP, Ng WP, Ferguson GG: Absence of microemboli on transcranial Doppler identifies low-risk patients with asymptomatic carotid stenosis. Stroke 2005;36:2373–2378.
61 Wong KS, Gao S, Lam WW, Chan YL, Kay R: A pilot study of microembolic signals in patients with middle cerebral artery stenosis. J Neuroimaging 2001;11:137–140.
62 Nabavi DG, Georgiadis D, Mumme T, Zunker P, Ringelstein EB: Detection of microembolic signals in patients with middle cerebral artery stenosis by means of a bigate probe. A pilot study. Stroke 1996;27:1347–1349.
63 Nakajima M, Kimura K, Shimode A, et al: Microembolic signals within 24 h of stroke onset and diffusion-weighted MRI abnormalities. Cerebrovasc Dis 2007;23:282–288.
64 Poppert H, Sadikovic S, Sander K, Wolf O, Sander D: Embolic signals in unselected stroke patients: prevalence and diagnostic benefit. Stroke 2006;37:2039–2043.
65 Gao S, Wong KS, Hansberg T, Lam WW, Droste DW, Ringelstein EB: Microembolic signal predicts recurrent cerebral ischemic events in acute stroke patients with middle cerebral artery stenosis. Stroke 2004;35:2832–2836.
66 Goertler M, Blaser T, Krueger S, Lutze G, Wallesch CW: Acetylsalicylic acid and microembolic events detected by transcranial Doppler in symptomatic arterial stenoses. Cerebrovasc Dis 2001; 11:324–329.
67 Goertler M, Blaser T, Krueger S, Hofmann K, Baeumer M, Wallesch CW: Cessation of embolic signals after antithrombotic prevention is related to reduced risk of recurrent arterioembolic transient ischaemic attack and stroke. J Neurol Neurosurg Psychiatry 2002;72:338–342.
68 Esagunde RU, Wong KS, Lee MP, et al: Efficacy of dual antiplatelet therapy in cerebrovascular disease as demonstrated by a decline in microembolic signals. A report of eight cases. Cerebrovasc Dis 2006;21:242–246.
69 Wong KS, Gao S, Chan YL, et al: Mechanisms of acute cerebral infarctions in patients with middle cerebral artery stenosis: a diffusion-weighted imaging and microemboli monitoring study. Ann Neurol 2002;52:74–81.
70 Droste DW, Junker K, Hansberg T, Dittrich R, Ritter M, Ringelstein EB: Circulating microemboli in 33 patients with intracranial arterial stenosis. Cerebrovasc Dis 2002;13:26–30.
71 Momjian-Mayor I, Baron JC: The pathophysiology of watershed infarction in internal carotid artery disease: review of cerebral perfusion studies. Stroke 2005; 36:567–577.
72 Dittrich R, Ritter MA, Kaps M, et al: The use of embolic signal detection in multicenter trials to evaluate antiplatelet efficacy: signal analysis and quality control mechanisms in the CARESS (Clopidogrel and Aspirin for Reduction of Emboli in Symptomatic carotid Stenosis) trial. Stroke 2006;37:1065–1069.
73 Markus H, Loh A, Israel D, Buckenham T, Clifton A, Brown MM: Microscopic air embolism during cerebral angiography and strategies for its avoidance. Lancet 1993;341:784–787.
74 Ackerstaff RG, Jansen C, Moll FL, Vermeulen FE, Hamerlijnck RP, Mauser HW: The significance of microemboli detection by means of transcranial Doppler ultrasonography monitoring in carotid endarterectomy. J Vasc Surg 1995; 21:963–969.
75 Ackerstaff RG, Moons KG, van de Vlasakker CJ, et al: Association of intraoperative transcranial doppler monitoring variables with stroke from carotid endarterectomy. Stroke 2000;31:1817–1823.
76 Babikian VL, Cantelmo NL: Cerebrovascular monitoring during carotid endarterectomy. Stroke 2000;31:1799–1801.
77 Gerraty RP, Bowser DN, Infeld B, Mitchell PJ, Davis SM: Microemboli during carotid angiography. Association with stroke risk factors or subsequent magnetic resonance imaging changes? Stroke 1996;27:1543–1547.
78 Gossetti B, Gattuso R, Irace L, et al: Embolism to the brain during carotid stenting and surgery. Acta Chir Belg 2007; 107:151–154.
79 Tedesco MM, Lee JT, Dalman RL, et al: Postprocedural microembolic events following carotid surgery and carotid angioplasty and stenting. J Vasc Surg 2007;46:244–250.
80 Wolf O, Heider P, Heinz M, et al: Microembolic signals detected by transcranial Doppler sonography during carotid endarterectomy and correlation with serial diffusion-weighted imaging. Stroke 2004;35:e373–e375.
81 Abbott AL, Levi CR, Stork JL, Donnan GA, Chambers BR: Timing of clinically significant microembolism after carotid endarterectomy. Cerebrovasc Dis 2007; 23:362–367.
82 de Borst GJ, Hilgevoord AA, de Vries JP, et al: Influence of antiplatelet therapy on cerebral micro-emboli after carotid endarterectomy using postoperative transcranial Doppler monitoring. Eur J Vasc Endovasc Surg 2007;34:135–142.
83 Saqqur M, Molina CA, Salam A, et al: Clinical deterioration after intravenous recombinant tissue plasminogen activator treatment: a multicenter transcranial Doppler study. Stroke 2007;38:69–74.
84 Pagola J, Ribo M, Alvarez-Sabin J, Lange M, Rubiera M, Molina CA: Timing of recanalization after microbubble-enhanced intravenous thrombolysis in basilar artery occlusion. Stroke 2007;38: 2931–2934.

85 Saqqur M, Uchino K, Demchuk AM, et al: Site of arterial occlusion identified by transcranial Doppler predicts the response to intravenous thrombolysis for stroke. Stroke 2007;38:948–954.
86 Alexandrov AV, Burgin WS, Demchuk AM, El-Mitwalli A, Grotta JC: Speed of intracranial clot lysis with intravenous tissue plasminogen activator therapy: sonographic classification and short-term improvement. Circulation 2001; 103:2897–2902.
87 Tsivgoulis G, Alexandrov AV: Ultrasound-enhanced thrombolysis in acute ischemic stroke: potential, failures, and safety. Neurotherapeutics 2007;4:420–427.
88 Alexandrov AV, Molina CA, Grotta JC, Garami Z, Ford SR, Alvarez-Sabin J, Montaner J, Saqqur M, Demchuk AM, Moyé LA, Hill MD, Wojner AW; CLOTBUST Investigators. Ultrasound-enhanced systemic thrombolysis for acute ischemic stroke. N Engl J Med 2004;351:2170–2178.
89 Alexandrov AV, Mikulik R, Ribo M, Sharma VK, Lao AY, Tsivgoulis G, Sugg RM, Barreto A, Sierzenski P, Malkoff MD, Grotta JC: A pilot randomized clinical safety study of sonothrombolysis augmentation with ultrasound-activated perflutren-lipid microspheres for acute ischemic stroke. Stroke 2008;39:1464–1469.

Vijay K. Sharma, MD
Yong Loo Lin School of Medicine
National University of Singapore
Division of Neurology, National University Hospital (Singapore)
E-Mail mdcvks@nus.edu.sg

Kim JS, Caplan LR, Wong KS (eds): Intracranial Atherosclerosis: Pathophysiology, Diagnosis and Treatment.
Front Neurol Neurosci. Basel, Karger, 2016, vol 40, pp 141–151 (DOI: 10.1159/000448310)

Antithrombotic Therapy

Sun U. Kwon · Jong S. Kim

Department of Neurology, Asan Medical Center, University of Ulsan, Seoul, Korea

Abstract

Symptomatic cerebral atherosclerosis including intracranial atherosclerosis (ICAS) is associated with a high risk of recurrent stroke. Antithrombotic agents are the mainstay of therapy in these patients. Several studies have found anticoagulation (warfarin) to increase the risk of bleeding events and have an efficacy no better than that of aspirin. Therefore, anticoagulants are not widely used unless patients develop recurrent ischemic symptoms despite receiving antiplatelet therapy. Because ICAS progression is not uncommon and the risk of stroke recurrence is high when aspirin monotherapy is used, dual antiplatelet agents may be needed at least in the early disease stage. The Trial of Cilostazol in Symptomatic Intracranial Stenosis (TOSS) found that aspirin plus cilostazol was significantly better than aspirin monotherapy in preventing progression (6.7 vs. 28.8%, $p = 0.008$). The TOSS II trial that compared aspirin plus cilostazol with aspirin plus clopidogrel found no significant difference in the progression rate (9.3% vs. 15.5%, $p = 0.092$). However, the overall changes in stenosis were more favorable (i.e., less progression and more regression) in the cilostazol group ($p = 0.049$). TOSS studies have limitations in that the end points were changes in magnetic resonance angiography results rather than clinical outcomes. Based on the Clopidogrel in High-Risk Patients with Acute Nondisabling Cerebrovascular Events (CHANCE) trial results, and the fair outcome found in patients enrolled in the SAMMPRIS (Stenting versus Aggressive Medical Therapy for Intracranial Arterial Stenosis) trial, aspirin plus clopidogrel has been recommended in the early stage of symptomatic ICAS. However, the combination of aspirin and clopidogrel did not show superiority over aspirin monotherapy in ICAS patients in a recent CHANCE substudy. Considering that ICAS is the major pathology leading to stroke worldwide, further studies are needed to identify the best medication strategy in ICAS patients. Until then, physicians may choose appropriate antiplatelet agents after careful consideration of the characteristics of both the patients (i.e., degree of stenosis, stroke mechanism, risk of stroke, and risk of bleeding) and the antiplatelet agent (e.g., side effect, cost).

Introduction

The prevalence of intracranial atherosclerosis (ICAS) is higher in Asians and Blacks. The stroke recurrence rate of patients with ICAS is reportedly

4–19% annually [1–4], which is comparable to the rate of symptomatic severe carotid stenosis [5]. Angioplasty, stenting, or bypass surgery is only occasionally performed in certain specific conditions, and antithrombotic medications remain the mainstay of therapy. However, there are no specific recommendations for the management of ICAS because few antithrombotic trials have focused on patients with ICAS. In this chapter we first briefly present a general overview of antithrombotic therapy for ischemic stroke. We then review the clinical trials performed with antithrombotic agents for patients with ICAS, and discuss future possible directions for better management strategies.

Antithrombotic Agents for Stroke: General Overview

Antiplatelet Agents and Their Mechanisms

Platelet activation and aggregation are crucial pathogenic events in the development of the ischemic heart disease or stroke [6, 7]. The activation and aggregation of platelets usually depend on the activation state of glycoprotein IIb-IIIa (GPIIb-IIIa), which is a bimolecular membrane complex that is specific to platelets and megakaryocytes [8–10] and is strictly regulated by a balance of activating signals from ADP, thrombin, and thromboxane A_2 (TXA_2) receptors and inhibitory signals from nitric oxide (NO) and prostacyclin receptors (fig. 1) [11]. This means that the following mechanisms can inhibit the activation and aggregation of platelets: inhibition of TXA_2 production, blocking of ADP, thrombin, and TXA_2 receptors, or activation of NO and prostacyclin receptors. Drugs such as aspirin, clopidogrel, ticagrelor, cilostazol, and dipyridamole have been developed for this purpose [11, 12]. Aspirin irreversibly inhibits cyclooxygenase (COX)-1 via the acetylation of serine-530, which is close to the active site of COX-1 [13]. Inhibition of COX-1 located in the platelets or endothelial cells prevents the conversion of arachidonic acid into various prostaglandin derivatives including TXA_2 and prostacyclin. Aspirin permanently inhibits platelet aggregation by blocking the production of TXA_2, since anucleated platelets can no longer synthesize the protein [13].

The $P2Y_{12}$ receptor, which is an ADP receptor on platelets, is irreversibly bound by the thienopyridine drugs clopidogrel and prasugrel [14]. Because this particular subtype of the ADP receptor is associated with amplification of platelet aggregation and secretion [14, 15], these drugs irreversibly inhibit ADP-mediated platelet activation. Ticagrelor is a newer form of thienopyridine that reversibly inhibits ADP-mediated platelet activation. Phosphodiesterase (PDE) is a key enzyme for regulating the activation of GPIIb-IIIa in the prostacyclin and NO agonist receptor system (fig. 1). Dipyridamole increases the level of cyclic GMP by inhibiting PDE in this pathway, and it also indirectly affects cyclic AMP levels and inhibits the cellular uptake and metabolism of adenosine. These mechanisms result in the inhibition of platelet function [16]. Cilostazol also exerts an antiplatelet action by increasing cyclic AMP through the inhibition of PDE in platelets [17].

Monotherapy with Antiplatelet Agents for Stroke Prevention

Aspirin

Based on clinical trials carried out in the 1970s and 1980s [18], the Antithrombotic Trialists' Collaboration concluded in 1988 that aspirin is effective in the secondary prevention of vascular diseases [19]. A meta-analysis of 65 clinical trials showed that aspirin reduced the risk of cardiovascular events by 23% compared to placebo [12]. The efficacy of aspirin is limited by the existence of alternative pathways for platelet activation and is partially offset by the inhibition of prostacyclin, a powerful endothelium-derived inhibitor of platelets. Platelet activation is not inhibited sufficiently in a significant proportion of aspirin

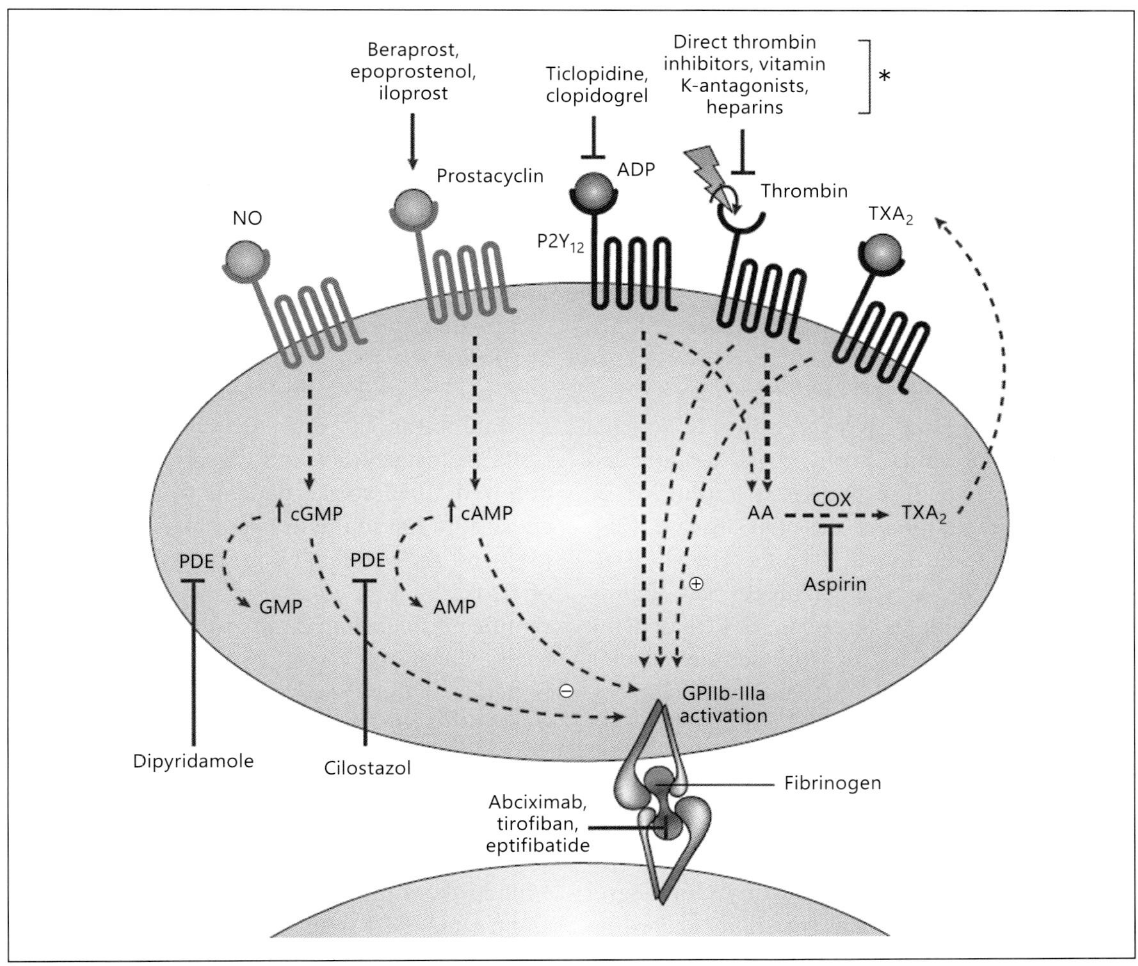

Fig. 1. Mechanisms underlying the effects of current antithrombotic drugs. The principal factor regulating the adhesiveness of platelets is the activation state of GPIIb-IIIa. The affinity status of this receptor is strictly regulated by a balance of activating signals (+ve; ADP, thrombin, and TXA_2) and inhibitory signals (–ve; prostacyclin and NO). Several of these regulatory pathways have been successfully targeted therapeutically, leading to the development of a diverse range of antithrombotic approaches. These include various surface-receptor antagonists (ADP $P2Y_{12}$ receptor: ticlopidine and clopidogrel; GPIIb-IIIa: abciximab, tirofiban, and eptifibatide), inhibitors of platelet signaling enzymes (COX: aspirin; cAMP PDE: cilostazol; and cGMP PDE: dipyridamole), receptor agonists (prostacyclin: iloprost), and soluble agonist inhibitors (thrombin: heparins, direct thrombin inhibitors, or vitamin-K antagonists). AA = Arachidonic acid; COX = cyclooxygenase; NO = nitric oxide; PDE = phosphodiesterase; TXA_2 = thromboxane A_2. Image courtesy of Jackson and Schoenwaelder [11].

users taking conventional doses of aspirin (so-called aspirin resistance), which reduces the efficacy of aspirin in stroke prevention [20–23]. The mechanisms underlying aspirin resistance include poor compliance, poor absorption, and drug interactions [20]. In addition, monocytes and macrophages are another source of TXA_2 – they can regenerate COX-1 enzyme after exposure to aspirin. COX-2 expression can be augmented by 10- to 20-fold in these nucleated cells in an inflammatory condition [23]. Therefore, a fixed dose of aspirin does not exert a constant antiplatelet effect over time. There has been increasing evidence of a relationship between aspirin resistance or variability in the effect of aspirin and the occurrence of thrombotic events. Aspirin resistance was found to increase the risk of death, myocardial infarction (MI), or stroke by more than threefold in a prospective study involving patients with stable cardiovascular diseases [24].

Clopidogrel and Newer Thienopyridines

The CAPRIE (Clopidogrel vs. Aspirin in Patients at Risk of Ischemic Event) trial randomized 19,185 patients with recent stroke, recent MI, or symptomatic peripheral vascular disease [25], and found that the annual risk of a cerebrovascular accident, MI, or vascular death was slightly lower in the clopidogrel group (5.32%) than in the aspirin group (5.83%). Because serious adverse effects were rare in patients treated with clopidogrel, this has become a popular antiplatelet agent for preventing cardiovascular events.

However, insensitivity to clopidogrel is a potential problem. Clopidogrel is a prodrug activated by hepatic cytochrome P450 (CYP) 3A4, and the extent of platelet inhibition by clopidogrel shows wide interindividual variability according to CYP3A4 activity [26]. The platelet responsiveness to clopidogrel among 544 patients with coronary diseases or stroke had a normal bell-shaped distribution when aggregation was induced by 5 μmol/l ADP [27]. Less inhibition of platelet aggregation by clopidogrel was associated with a higher incidence of recurrent cardiovascular events after percutaneous coronary interventions [28, 29].

The newer antiplatelet agents prasugrel and ticagrelor are not widely administered to stroke patients because they are associated with an increased risk of bleeding events that may offset the beneficial effect of a lower probability of resistance. There are currently ongoing trials into the use of these new drugs in stroke patients.

Dipyridamole and Cilostazol

Dipyridamole was used for a long time to prevent atherothrombotic diseases. However, a Cochrane Review of 18 clinical trials found that there was no evidence of dipyridamole reducing vascular events [30]. The requirement for four daily doses due to its short-lasting effect and the occurrence of frequent headaches due to its vasodilatory effects may have resulted in poor compliance and contributed to the reported lack of efficacy.

A clinical study found that cilostazol, another PDE inhibitor, can prevent ischemic stroke: the CSPS (Cilostazol Stroke Prevention Study) randomized 1,052 stroke patients to receive either cilostazol (200 mg daily) or a matching placebo [31], and showed that cilostazol reduced the risk of stroke by 42% compared to placebo without significant bleeding events. Two large clinical trials, Cilostazol versus Aspirin for Secondary Ischemic Stroke Prevention (CASISP) and Cilostazol Stroke Prevention Study 2 (CSPS2), evaluated the safety and efficacy of cilostazol compared to aspirin in preventing recurrent stroke in Chinese and Japanese stroke patients. The CASISP study randomized 720 patients with ischemic stroke within 1–6 months of the index event, and treated them with either cilostazol or aspirin for 12–18 months. Stroke recurred in 12 patients in the cilostazol group and 20 in the aspirin group (hazard ratio [HR] = 0.62, 95% confidence interval [CI] = 0.30–1.26, p = 0.185). The CSPS2 treated 2,757 patients for more than 2 years, with a mean follow-up of 29 months. The annual incidence of the primary end point (the first occurrence of stroke including cerebral infarction, cerebral hemorrhage, or subarachnoid hemorrhage) was 2.76% (n = 82) in the cilostazol group and 3.71% (n = 119) in the aspirin group (HR = 0.743, 95% CI = 0.564–0.981, p = 0.0357), and there were also fewer major hemorrhagic events in the cilostazol group (HR = 0.458, 95% CI = 0.296–0.711, p = 0.0004).

Combined Use of Antiplatelet Agents

As discussed above, activation of alternative pathways during antiplatelet therapy is one of important causes of insensitivity or resistance to antiplatelet agents. Adding another antiplatelet agent that acts via a different mechanism may thereby result in more-complete inhibition of platelet activation. The combined use of aspirin and clopidogrel has apparent benefits over aspirin monotherapy for the management of acute coronary syndrome, as shown by two large clinical trials: the CURE (Clopidogrel in Unstable angina to prevent Recurrent Events) trial [32] and the CREDO (Clopidogrel for the Reduction of Events During Observation) trial [33]. Combination therapy may also be beneficial in managing stroke patients. The Clopidogrel and Aspirin for Reduction of Emboli in Symptomatic Carotid Stenosis (CARESS) trial showed that combining aspirin and clopidogrel significantly reduced microemboli detected on transcranial Doppler (TCD) ultrasonography and the incidence of clinical events during the acute period relative to aspirin monotherapy in patients with symptomatic carotid stenosis [34]. The ESPS-2 (European Stroke Prevention Study 2) and European/Australasian Stroke Prevention in Reversible Ischaemia Trial (ESPRIT) showed the positive effects of combination low-dose aspirin and dipyridamole over aspirin monotherapy [35]. However, another large clinical trial, PROFESS (Prevention Regimen For Effectively avoiding Second Strokes), which recruited more than 20,000 patients with ischemic stroke, failed to show a beneficial effect of low-dose aspirin plus dipyridamole (Aggrenox) compared to clopidogrel monotherapy [36].

Polytherapy is not always more effective than monotherapy, and may also significantly increase the risk of adverse effects. The Management of ATherothrombosis with Clopidogrel in High-risk patients (MATCH) study randomized 7,599 patients with recent ischemic stroke or transient ischemic attacks (TIAs) to receive either clopidogrel alone or clopidogrel plus aspirin for 18 months [37]. The combination of aspirin and clopidogrel failed to reduce the occurrence of major cardiovascular events (ischemic stroke, MI, vascular death, or rehospitalization for acute ischemia) compared to clopidogrel monotherapy (15.7 vs. 16.7%; relative risk reduction = 6%, 95% CI = –4.6 to 16.3%), and it was associated with a significant increase in major bleeding events. The CHARISMA (Clopidogrel for High Atherothrombotic Risk and Ischemic Stabilization, Management, and Avoidance) trial randomly assigned more than 15,000 patients with cardiovascular diseases or multiple vascular risk factors to aspirin plus clopidogrel or aspirin monotherapy, and found similar clinical outcomes between the two groups [38]. Furthermore, the recent clinical SPS3 trial (Secondary Prevention of Small Subcortical Strokes trial) was terminated prematurely due to significant increases in the risk of bleeding and death in patients treated by aspirin and clopidogrel as compared to aspirin monotherapy. Investigators treated 3,020 patients with recent symptomatic lacunar infarcts for 3.4 years, and found that the annual risk of recurrent stroke did not differ between dual antiplatelet therapy and aspirin alone (2.5 vs. 2.7%; HR = 0.92, 95% CI = 0.72–1.16), with a doubled risk of major bleeding events and mortality in the combination therapy group.

Thus, the combined use of aspirin and clopidogrel treatment may have to be applied to those patients who have both a high risk of secondary ischemic events and a low risk of bleeding. With this background, the Clopidogrel in High-Risk Patients with Acute Nondisabling Cerebrovascular Events (CHANCE) randomized, double-blind, placebo-controlled trial [39] assigned 5,170 patients within 24 h of the onset of a minor ischemic stroke or high-risk TIA to combination therapy of clopidogrel and aspirin or aspirin monotherapy. The results showed that the primary end point (any type of stroke within 90 days) occurred in 8.2% of patients in the clopidogrel plus aspirin group, and in 11.7% of those in the aspirin group (HR = 0.68, 95% CI = 0.57–0.81, p < 0.001). The rates of severe hemorrhage and hemorrhagic stroke did not differ between the groups. That study illustrates that the combination of clopidogrel and aspirin is superior to aspirin alone for reducing the risk of stroke in the early period of stroke in patients with TIA or minor stroke, and without increasing the risk of hemorrhage.

Antiplatelet Therapy for ICAS

Anticoagulants for ICAS

Retrospective studies have suggested that anticoagulation is effective in reducing the risk of stroke in patients with ICAS compared to placebo or aspirin [40–42]. Three large multicenter randomized trials were performed in the 1990s to evaluate the role of anticoagulation in secondary stroke prevention: the Warfarin-Aspirin Recurrent Stroke Study (WARSS), the Stroke Prevention in Reversible Ischemia Trial (SPIRIT), and the ESPRIT. The WARSS compared the effects of warfarin (target international normalized ratio [INR] = 1.4–2.8) and aspirin (325 mg/day) in patients with a prior noncardioembolic ischemic stroke. Over a 2-year period the composite primary end point of recurrent stroke or death did not differ significantly between patients treated with warfarin or aspirin (17.8 vs. 16.0%, p = 0.25).

The SPIRIT compared the effects of higher intensity anticoagulation (target INR = 3.0–4.5) and aspirin (30 mg/day) on the composite primary end point of vascular death, nonfatal stroke, nonfatal MI, or nonfatal major bleeding events in patients with a history of TIA or noncardioembolic ischemic stroke. The trial was stopped after the first interim analysis revealed that the primary event rate was significantly higher in patients treated with anticoagulation than with aspirin (HR = 2.3, 95% CI = 1.6–3.5). Over a mean follow-up of 14 months, there were 53 major bleeding events in the anticoagulation group compared with only 6 in the aspirin group. The ESPRIT evaluated the effects of anticoagulation (target INR = 2.0–3.0), aspirin (30–325 mg/day), and aspirin (30–325 mg/day) plus dipyridamole (200 mg twice daily) on the composite primary end point of vascular death, nonfatal stroke, nonfatal MI, or major bleeding event in patients with a history of TIA or minor stroke of presumed arterial origin. The ESPRIT was also stopped after the first interim analysis revealed that the combination of aspirin and dipyridamole was more effective than aspirin alone. Over a mean follow-up of 4.6 years, the occurrence of the primary end point did not differ significantly between patients treated with anticoagulants and all patients treated with aspirin (HR = 1.02, 95% CI = 0.77–1.35). However, these trials did not specifically evaluate the role of anticoagulation in patients with intracranial arterial stenosis.

Based on the above-described results, a double-blind, randomized, controlled trial was performed to compare the efficacies of warfarin and aspirin in patients with symptomatic intracranial artery stenosis: the WASID (Warfarin-Aspirin Symptomatic Intracranial Disease) trial [5]. This trial planned to recruit 806 patients with TIAs or nondisabling stroke caused by angiographically verified stenosis of 50–99% in a major intracranial artery within 90 days of the events. However, the safety monitoring committee recommended stopping enrollment after enrolling 569 patients because of concerns about the safety of those patients assigned to receive warfarin. During a mean follow-up period of 1.8 years, the primary end point (defined as ischemic stroke, brain hemorrhage, or vascular death) occurred in 22.1% of those in the aspirin group and 21.8% of those in the warfarin group (HR = 1.04, p = 0.83). The incidence of major hemorrhage was significantly lower in the aspirin group than in the warfarin group (3.2 vs. 8.3%; HR = 0.39, 95% CI = 0.18–0.84, p = 0.01) along with a lower annual mortality rate (2.4 vs.

5.2%; HR = 0.46, 95% CI = 0.23–0.90, p = 0.02). Based on these results, oral anticoagulation is nowadays rarely recommended in patients with ICAS.

However, the Fraxiparine in Ischemic Stroke (FISS) study suggested that low-molecular-weight heparin (LMWH) may be effective in the management of acute ischemic stroke [43]. Unfortunately, the subsequent larger clinical trials involving different ethnic groups or using different kinds of LMWH failed to reproduce the beneficial effects on the management of acute ischemic stroke [44, 45], which resulted in no type of anticoagulants being recommended for the management of acute ischemic stroke. However, there is still debate about whether the positive results of the FISS study were a chance finding or illustrated actual ethnicity differences in the underlying pathophysiological mechanism of ischemic stroke, because the study was conducted in an area with a high prevalence of ICAS. The investigators of the FISS-tris study assumed that the predominance of ICAS in Asian stroke patients could explain the discrepancy in the beneficial effects of LMWH. To demonstrate this, the FISS-tris study randomly assigned 353 patients with acute ischemic stroke to receive either subcutaneous nadroparin or oral aspirin for 10 days [46]. Because the FISS-tris study exclusively recruited patients with large-artery occlusive disease, 97% of them had ICAS (300 had ICAS only and 42 had both intracranial and extracranial diseases). The results were equivocal: although the primary end point (the proportion of patients exhibiting a Barthel index of ≥85 after 6 months) did not differ significantly between the two groups, the outcome on the measured modified Rankin score – the proportion of patients with modified Rankin scores of 0 or 1 at 6 months – was better in the LMWH group (odds ratio = 1.55, 95% CI = 1.02–2.35). Thus, further larger trials are required to clarify the possible role of anticoagulation in acute ischemic stroke patients with ICAS.

Antiplatelet Therapy for ICAS

Annually 7–19% of ICAS patients reportedly develop recurrent stroke when taking an antiplatelet agent. Therefore, the combined use of antiplatelet agents might be considered for managing symptomatic ICAS. There are factors that should be considered when managing ICAS. In patients with extracranial arterial diseases, strokes or TIAs are usually caused by artery-to-artery embolism, and this mechanism is closely related to platelet aggregation and thrombus formation in the diseased artery. Therefore, strong antiplatelet agents (e.g., achieved by applying dual antiplatelet agents) may be beneficial at least in the early stage of stroke. In these patients, unstable and vulnerable plaque is more important than the degree of stenosis for generation of clinical events. On the other hand, ICAS results in clinical stroke with more diverse mechanisms as described in Chapter 5. It also has been shown that stenosis of intracranial arteries frequently progresses [47, 48], which may be a more serious event than in extracranial arteries; unlike extracranial arteries, hemodynamic disturbances caused by ICAS cannot be compensated for through collateral circulation via the circle of Willis. Previous studies have demonstrated a close relationship between ICAS progression and clinical stroke recurrence [47, 48]. Based on this information, we thought that drugs having actions beyond the simple antiplatelet function – such as inhibition of atherosclerosis progression, suppression of inflammation, or smooth-muscle proliferation – should be considered in the management of symptomatic ICAS. One such drug is cilostazol.

Cilostazol exerts vasodilating and anti-inflammatory effects in addition to an antiplatelet effect, and has been shown to be effective in improving symptomatic intermittent claudication [49, 50], preventing restenosis after coronary stenting, and decreasing the progression of carotid intima medial thickening in diabetic patients [51]. Moreover, because the risk of bleeding events is significantly lower for cilostazol than for other antiplatelet agents, it can be safely used in stroke patients. A meta-analysis of 13 placebo-controlled, randomized trials involving a total 6,165 patients showed that cilostazol reduced the incidence of vascular events by 16% compared with placebo, with no increase in the incidence of serious bleeding events (1.4 vs. 1.5%) [52].

These results prompted the Trial of Cilostazol in Symptomatic Intracranial Stenosis (TOSS) investigators to hypothesize that adding cilostazol to aspirin would be beneficial in the management of ICAS by reducing the progression of symptomatic ICAS without increasing the risk of bleeding events. The TOSS I study [53] randomized 135 Korean patients with acute symptomatic stenosis in the middle cerebral artery or the basilar artery into either the cilostazol or placebo group. Aspirin (100 mg/day) was also administered to all of the patients. The degree of stenosis was assessed at the time of enrollment and at 6 months after treatment using magnetic resonance angiography and TCD. Progression of symptomatic stenosis occurred in 6.7% of patients in the cilostazol plus aspirin group, and in 28.8% of those in the aspirin monotherapy group. Furthermore, the regression rate was higher in the cilostazol group (24.4%) than in the placebo group (15.4%). The differences were significant for both stenosis progression ($p = 0.008$) and the overall changes in stenosis ($p = 0.018$).

After the TOSS results, there still remained questions regarding the best choice of antiplatelet agents in patients with symptomatic ICAS. One of the other options could be aspirin plus clopidogrel, since this combination was more effective in reducing microembolic signals than aspirin monotherapy in the CARESS trial [31]. One concern is the increased risk of bleeding events. Overall, the rates of major bleeding events for combined aspirin and clopidogrel found in major clinical trials are 1.2–2.6%. However, the increased risk of bleeding events in the MATCH trial was partially due to the inclusion of z large number of patients with lacunar infarcts, whereas patients with major-vessel atherosclerosis are expected to experience bleeding events less often. Thus, combination therapy with aspirin and clopidogrel in the early stage of symptomatic ICAS is worth examining.

The TOSS II study compared the efficacies of dual antiplatelet therapies (aspirin plus cilostazol versus aspirin plus clopidogrel) in managing symptomatic ICAS [54]. The treatment was applied for 7 months, and the progression of intracranial stenosis was assessed. The rate of progression did not differ significantly between the cilostazol group (n = 20, 9.3%) and the clopidogrel group (n = 32, 15.5%; $p = 0.092$). However, the overall changes in stenosis were more favorable (i.e., less progression and more regression) in the cilostazol group ($p = 0.049$).

While these results indicate that cilostazol is effective in preventing the progression of stenosis in patients with symptomatic ICAS, the TOSS I and TOSS II trials had limitations: they included relatively few patients, all of the patients were Asians (majority were Koreans), and most importantly, the main end point was the progression of ICAS rather than the clinical outcome. Nevertheless, because the progression of arterial stenosis is closely related to clinical recurrence, cilostazol is widely used for patients with ICAS in some parts of the world (mostly Asia).

The SAMMPRIS (Stenting versus Aggressive Medical Therapy for Intracranial Arterial Stenosis) trial [3] enrolled patients who had symptomatic ICAS (70–99%). That trial compared aggressive medical management using aspirin plus clopidogrel with the combination of medical management and stenting therapy. The outcome in the medical-management group was relatively favorable; patients had a much lower rate of stroke (5.8% at 30 days and 12.2% at 1 year) compared with patients in the WASID trial who met the SAMMPRIS entry criteria and received either aspirin or warfarin (10.7% at 30 days and 25% at 1 year). After adjustment for different baseline characteristics, stroke recurrence was about 2-fold higher in WASID patients [55].

Based on this result, the combination of aspirin and clopidogrel is widely used in some parts of the world. However, SAMMPRIS was not a study that compared the efficacy of certain antiplatelets, and the relatively fair prognosis in these patients may be related to the better management of stroke risk factors (i.e., hypertension, LDL cholesterol, etc.) rather than antipletelets. Moreover, in the more recent CHANCE substudy of 481 patients with ICAS [56], although there was a trend for the recurrence rate of stroke at 90 days to be lower in the clopidogrel plus aspirin group than in the aspirin monotherapy group (11.3 vs. 13.6%), the difference was not statistically significant.

Therefore, further studies are required that examine clinical end points and include larger numbers of ICAS patients with diverse ethnicities. At the present time, physicians may choose appropriate antiplatelet agents based on available data after careful consideration of the characteristics of both the patients (i.e., degree of stenosis, stroke mechanism, risk of stroke, and risk of bleeding) and the antiplatelet agent (e.g., side effect, cost).

References

1 Kern R, Steinke W, Daffertshofer M, Prager R, Hennerici M: Stroke recurrences in patients with symptomatic vs asymptomatic middle cerebral artery disease. Neurology 2005;65:859–864.

2 Mazighi M, Tanasescu R, Ducrocq X, Vicaut E, Bracard S, Houdart E, Woimant F: Prospective study of symptomatic atherothrombotic intracranial stenoses: the gesica study. Neurology 2006;66:1187–1191.

3 Chimowitz MI, Lynn MJ, Derdeyn CP, Turan TN, Fiorella D, Lane BF, Janis LS, Lutsep HL, Barnwell SL, Waters MF, Hoh BL, Hourihane JM, Levy EI, Alexandrov AV, Harrigan MR, Chiu D, Klucznik RP, Clark JM, McDougall CG, Johnson MD, Pride GL Jr, Torbey MT, Zaidat OO, Rumboldt Z, Cloft HJ, Investigators ST: Stenting versus aggressive medical therapy for intracranial arterial stenosis. N Engl J Med 2011;365:993–1003.

4 Jung JM, Kang DW, Yu KH, Koo JS, Lee JH, Park JM, Hong KS, Cho YJ, Kim JS, Kwon SU: Predictors of recurrent stroke in patients with symptomatic intracranial arterial stenosis. Stroke 2012;43:2785–2787.

5 Chimowitz MI, Lynn MJ, Howlett-Smith H, Stern BJ, Hertzberg VS, Frankel MR, Levine SR, Chaturvedi S, Kasner SE, Benesch CG, Sila CA, Jovin TG, Romano JG: Comparison of warfarin and aspirin for symptomatic intracranial arterial stenosis. N Engl J Med 2005;352:1305–1316.

6 Fuster V, Badimon L, Badimon JJ, Chesebro JH: The pathogenesis of coronary artery disease and the acute coronary syndromes (1). N Engl J Med 1992;326:242–250.

7 Falk E, Shah PK, Fuster V: Coronary plaque disruption. Circulation 1995;92:657–671.

8 Phillips DR, Charo IF, Scarborough RM: GPIIb-IIIa: the responsive integrin. Cell 1991;65:359–362.

9 Du X, Ginsberg MH: Integrin alpha iib beta 3 and platelet function. Thromb Haemost 1997;78:96–100.

10 Plow EF, D'Souza SE, Ginsberg MH: Ligand binding to GPIIb-IIIa: a status report. Semin Thromb Hemost 1992;18:324–332.

11 Jackson SP, Schoenwaelder SM: Antiplatelet therapy: in search of the 'magic bullet'. Nat Rev Drug Discov 2003;2:775–789.

12 Collaborative meta-analysis of randomised trials of antiplatelet therapy for prevention of death, myocardial infarction, and stroke in high risk patients. BMJ 2002;324:71–86.

13 Schror K: Aspirin and platelets: the antiplatelet action of aspirin and its role in thrombosis treatment and prophylaxis. Semin Thromb Hemost 1997;23:349–356.

14 Hollopeter G, Jantzen HM, Vincent D, Li G, England L, Ramakrishnan V, Yang RB, Nurden P, Nurden A, Julius D, Conley PB: Identification of the platelet adp receptor targeted by antithrombotic drugs. Nature 2001;409:202–207.

15 Fontana P, Dupont A, Gandrille S, Bachelot-Loza C, Reny JL, Aiach M, Gaussem P: Adenosine diphosphate-induced platelet aggregation is associated with P2Y12 gene sequence variations in healthy subjects. Circulation 2003;108:989–995.

16 Movsesian MA: Therapeutic potential of cyclic nucleotide phosphodiesterase inhibitors in heart failure. Expert Opin Investig Drugs 2000;9:963–973.

17 Umekawa H, Tanaka T, Kimura Y, Hidaka H: Purification of cyclic adenosine monophosphate phosphodiesterase from human platelets using new-inhibitor sepharose chromatography. Biochem Pharmacol 1984;33:3339–3344.

18 Genton E, Barnett HJ, Fields WS, Gent M, Hoak JC: XIV. Cerebral ischemia: the role of thrombosis and of antithrombotic therapy. Study group on antithrombotic therapy. Stroke 1977;8:150–175.

19 Secondary prevention of vascular disease by prolonged antiplatelet treatment. Antiplatelet trialists' collaboration. Br Med J (Clin Res Ed) 1988;296:320–331.

20 Bhatt DL: Aspirin resistance: more than just a laboratory curiosity. J Am Coll Cardiol 2004;43:1127–1129.

21 Jilma B: Therapeutic failure or resistance to aspirin. J Am Coll Cardiol 2004; 43:1332;author reply 1332–1333.
22 Pulcinelli FM, Pignatelli P, Celestini A, Riondino S, Gazzaniga PP, Violi F: Inhibition of platelet aggregation by aspirin progressively decreases in long-term treated patients. J Am Coll Cardiol 2004; 43:979–984.
23 Eikelboom JW, Hirsh J, Weitz JI, Johnston M, Yi Q, Yusuf S: Aspirin-resistant thromboxane biosynthesis and the risk of myocardial infarction, stroke, or cardiovascular death in patients at high risk for cardiovascular events. Circulation 2002;105:1650–1655.
24 Gum PA, Kottke-Marchant K, Welsh PA, White J, Topol EJ: A prospective, blinded determination of the natural history of aspirin resistance among stable patients with cardiovascular disease. J Am Coll Cardiol 2003;41:961–965.
25 A randomised, blinded, trial of clopidogrel versus aspirin in patients at risk of ischaemic events (caprie). Caprie steering committee. Lancet 1996;348:1329–1339.
26 Lau WC, Gurbel PA, Watkins PB, Neer CJ, Hopp AS, Carville DG, Guyer KE, Tait AR, Bates ER: Contribution of hepatic cytochrome p450 3a4 metabolic activity to the phenomenon of clopidogrel resistance. Circulation 2004;109: 166–171.
27 Serebruany VL, Steinhubl SR, Berger PB, Malinin AI, Bhatt DL, Topol EJ: Variability in platelet responsiveness to clopidogrel among 544 individuals. J Am Coll Cardiol 2005;45:246–251.
28 Matetzky S, Shenkman B, Guetta V, Shechter M, Beinart R, Goldenberg I, Novikov I, Pres H, Savion N, Varon D, Hod H: Clopidogrel resistance is associated with increased risk of recurrent atherothrombotic events in patients with acute myocardial infarction. Circulation 2004;109:3171–3175.
29 Gurbel PA, Bliden KP, Hiatt BL, O'Connor CM: Clopidogrel for coronary stenting: response variability, drug resistance, and the effect of pretreatment platelet reactivity. Circulation 2003;107: 2908–2913.
30 De Schryver EL, Algra A, van Gijn J: Cochrane review: dipyridamole for preventing major vascular events in patients with vascular disease. Stroke 2003; 34:2072–2080.
31 Gotoh F, Tohgi H, Hirai S, Terashi A, Fukuuchi Y, Otomo E, Shinohara Y, Itoh E, Matsuda T, Sawada T, Yamaguchi T, Nishimaru K, Ohashi Y: Cilostazol stroke prevention study: a placebo-controlled double-blind trial for secondary prevention of cerebral infarction. J Stroke Cerebrovasc Dis 2000;9:147–157.
32 Fox KA, Mehta SR, Peters R, Zhao F, Lakkis N, Gersh BJ, Yusuf S: Benefits and risks of the combination of clopidogrel and aspirin in patients undergoing surgical revascularization for non-st-elevation acute coronary syndrome: the clopidogrel in unstable angina to prevent recurrent ischemic events (cure) trial. Circulation 2004;110:1202–1208.
33 Steinhubl SR, Berger PB, Mann JT, 3rd, Fry ET, DeLago A, Wilmer C, Topol EJ: Early and sustained dual oral antiplatelet therapy following percutaneous coronary intervention: a randomized controlled trial. JAMA 2002;288:2411–2420.
34 Markus HS, Droste DW, Kaps M, Larrue V, Lees KR, Siebler M, Ringelstein EB: Dual antiplatelet therapy with clopidogrel and aspirin in symptomatic carotid stenosis evaluated using doppler embolic signal detection: the clopidogrel and aspirin for reduction of emboli in symptomatic carotid stenosis (caress) trial. Circulation 2005;111:2233–2240.
35 Diener HC, Cunha L, Forbes C, Sivenius J, Smets P, Lowenthal A: European stroke prevention study. 2. Dipyridamole and acetylsalicylic acid in the secondary prevention of stroke. J Neurol Sci 1996;143:1–13.
36 Diener HC, Sacco R, Yusuf S: Rationale, design and baseline data of a randomized, double-blind, controlled trial comparing two antithrombotic regimens (a fixed-dose combination of extended-release dipyridamole plus asa with clopidogrel) and telmisartan versus placebo in patients with strokes: the prevention regimen for effectively avoiding second strokes trial (profess). Cerebrovasc Dis 2007;23:368–380.
37 Diener HC, Bogousslavsky J, Brass LM, Cimminiello C, Csiba L, Kaste M, Leys D, Matias-Guiu J, Rupprecht HJ: Aspirin and clopidogrel compared with clopidogrel alone after recent ischaemic stroke or transient ischaemic attack in high-risk patients (match): randomised, double-blind, placebo-controlled trial. Lancet 2004;364:331–337.
38 Bhatt DL, Fox KA, Hacke W, Berger PB, Black HR, Boden WE, Cacoub P, Cohen EA, Creager MA, Easton JD, Flather MD, Haffner SM, Hamm CW, Hankey GJ, Johnston SC, Mak KH, Mas JL, Montalescot G, Pearson TA, Steg PG, Steinhubl SR, Weber MA, Brennan DM, Fabry-Ribaudo L, Booth J, Topol EJ: Clopidogrel and aspirin versus aspirin alone for the prevention of atherothrombotic events. N Engl J Med 2006;354:1706–1717.
39 Wang Y, Wang Y, Zhao X, Liu L, Wang D, Wang C, Wang C, Li H, Meng X, Cui L, Jia J, Dong Q, Xu A, Zeng J, Li Y, Wang Z, Xia H, Johnston SC, Investigators C: Clopidogrel with aspirin in acute minor stroke or transient ischemic attack. N Engl J Med 2013;369:11–19.
40 Olsson JE, Brechter C, Backlund H, Krook H, Muller R, Nitelius E, Olsson O, Tornberg A: Anticoagulant vs antiplatelet therapy as prophylactic against cerebral infarction in transient ischemic attacks. Stroke 1980;11:4–9.
41 Whisnant JP, Cartlidge NE, Elveback LR: Carotid and vertebral-basilar transient ischemic attacks: effect of anticoagulants, hypertension, and cardiac disorders on survival and stroke occurrence – a population study. Ann Neurol 1978;3:107–115.
42 Chimowitz MI, Kokkinos J, Strong J, Brown MB, Levine SR, Silliman S, Pessin MS, Weichel E, Sila CA, Furlan AJ, et al: The warfarin-aspirin symptomatic intracranial disease study. Neurology 1995;45:1488–1493.
43 Kay R, Wong KS, Yu YL, Chan YW, Tsoi TH, Ahuja AT, Chan FL, Fong KY, Law CB, Wong A: Low-molecular-weight heparin for the treatment of acute ischemic stroke. N Engl J Med 1995;333: 1588–1593.
44 Low molecular weight heparinoid, org 10172 (danaparoid), and outcome after acute ischemic stroke: A randomized controlled trial. The publications committee for the trial of org 10172 in acute stroke treatment (toast) investigators. JAMA 1998;279:1265–1272.
45 Bath PM, Lindenstrom E, Boysen G, De Deyn P, Friis P, Leys D, Marttila R, Olsson J, O'Neill D, Orgogozo J, Ringelstein B, van der Sande J, Turpie AG: Tinzaparin in acute ischaemic stroke (taist): a randomised aspirin-controlled trial. Lancet 2001;358:702–710.

46 Wong KS, Chen C, Ng PW, Tsoi TH, Li HL, Fong WC, Yeung J, Wong CK, Yip KK, Gao H, Wong HB: Low-molecular-weight heparin compared with aspirin for the treatment of acute ischaemic stroke in asian patients with large artery occlusive disease: a randomised study. Lancet Neurol 2007;6:407–413.
47 Wong KS, Li H, Lam WW, Chan YL, Kay R: Progression of middle cerebral artery occlusive disease and its relationship with further vascular events after stroke. Stroke 2002;33:532–536.
48 Arenillas JF, Molina CA, Montaner J, Abilleira S, Gonzalez-Sanchez MA, Alvarez-Sabin J: Progression and clinical recurrence of symptomatic middle cerebral artery stenosis: a long-term follow-up transcranial doppler ultrasound study. Stroke 2001;32:2898–2904.
49 Robless P, Mikhailidis DP, Stansby GP: Cilostazol for peripheral arterial disease. Cochrane Database Syst Rev 2007: CD003748.
50 Thompson PD, Zimet R, Forbes WP, Zhang P: Meta-analysis of results from eight randomized, placebo-controlled trials on the effect of cilostazol on patients with intermittent claudication. Am J Cardiol 2002;90:1314–1319.
51 Douglas JS Jr, Holmes DR Jr, Kereiakes DJ, Grines CL, Block E, Ghazzal ZM, Morris DC, Liberman H, Parker K, Jurkovitz C, Murrah N, Foster J, Hyde P, Mancini GB, Weintraub WS: Coronary stent restenosis in patients treated with cilostazol. Circulation 2005;112:2826–2832.
52 Uchiyama S, Demaerschalk BM, Goto S, Shinohara Y, Gotoh F, Stone WM, Money SR, Kwon SU: Stroke prevention by cilostazol in patients with atherothrombosis: meta-analysis of placebo-controlled randomized trials. J Stroke Cerebrovasc Dis 2009;18:482–490.
53 Kwon SU, Cho YJ, Koo JS, Bae HJ, Lee YS, Hong KS, Lee JH, Kim JS: Cilostazol prevents the progression of the symptomatic intracranial arterial stenosis: the multicenter double-blind placebo-controlled trial of cilostazol in symptomatic intracranial arterial stenosis. Stroke 2005;36:782–786.
54 Kwon SU, Hong KS, Kang DW, Park JM, Lee JH, Cho YJ, Yu KH, Koo JS, Wong KS, Lee SH, Lee KB, Kim DE, Jeong SW, Bae HJ, Lee BC, Han MK, Rha JH, Kim HY, Mok VC, Lee YS, Kim GM, Suwanwela NC, Yun SC, Nah HW, Kim JS: Efficacy and safety of combination antiplatelet therapies in patients with symptomatic intracranial atherosclerotic stenosis. Stroke 2011;42:2883–2890.
55 Chaturvedi S, Turan TN, Lynn MJ, Derdeyn CP, Fiorella D, Janis LS, Chimowitz MI, Investigators ST: Do patient characteristics explain the differences in outcome between medically treated patients in sammpris and wasid? Stroke 2015;46:2562–2567.
56 Liu L, Wong KS, Leng X, Pu Y, Wang Y, Jing J, Zou X, Pan Y, Wang A, Meng X, Wang C, Zhao X, Soo Y, Johnston SC, Wang Y, Investigators C: Dual antiplatelet therapy in stroke and icas: subgroup analysis of chance. Neurology 2015;85: 1154–1162.

Sun U. Kwon, MD, PhD
Department of Neurology, Asan Medical Center, University of Ulsan
Asanbyeongwon-gil 86, Songpa-gu
Seoul 138-736 (Korea)
E-Mail sukwon@amc.seoul.kr

Kim JS, Caplan LR, Wong KS (eds): Intracranial Atherosclerosis: Pathophysiology, Diagnosis and Treatment.
Front Neurol Neurosci. Basel, Karger, 2016, vol 40, pp 152–163 (DOI: 10.1159/000448311)

Angioplasty and Stenting

Thomas W. Leung[a] • Ashley M. Wabnitz[b] • Zhongrong Miao[c] • Marc I. Chimowitz[b]

[a]Department of Medicine and Therapeutics, The Prince of Wales Hospital, The Chinese University of Hong Kong, Hong Kong, SAR, China; [b]Department of Neurosciences, Medical University of South Carolina, Charleston, S.C., USA; [c]Department of Interventional Neuroradiology, Beijing Tiantan Hospital, Capital Medical University, Beijing, China

Abstract

The high rate of recurrent strokes in patients with intracranial atherosclerotic disease (ICAS) despite medical therapy prompted intracranial angioplasty and/or stenting an adjunctive treatment option. The minute calibers of cerebral arteries, the relative paucity of supporting medial and adventitia layers, the presence of end-anastomosing perforator branches, and the vascular tortuosity from groin to head all demand specialized operative skills and dedicated tools. Since the stroke mechanism of ICAS is diverse, patient selection for endovascular treatment requires a sound understanding of the underlying pathophysiology. Patients with territorial cerebral hypo-perfusion associated with a high-grade steno-occlusive lesion may benefit most from endovascular revascularization. On the other hand, patients with atheromatous branch disease may stand a higher risk of perforator stroke from 'snow plowing' effect if angioplasty or stenting is inadvertently performed. A joint evaluation on the indication, procedural risks and benefits, and an individualized perioperative care plan by a stroke neurologist and a neurointerventionist is crucial prior to a procedure. Currently, the U.S. Food and Drug Administration approved Wingspan for patients who have developed two or more strokes despite aggressive medical management. The treatment indication will likely evolve in parallel with the advancement of endovascular techniques and our understanding of ICAS.

Introduction

The prognosis of intracranial atherosclerotic disease (ICAS) is unfavorable despite medical therapy. In WASID (Warfarin-Aspirin Symptomatic Intracranial Disease trial), the risks of stroke or death in the first year after a stroke attributed to ICAS (50–99% stenosis) were 15% and 17% when treated by aspirin or warfarin [1, 2]. In the recent CHANCE study (Clopidogrel in High-risk patients with Acute Non-disabling Cerebrovascular Events), among patients with non-cardioembolic stroke or transient ischemic attacks, ICAS patients had significantly higher rates of recurrent stroke at 90 days than those without (12.5 vs. 5.4%; $p < 0.0001$), irrespective of the antiplatelet regimen assigned [3]. The excessive risk of recurrent stroke in ICAS patients prompted consideration for an adjunctive therapy, notably stenting and/or angioplasty. This chapter reviews the evolution of endovascular treatment for symptomatic ICAS and the current controversy regarding the benefit of this procedure.

The History of Angioplasty and Stenting for ICAS

Intracranial angioplasty and stenting aims to improve cerebral perfusion and restore luminal patency through a minimally invasive approach. Through a vascular sheath at the femoral artery, guide-wires, micro-catheters, balloons and stents swiftly gain access to cerebral arteries and rectify steno-occlusive lesions. Dated back in 1980, Sundt et al. [4] first reported successful balloon angioplasty in 2 patients with refractory basilar artery stenosis. Since then, many case reports and series have described the technical feasibility of balloon angioplasty in ICAS [5–7]. However, procedural complications such as intimal dissection, thrombosis, recoiling and vessel rupture were frequent in those early series. Subsequently, Connors and Wojak advocated slow and submaximal balloon dilatation in 1999 to reduce vascular trauma, and this has now become a widely adopted practice [8, 9].

Although revascularization by balloon angioplasty alone was technically less demanding, recoiling and dissection are significant problems in the absence of mechanical support by a stent. In 1996, Feldman et al. [10] reported off-label use of coronary balloon-expandable stent (Palmaz-Schatz) for stenosis in the intracranial segment of the internal carotid artery (ICA). Many case reports and series on stenting then followed [11–14]. To reduce the complication rates, Levy et al. [15] introduced the staged treatment approach; and de Rochemont Rdu et al. [16] evaluated the safety and efficacy of undersized stents. Jiang et al. [17–19] explored three factors (lesion location, morphology and vascular tortuosity) that could be associated with technical success and procedural complications. Drug-eluted stents were also employed in a small cohort of ICAD patients [20]. Prospective multi-center study was not available until in 2004, when SSYLVIA (Stenting of SYmptomatic atherosclerotic Lesions in the Vertebral or Intracranial Arteries) showed the feasibility of Neurolink intracranial stent system, a balloon-expandable stent system (Guidant Corp: Indianapolis, IN) for intracranial ICA, middle cerebral artery (MCA) and vertebro-basilar stenoses in a non-randomized study [21]. So far, however, no study has prospectively compared balloon angioplasty versus stenting in the treatment of ICAS. A retrospective study showed that stenting was more effective than angioplasty alone in terms of the initial and late gains in diameter for the petrous and cavernous segment ICA stenosis [22].

The application of balloon-expandable stents in intracranial vasculature has certain limitations and risks. First, the relatively high profile of balloon-mounted stent limits the trackability of the stent system in negotiating tight stenosis. Plaque and stent dislodgement may occur while advancing a tortuous route. Moreover, the high nominal pressure of balloon-expandable stents may aggravate vascular trauma cause dissection. Furthermore, although the uniform post-deployment diameter of balloon-expandable stent may improve the immediate luminal gain and help reduce the restenosis rate [23], failure of the stent to conform to the natural tapering or anatomic curvature of the parent artery may result in over-dilatation or poor stent-to-wall apposition [24].

Wingspan stent system was designed to overcome the shortcomings of balloon-mounted stents, which involves submaximal balloon angioplasty (Gateway balloon), followed by deployment of a self-expandable stent (Wingspan) that is pre-loaded in a 3.5F multi-lumen over-the-wire delivery catheter [25, 26]. The nitinol stent provides more than twice the radial outward strength of a Neuroform III stent (Boston Scientific).

Based on the European Wingspan pilot study, the US Food and Drug Administration approved the Wingspan stent system under the Humanitarian Device Exemption for treatment in patients with symptomatic ICAS ≥50% and are refractory to medical treatment [25, 26].

Peri-Operative Care and Technical Nuance

A joint pre-operative evaluation by stroke neurologists, neuro-radiologists and neuro-interventionists is crucial. The multidisciplinary team should analyze the stroke etiology and mechanism, tabulate the procedural risk and benefit, and formulate a customized treatment plan if the procedure is deemed indicated and feasible (see 'Patient Selection' below). Stringent control of cardiovascular risks is essential. Dual antiplatelet agents (commonly aspirin plus clopidogrel) are prescribed from one week before till 3 months after stent implantation.

Intracranial angioplasty and/or stenting can be performed under general or local anesthesia. While general anesthesia minimizes anxiety and untoward movements during the procedure, one advantage of local anesthesia is instantaneous neurologic evaluations throughout. In a transfemoral approach, a guide catheter (usually 6F) will perch at the distal cervical segment of an ICA for MCA stenosis; or distal V2 segment of a vertebral artery (VA) for basilar artery stenosis. In patients with a singular VA, or if the target VA is <3.0 mm in diameter or severely tortuous, the guide catheter, preferably an 8F catheter for stronger support, may need to be positioned in the subclavian artery.

Guided by activated clotting time (ACT), anti-coagulation is maintained intra-operatively by an intravenous bolus of conventional heparin at the beginning, followed by either a continuous infusion or another bolus of heparin one hour later. The optimal anti-coagulation intensity for intracranial stenting remains uncertain. Two regimens have been tested out. In one regimen, heparin was given in a bolus of 3,000 units followed by 800 units/h to maintain an ACT between 250–300 s. Another regimen involved a lower dose of heparin, in which the bolus and infusion were 2,000 and 500 units/h, respectively, aiming at an ACT of 160–220 s (same as what was used in PROACT II Study) [27]. It was found that the rate of intracranial bleeding was 7.4% (5/68) in the high dose regimen and 1.0% (1/101) in the low dose regimen, whereas thrombotic event rate was 2.9% (2/68) in the high dose regimen and 4.0% (4/101) in the low dose regimen. Univariate analysis showed that the high dose regimen was significantly associated with ICH, but did not significantly reduce target-lesion thrombosis [19].

To minimize vascular trauma, submaximal balloon angioplasty (i.e. 80% of the parent artery diameter) with a slow balloon inflation rate has been widely adopted. Technical success is commonly defined as residual stenosis ≤50% coupled with good anterograde flow. Readers interested in the evolution of the technique may refer to the pertinent references, regarding angioplasty with undersized balloon with a slow inflation [8], staged stent placement [15], and angioplasty with undersized stent [16].

The anatomic features of cerebral arteries require a distinct set of endovascular techniques when compared with coronary angioplasty [28, 29]. First, cranio-cervical arteries are tortuous and the target lesions are much farther away from the femoral sheath or the tip of the guide catheter. Establishing a stable and functional endovascular conduit from the groin to the cerebral lesion is of paramount importance. A floppy-tipped microwire is often needed to first negotiate a tortuous and tight vascular access (such as Transcend 300 floppy, 0.014, 205 cm, Boston Scientific) before replacement by an exchange-length microwire (such as Xynchro-2, 0.014, 300 cm, Stryker) through a microcatheter.

Second, perforating arteries emanating within the target stenotic segment are end-anastomosing arteries supplying the basal ganglia or brain stem, and it is critical to preserve their patency. Since conventional digital subtraction angiogram (DSA) may not depict these branches or the patho-anatomy in details, a pre-operative 3-dimensional rotational angiogram (3DRA) offers an appreciation of the angio-architecture in a much higher resolution and from almost an infinite number of planes. Ostial stenosis of a perforator may signify risk of branch occlusion or perforator stroke during stenting. A meticulous study of the anatomy minimizes inadvertent advancement of microwire or microcatheter into these small branches that may result in perforator rupture and intracranial hemorrhage. In negotiating a tight stenosis, a deformed microwire tip would mean confronting to an atherosclerotic plaque or a side branch orifice, and should demand immediate retreat and adjustment of the guide-wire tip orientation.

Third, cerebral arteries are in the subarachnoid space and 'anchored' to the brain by small penetrating branches. Therefore, abrupt inattentive endovascular manipulations of wire, catheter, balloon or stent system may stretch the major cerebral arteries and avulse the small penetrating branches, causing catastrophic hemorrhage. The distal end of devices dedicated for neuro-intervention should be highly pliable and flexible, while the proximal part should provide sufficient mechanical support. Precaution is much needed when coronary devices are used 'off-label' for ICAS.

Fourth, a functionally less important vessel should be selected for distal access of the microwire. For instance, in M1 MCA angioplasty, the microwire may perch in the inferior division of MCA, or more preferably, in the temporo-occipital branch as vascular complication arising in this territory is relatively less catastrophic than those of the superior division. Likewise, in basilar artery stenting, it is advisable to place the microwire in the P4 segment of posterior cerebral artery (PCA) because the prognosis of supra-tentorium bleeding or distal occlusion of PCA caused by the microwire tip would be relatively benign as compared to infra-tentorium bleeding or proximal PCA occlusion.

Lastly, the wall of cerebral arteries is thinner than that of coronary arteries, due to the paucity of vasa vasorum, the absence of external elastic membranes, and near absence of the adventitia. The tunica media is composed principally of a thin smooth muscle layer. Thus, submaximal angioplasty with a slow inflation rate should be applied in the intracranial vasculature to avoid dissection or vascular rupture.

In operation with Wingspan stent and Gateway balloon, the microwire and guiding catheter should perch at a site that can stably support the delivery of the stent system. A dilatation with Gateway balloon (at a nominal pressure of 6 atmospheric pressures) is performed before stent placement (the recommended Gateway balloon diameter is 80% or less of the native vessel diameter, on either side of the stenosis whichever is smaller). Stent selection is based on the normal adjacent vessel diameter (fully expanded stent diameter is 0.5 mm to 1.0 mm greater than the diameter of normal adjacent vessel [on either side of the stenosis whichever is larger]) and the length of the stenotic lesion (deployed stent to extend at least 3 mm on either side of the lesion). The Wingspan stent is available in 5 diameters [2.5 mm to 4.5 mm] and 3 lengths [9, 15, 20 mm]. A continuous heparinized saline flush to the Wingspan stent system and Gateway catheter is recommended.

Treatment for Tandem or Multifocal Stenoses

Multi-focal cranio-cervical stenoses can occur either ipsilaterally (i.e. commonly extracranial and intracranial stenoses in the same vascular territory, coined tandem stenoses); or in different vascular territories (i.e. bilaterally, or concurrent carotid and vertebra-basilar stenoses). Each scenario may require customized endovascular strategy [30].

For ipsilateral tandem lesions, dilatation of the proximal stenosis should be performed prior to the distal lesion as improved distal runoff after stenting of the proximal lesion may enhance the clearance of microemboli during treatment for the distal lesion. Moreover, stenting of the proximal lesion first also makes room for advancement of guide catheter to perch more distally, increasing the stability of the endovascular conduit during the intracranial procedure.

In cases of stenoses distributing in different vascular territories, simultaneous revascularization of bilateral stenoses at the same session appears feasible and cost-effective, and may reduce the procedural burden [30, 31]. If only one of the high-grade lesions is treated, blood pressure control could be difficult post-operatively. Ischemic symptoms from the untreated territories may occur due to hypo-perfussion when systolic blood pressure is brought to a lower target for the prevention of hyperperfusion syndrome. The unbalanced cerebral hemodynamics may also accelerate steno-occlusion of the untreated vascular territory [30].

Patient Selection Based on Stroke Mechanism

Selection of ICAS patients for endovascular treatment should be based on an understanding of the cause of vascular lesion and individual stroke mechanism in addition to the degree of stenosis [32]. In fact, angioplasty or stenting does not have a role in cerebral occlusive vasculopathy caused by Moyamoya disease or vasculitis of infective or autoimmune origin. A high-grade intracranial stenosis could be a by-stander in strokes caused by small vessel disease or cardioembolism. Angioplasty/stenting is generally not performed in asymptomatic ICAS. It is also imperative to consider the stroke mechanism of the culprit ICAS, i.e., artery-to-artery thromboembolism, occlusion of penetrating artery ostium by a clot or atheroma, hypoperfusion or a combination of these (e.g. thromboembolism with impaired washout at borderzones) [33–38] (see Chapter 3 for detail). Obviously, not all these scenarios may benefit from angioplasty or stenting. An important predictor of subsequent stroke is cerebral perfusion failure from progressive ICAS (70–99% stenosis) without adequate collateralization [38]. Hence, ICAS patients with relevant regional hypo-perfusion may benefit most from endovascular revascularization. For patients with unstable plaque that leads to local thrombosis or artery-to-artery thromboembolism, treatment strategy should primarily focus on plaque stabilization and antithrombosis rather than revascularization [39]. In ICAD patients who have perforator occlusion from atheromatous branch disease [40], stenting cannot revascularize the occluded perforators, and may even exacerbate perforator occlusion as a result of 'snow plowing' effect.

Complications of Intracranial Stenting

Peri-operative complications of intracranial stenting remain a prime concern as they may offset the potential benefit of the procedure. Reported vascular complications are diverse, which include intracranial hemorrhage (ICH), stent thrombosis, perforator stroke, embolic stroke and vessel dissection.

Hyperperfusion and vessel perforation are the two major causes of ICH after intracranial stenting [19, 41]. Currently, aggressive systemic blood pressure control (i.e. systolic blood pressure <140 mm Hg) appears to be a feasible approach to prevent and treat hyperperfusion syndrome. A single stenosis is best straddled by a single stent as tandem stenting for a single stenosis may be an independent risk factor of ICH [19]. It appears that in tandem stenting, the stent struts may perforate the arterial wall when the distal stent is impinged by the proximal stent. In addition, the advancement of the second stent system may catch the deployed stent and drag on the major cerebral arteries, leading to avulsion or rupture of the fragile perforators.

To minimize thrombotic complication, preprocedural dual anti-platelet treatment is mandatory. Non-compliance with anti-platelet therapy was found to be associated with a higher frequency of stent thrombosis [19]. Patients with pre-operative perforator infarct adjacent to the stenotic segment may have a higher rate of perforator stroke after elective stening [18], probably related to atheroma displacing into the perforator ostia by the stent, or stent struts covering the perforator ostia.

Compared to vertebral artery angioplasty, basilar artery stenting is associated with a higher risk of the post-stent stroke in relation to its larger number of perforators and a more distal access of the stent system during stenting [42].

SAMMPRIS and On-Going Debates

SAMMPRIS (The Stenting and Aggressive Medical Management for Preventing Recurrent stroke in Intracranial Stenosis) was a large randomized clinical trial evaluating whether intracranial angioplasty combined with stenting (i.e. the Gateway-Wingspan system) would add benefit to aggressive medical therapy alone for preventing stroke in patients with high-grade (70–99%) symptomatic intracranial arterial stenosis [43]. All patients were enrolled within 30 days after a transient ischemic attack or non-disabling stroke. Aggressive medical management consisted of aspirin 325 mg daily for the entire follow-up, clopidogrel 75 mg/day for 90 days after enrollment, systolic blood pressure <140 mm Hg and low-density lipoprotein (LDL) <70 mg/dl.

In April 2011, the National Institute of Neurological Disorders and Stroke (NINDS) stopped recruitment of the study after 451 of the planned 764 patients had been enrolled in 50 participating centers in the US [44]. According to the clinical alert, 14% of patients in the stent arm experienced a stroke or died within the 30 days after enrollment, compared with 5.8% of patients treated with medical therapy alone. NINDS and the SAMMPRIS investigators opined, 'Aggressive medical management alone is superior to angioplasty combined with stenting in patients with recent symptoms and high grade intracranial arterial stenosis'.

Based on SAMMPRIS, the U.S. Food and Drug Administration now approved Wingspan only for patients who are between 22 and 80 years old and who meet all of the following criteria:

(1) two or more strokes despite aggressive medical management;

(2) whose most recent stroke occurred more than 7 days prior to planned treatment with Wingspan;

(3) who have 70–99% stenosis due to atherosclerosis of the intracranial artery related to the recurrent strokes; and

(4) who have made good recovery from previous stroke and have modified Rankin score of 3 or less prior to Wingspan treatment.

After SAMMPRIS, there is an on-going debate on whether we should stop the use of stenting for ICAS. The arguments below are put forward for the interests of the readers. The debate will likely continue along the advancement of endovascular techniques and our improving understanding of the pathogenic mechanisms of ICAS.

Stenting May Still be Needed in ICAS Patients

Zhongrong Miao, MD

Intracranial atherosclerotic disease (ICAS) is an important cause of ischemic stroke [45, 46]. ICAS is particularly prevalent in black, Asian, Hispanic, and some Arabic countries, which suggests that the global burden of stroke from ICAS is likely to grow as populations continue to expand in these regions [47].

Although intracranial angioplasty and stenting showed initial promise for the treatment of severe symptomatic ICAD [48], the SAMMPRIS (Stenting and Aggressive Medical Management for Preventing Recurrent Stroke) trial and the VISSIT (Vitesse Intracranial Stent Study for Ischemic Stroke Therapy) trial revealed negative results for patients treated with the Gateway and Wingspan system (Boston Scientific, Natick, Mass., USA) or Pharos Vitesse balloon-expandable neurovascular stent system (Codman Neurovascular, Raynham, Massachusetts, USA) [49–51]. These two multi-center randomized trials suggest that endovascular therapy should not be the primary treatment for symptomatic ICAS. In addition, a post-hoc analysis of the SAMMPRIS dataset failed to show any subgroup of patients with ICAS who benefited from stenting, including subgroups at a particularly high risk of stroke [52].

Despite the continuing debates [53–56], these results have changed treatment preferences of neurologists and neurointerventionists worldwide. The percentage of neurointerventionists in USA who recommended angioplasty/stenting in >25% of ICAS patients decreased from post-WASID (49%) to post-SAMMPRIS surveys (17%) [57], and a similar tendency occurred in European and Asian countries.

However, it is not a time to say no for angioplasty/stenting in patients with symptomatic severe ICAS. Patients in the SAMMPRIS study who were managed with dual antiplatelet therapy for 90 days followed by aspirin alone plus intensive risk factor management had a primary endpoint rate of 12.2% at 1 year [49], which implies that a subgroup of these patients still had a risk of stroke at 1 year that exceeds 12.2% [58]. For these cohorts with a high risk of recurrent stroke, a modified endovascular approach may remain a promising therapy if lower complication rate are achieved [59].

In recent prospective, single or multicenter registry studies using a tailored endovascular treatment, the threshold of a 4% rate of peri-procedural stroke and/or death was reported in patients with symptomatic ICAS combined with hemodynamic comprise [59–61]. Nonetheless, the weight of these studies cannot be compared with that of randomized clinical trials [55]. Randomized clinical trials are thus warranted to confirm or refute these findings.

The new trials should differ from SAMMPRIS and VISSIT regarding the following aspects:

First, patient selection should be based on the stroke mechanism. There are at least four likely mechanisms of stroke based on the infarct patterns at baseline in the 136 patients based on the Warfarin-Aspirin Symptomatic Intracranial Disease (WASID) trial data, including artery to artery embolism (n = 69; 50.7%), perforator occlusion (n = 34; 25%), hypoperfusion (n = 12; 8.8%), and mixed (n = 21; 15.5%) [62].

The new trial should be limited to patients with perfusion disturbances. Due to poor collaterals, these patients are highly likely to fail with medical therapy and would benefit from revascularization [63, 64]. Patients with perforator strokes or those with artery-to-artery thromboembolism without perfusion defect may have to be excluded from this trial. Perforator stroke is one of the most common complications of endovascular treatment for ICAS [64]. For example, patients with pontine infarction associated with basilar artery stenosis are at high risks of peri-procedural complications related to occlusion of perforators. These patients may be better treated with medical therapy to stabilize the atherosclerotic plaque and to prevent further progression of local disease. Interestingly, although SAMMPRIS results did not provide evidence to support the use of Wingspan stent system compared with medical treatment in patients with qualifying events with presumable hypoperfusion symptoms, there was a numeric difference in the outcome between the two groups (18 cases in stenting group with 2 years probability of 5.6% [0.8–33.4] vs. 31 case in medical management group with 2 years probability of 7.0% [1.8–25.3], p = 0.5780) [52].

Second, the endovascular approach should be customized (i.e. assigning patients to balloon mounted stents, angioplasty alone and angioplasty and stenting with self-expanding stent based on the vascular access and lesion morphology) as each device has its own merits and weaknesses. For example, balloon-mounted stents are rigid and of a high profile, and thus navigation along tortuous vessels could be difficult; whereas self-expanding stents have a lower radial force, thus are less suitable to achieve good luminal gain in calcified lesions. For patients with a tortuous arterial access, a short lesion length, or a small target vessel diameter (<2.5 mm), direct balloon angioplasty alone may have the advantage of having the smallest profile with much flexibility compared with other devices. Considering the complexity of ICAS in real world, the study protocol should allow device selection based on the experience and preference of an operator and the morphologic and anatomic features of the lesion, rather than specify a single device.

Third, endovascular treatment should be performed beyond the acute stage of stroke. In previous studies that showed a favorable result, the recommended time interval between the last ischemic event and the procedure was three weeks [60, 61]. A longer interim period may allow plaque stabilization, dissolution of overlying thrombus, as well as a reduced risk of hemorrhagic conversion of the infarct when dual antiplatelets and heparin are administered peri-operatively.

Fourth, the endovascular treatment should be performed by experienced neuro-interventionists who surpassed the initial steep portion of the learning curve [65]. A set of more stringent credentialing criteria than that used in the previous trials may decrease the procedural complication associated with the lack of experience.

In conclusion, customized endovascular treatment of ICAS using balloon mounted stents, angioplasty alone and plus self-expanding stents based on anatomical features and lesion morphology may yield a lower complication rate in patients with perfusion abnormalities and poor collateral flow. Future randomized clinical trials may have to focus on this particular patient subgroup.

Stenting Is Not Needed in ICAS Patients

Ashley M. Wabnitz, MD, and
Marc I. Chimowitz, MD

ICAS is a common cause of stroke worldwide that is associated with a high risk of recurrent stroke [1]. Randomized trials that have evaluated various antithrombotic regimens have shown high recurrent ischemic event rates [1, 66], particularly in patients with severe (70–99%) stenosis whose rate of stroke in the same territory of the stenotic artery was as high as 18% at one year [2]. This high rate of stroke prompted interest in evaluating the role of intracranial stenting as an alternative treatment, which ultimately led to two randomized trials comparing stenting with medical therapy in high-risk patients with ICAS. The first trial was the Stenting and Aggressive Medical Management for Preventing Recurrent Ischemic Stroke (SAMMPRIS) trial, which was funded by the National Institutes of Health and performed at 50 sites in the USA [49]. The second trial was the Vitesse Intracranial Stent Study for Ischemic Stroke Therapy (VISSIT), which was an industry-funded trial that included sites in China and Europe [50].

Both SAMMPRIS and VISSIT had similar eligibility criteria and medical and risk factor management but they differed in the endovascular device used – the SAMMPRIS trial used a self-expanding stent, whereas the VISSIT trial utilized a balloon-mounted stent. The medical management in all treatment groups in both trials included antithrombotic treatment with aspirin 81 mg-325 mg per day (SAMMPRIS required 325 mg per day) for the duration of follow-up as well as clopidogrel 75 mg per day for 90 days after enrollment only. Risk factor management included targeting a systolic blood pressure of less than 140 mm Hg in both trials (<130 mm Hg if diabetic in SAMMPRIS) and low-density lipoprotein [LDL] cholesterol targets of <70 mg/dl in SAMMPRIS and <100 mg/dl in VISSIT [48, 49]. Patients in SAMMPRIS also participated in a lifestyle modification program [49].

Enrollment in SAMMPRIS was stopped early after 451 patients had been randomized because of the higher than expected rate of peri-procedural stroke in the stenting group (14.7% at 30 days: 10.3% ischemic stroke, 4.5% hemorrhagic stroke) and a 50% lower than projected rate of stroke on aggressive medical therapy [49]. The absolute reduction in the risk of stroke from medical therapy alone was 8.9% at 30 days and 9.0% at 3 years, indicating there was no benefit from stenting even beyond the peri-procedural period [49, 51].

Enrollment in VISSIT was also stopped early after only 112 patients were randomized and the peri-procedural stroke rate (25.8% at 30 days: 17.2% ischemic stroke, 8.6% hemorrhagic stroke) was even higher than in SAMMPRIS. Additionally, in VISSIT there was a much higher rate of ischemic stroke in the stenting group than in the medical group beyond the 30-day peri-procedural period, resulting in an absolute increase in the rate of ischemic stroke in the same territory from stenting of 25.1% at one year. Combining the 30-day hemorrhagic strokes with the ischemic strokes within one year in VISSIT resulted in an increase in the absolute risk of ischemic or hemorrhagic stroke from stenting at one year of 33.7%, which is equivalent to a number needed to harm from stenting of only three [50].

These two trials, which are the only completed multi-center randomized trials on intracranial stenting for ICAS, raise serious concerns about the peri-procedural risk of stroke from stenting and fail to show any long-term benefit of stenting in patients with severe ICAS. While there are data from non-randomized studies showing lower peri-procedural stroke rates after intracranial stenting [61, 65, 67], this was also true of stenting registries in the USA preceding SAMMPRIS [48, 68]. One important reason for this discrepancy is that randomized clinical trials typically rely on a rigorous protocol for evaluating potential endpoints such as the evaluation of all events by non-endovascular neurologists, final adjudication of events by external blinded evaluators, and site monitoring to ensure that all potential endpoints are reported. These protocol requirements are not typically performed in registries or case series, which likely leads to an underestimate of stroke rates.

It has also been suggested that a factor contributing to the higher rate of peri-procedural stroke in SAMMPRIS was inexperience of US interventionists with intracranial stenting [53, 65]. However, arguing against that viewpoint are the following: the interventionists who participated in SAMMPRIS were carefully credentialed to participate in the trial [69] and most had participated in the stenting registries preceding SAMMPRIS that had reported lower peri-procedural stroke rates [48, 68]; the most senior and experienced interventionists did not have lower peri-procedural stroke rates than other interventionists in SAMMPRIS [57]; there was no difference in peri-procedural stroke rates between the highest and lowest enrolling sites in SAMMPRIS; and the peri-procedural stroke rate did not decline over the course of the enrollment period [49]. Moreover, the VISSIT trial included some sites in China and Europe that were amongst the six highest enrolling sites and the peri-procedural stroke rate was even higher than in SAMMPRIS [48].

Stenting proponents will argue that there is still a role for stenting in subgroups of ICAS patients that are at high-risk of stroke despite aggressive medical therapy [70]. However, a post-hoc analysis of the SAMMPRIS dataset failed to show any subgroup of patients with ICAS who benefited from stenting, including subgroups at particularly high risk of stroke on aggressive medical therapy [52]. The explanation for this is that subgroups at higher risk of stroke on medical therapy are also at higher risk of peri-procedural stroke after stenting [51, 52]. Additionally, given that most of the peri-procedural strokes in SAMMPRIS were perforator infarcts (presumably from 'snow-plowing' atherosclerotic plaque into perforators during balloon dilation or stent placement) or reperfusion hemorrhages after technically sound procedures [64, 71], it will be challenging to lower these complications using different stents or even with angioplasty alone. Moreover, since there was no benefit from stenting in SAMMPRIS or VISSIT beyond the peri-procedural period, even if the peri-procedural risk of stroke could be lowered to 5%, as originally anticipated in SAMMPRIS, stenting would still not provide any long term benefit over well implemented aggressive medical therapy.

In conclusion, aggressive medical therapy should be the standard of care for patients with symptomatic ICAS. Currently, there is no proven role for endovascular therapy, even in subgroups of patients at high-risk of stroke on aggressive medical therapy [72]. Future research is needed to develop safer and more effective therapies for these high-risk patients. Promising options include remote limb ischemic conditioning, which was shown to be more effective than usual medical management in two small randomized trials performed in China [73, 74], and a neurosurgical procedure (called encephaloduroarteriosynangiosis) to deliver flow distal to an intracranial stenosis [75].

References

1 Chimowitz MI, Lynn MJ, Howlett-Smith H, et al: Comparison of warfarin and aspirin for symptomatic intracranial arterial stenosis. N Engl J Med 2005;352: 1305–1316.

2 Kasner SE, Chimowitz MI, Lynn MJ, et al: Predictors of ischemic stroke in the territory of a symptomatic intracranial arterial stenosis. Circulation 2006;113: 555–563.

3 Liu L, Wong KS, Leng X, et al: Dual antiplatelet therapy in stroke and ICAS: subgroup analysis of CHANCE. Neurology: Published online before print August 28, 2015.

4 Sundt TM Jr, Smith HC, Campbell JK, Vlietstra RE, Cucchiara RF, Stanson AW: Transluminal angioplasty for basilar artery stenosis. Mayo Clin Proc 1980; 55:673–680.

5 Higashida RT, Tsai FY, Halbach VV, et al: Transluminal angioplasty for atherosclerotic disease of the vertebral and basilar arteries. J Neurosurg 1993;78: 192–198.

6 Yokote H, Terada T, Ryujin K, et al: Percutaneous transluminal angioplasty for intracranial arteriosclerotic lesions. Neuroradiology 1998;40:590–596.

7 Mori T, Fukuoka M, Kazita K, Mori K: Follow-up study after intracranial percutaneous transluminal cerebral balloon angioplasty. AJNR Am J Neuroradiol 1998;19:1525–1533.

8 Connors JJ 3rd, Wojak JC: Percutaneous transluminal angioplasty for intracranial atherosclerotic lesions: evolution of technique and short-term results. J Neurosurg 1999;91:415–423.

9 Marks MP, Wojak JC, Al-Ali F, et al: Angioplasty for symptomatic intracranial stenosis: clinical outcome. Stroke 2006;37:1016–1020.

10 Feldman RL, Trigg L, Gaudier J, Galat J: Use of coronary Palmaz-Schatz stent in the percutaneous treatment of an intracranial carotid artery stenosis. Cathet Cardiovasc Diagn 1996;38:316–319.

11 Gomez CR, Misra VK, Liu MW, et al: Elective stenting of symptomatic basilar artery stenosis. Stroke 2000;31:95–99.

12 Mori T, Kazita K, Chokyu K, Mima T, Mori K: Short-term arteriographic and clinical outcome after cerebral angioplasty and stenting for intracranial vertebrobasilar and carotid atherosclerotic occlusive disease. AJNR Am J Neuroradiol 2000;21:249–254.

13 Levy EI, Horowitz MB, Koebbe CJ, et al: Transluminal stent-assisted angiplasty of the intracranial vertebrobasilar system for medically refractory, posterior circulation ischemia: early results. Neurosurgery 2001;48:1215–1221; discussion 1221–1213.

14 Lylyk P, Cohen JE, Ceratto R, Ferrario A, Miranda C: Angioplasty and stent placement in intracranial atherosclerotic stenoses and dissections. AJNR Am J Neuroradiol 2002;23:430–436.

15 Levy EI, Hanel RA, Boulos AS, et al: Comparison of periprocedure complications resulting from direct stent placement compared with those due to conventional and staged stent placement in the basilar artery. J Neurosurg 2003;99:653–660.

16 de Rochemont Rdu M, Turowski B, Buchkremer M, Sitzer M, Zanella FE, Berkefeld J: Recurrent symptomatic high-grade intracranial stenoses: safety and efficacy of undersized stents – initial experience. Radiology 2004;231: 45–49.

17 Jiang WJ, Wang YJ, Du B, et al: Stenting of symptomatic M1 stenosis of middle cerebral artery: an initial experience of 40 patients. Stroke 2004;35:1375–1380.

18 Jiang WJ, Srivastava T, Gao F, Du B, Dong KH, Xu XT: Perforator stroke after elective stenting of symptomatic intracranial stenosis. Neurology 2006;66:1868–1872.
19 Jiang WJ, Du B, Leung TW, Xu XT, Jin M, Dong KH: Symptomatic intracranial stenosis: cerebrovascular complications from elective stent placement. Radiology 2007;243:188–197.
20 Abou-Chebl A, Bashir Q, Yadav JS: Drug-eluting stents for the treatment of intracranial atherosclerosis: initial experience and midterm angiographic follow-up. Stroke 2005;36:e165–e168.
21 Stenting of Symptomatic Atherosclerotic Lesions in the Vertebral or Intracranial Arteries (SSYLVIA): study results. Stroke 2004;35:1388–1392.
22 Terada T, Tsuura M, Matsumoto H, et al: Endovascular therapy for stenosis of the petrous or cavernous portion of the internal carotid artery: percutaneous transluminal angioplasty compared with stent placement. J Neurosurg 2003;98:491–497.
23 Suh DC, Kim JK, Choi JW, et al: Intracranial stenting of severe symptomatic intracranial stenosis: results of 100 consecutive patients. AJNR Am J Neuroradiol 2008;29:781–785.
24 Hartmann M, Jansen O: Angioplasty and stenting of intracranial stenosis. Curr Opin Neurol 2005;18:39–45.
25 Stryker Wingspan Stent System: Safety Communication – Narrowed Indications for Use http://www.fda.gov/safety/medwatch/safetyinformation/safetyalertsforhumanmedicalproducts/ucm314836.htm. Accessed 3 February 2016.
26 Bose A, Hartmann M, Henkes H, et al: A novel, self-expanding, nitinol stent in medically refractory intracranial atherosclerotic stenoses: the Wingspan study. Stroke 2007;38:1531–1537.
27 Furlan A, Higashida R, Wechsler L, et al: Intra-arterial prourokinase for acute ischemic stroke. The PROACT II study: a randomized controlled trial. Prolyse in Acute Cerebral Thromboembolism. JAMA 1999;282:2003–2011.
28 Schumacher HC, Khaw AV, Meyers PM, Gupta R, Higashida RT: Intracranial angioplasty and stent placement for cerebral atherosclerosis. J Vasc Interv Radiol 2004;15:S123–S132.
29 Levy EI, Kim SH, Bendok BR: Interventional neuroradiologic therapy; in Mohr JP, Choi DW, Weir B, Wolf PA (eds): Stroke: Pathophysiology, Diagnosis, and Management, ed 4. Churchill Livingstone, 2004, pp 1475–1520.
30 Pyun HW, Suh DC, Kim JK, et al: Concomitant multiple revascularizations in supra-aortic arteries: short-term results in 50 patients. AJNR Am J Neuroradiol 2007;28:1895–1901.
31 Henry M, Gopalakrishnan L, Rajagopal S, Rath PC, Henry I, Hugel M: Bilateral carotid angioplasty and stenting. Catheter Cardiovasc Interv 2005;64:275–282.
32 Leng X, Wong KS, Liebeskind DS: Evaluating intracranial atherosclerosis rather than intracranial stenosis. Stroke 2014;45:645–651.
33 Wong KS, Gao S, Chan YL, et al: Mechanisms of acute cerebral infarctions in patients with middle cerebral artery stenosis: a diffusion-weighted imaging and microemboli monitoring study. Ann Neurol 2002;52:74–81.
34 Man BL, FU YP, Chan YY, et al: Lesion Patterns and Stroke Mechanisms in Concurrent Atherosclerosis of Intracranial and Extracranial Vessels. Stroke 2009;40:3211–3215.
35 Dubow JS, Salamon E, Greenberg E, Patsalides A: Mechanism of acute ischemic stroke in patients with severe middle cerebral artery atherosclerotic disease. J Stroke Cerebrovasc Dis 2014;23:1191–1194.
36 Lee DK, Kim JS, Kwon SU, et al: Lesion patterns and stroke mechanism in atherosclerotic middle cerebral artery disease: early diffusion-weighted imaging study. Stroke 2005;36:2583–2588.
37 Caplan LR, Wong KS, Gao S, Hennerici MG: Is hypoperfusion an important cause of strokes? If so, how? Cerebrovasc Dis 2006;21:145–153.
38 López-Cancio E, Matheus MG, Romano JG, et al: Infarct patterns, collaterals and likely causative mechanisms of stroke in symptomatic intracranial atherosclerosis. Cerebrovasc Dis 2014;37:417–422.
39 Leung TW, Wang L, Soo YOY, et al: Evolution of intracranial atherosclerotic disease under modern medical therapy. Ann Neurol 2015;77:478–486.
40 Caplan LR: Intracranial branch atheromatous disease: a neglected, understudied, and underused concept. Neurology 1989;39:1246–1250.
41 Abou-Chebl A, Yadav JS, Reginelli JP, Bajzer C, Bhatt D, Krieger DW: Intracranial hemorrhage and hyperperfusion syndrome following carotid artery stenting: risk factors, prevention, and treatment. J Am Coll Cardiol 2004;43:1596–1601.
42 Jiang WJ, Xu XT, Du B, et al: Long-term outcome of elective stenting for symptomatic intracranial vertebrobasilar stenosis. Neurology 2007;68:856–858.
43 Stenting vs Aggressive Medical Management for Preventing Recurrent Stroke in Intracranial Stenosis (SAMMPRIS). http://clinicaltrials.gov/ct2/show/NCT00576693.
44 http://www.nlm.nih.gov/databases/alerts/intracranial_arterial_stenosis.html. (Accessed 11 February 2016).
45 Redon J, Olsen MH, Cooper RS, et al: Stroke mortality and trends from 1990 to 2006 in 39 countries from Europe and Central Asia: implications for control of high blood pressure. Eur Heart J 2011;32:1424–1431.
46 Wong KS, Li H, Lam WW, Chan YL, Kay R: Progression of middle cerebral artery occlusive disease and its relationship with further vascular events after stroke. Stroke 2002;33:532–536.
47 Gorelick PB, Wong KS, Bae HJ, Pandey DK: Large artery intracranial occlusive disease: a large worldwide burden but a relatively neglected frontier. Stroke 2008;39:2396–2399.
48 Zaidat OO, Klucznik R, Alexander MJ, et al; NIH Multi-center Wingspan Intracranial Stent Registry Study Group. The NIH registry on use of the wingspan stent for symptomatic 70–99% intracranial arterial stenosis. Neurology 2008;70:1518–1524.
49 Chimowitz MI, Lynn MJ, Derdeyn CP, et al; for the SAMMPRIS Trial Investigators. Stenting versus aggressive medical therapy for intracranial arterial stenosis. N Engl J Med 2011;365:993–1003.
50 Zaidat OO, Fitzsimmons BF, Woodward BK; VISSIT Trial Investigators: Effect of a balloon-expandable intracranial stent vs medical therapy on risk of stroke in patients with symptomatic intracranial stenosis: the VISSIT randomized clinical trial. JAMA 2015;313:1240–1248.

51 Derdeyn CP, Chimowitz MI, Lynn MJ, et al: Stenting and aggressive medical management for preventing recurrent stroke in intracranial stenosis trial investigators: Aggressive medical treatment with or without stenting in high-risk patients with intracranial artery stenosis (SAMMPRIS): the final results of a randomised trial. Lancet 2014;383:333–341.
52 Lutsep HL, Lynn MJ, Cotsonis GA, et al: SAMMPRIS Investigators. Does the stenting versus aggressive medical therapy trial support stenting for subgroups with intracranial stenosis? Stroke 2015;46:3282–3284.
53 Abou-Chebl A, Steinmetz H: Critique of 'Stenting versus Aggressive Medical Therapy for Intracranial Arterial Stenosis' by Chimowitz et al in the New England Journal of Medicine. Stroke 2012;43:616–620.
54 Chimowitz MI, Fiorella D, Derdeyn CP, et al: Response to critique of the Stenting and Aggressive Medical Management for Preventing Recurrent Stroke in Intracranial Stenosis (SAMMPRIS) trial by Abou-Chebl and Steinmetz. Stroke 2012;43:2806–2809.
55 Miao Z: Intracranial Angioplasty and Stenting before and after SAMMPRIS: 'From Simple to Complex Strategy – The Chinese Experience'. Front Neurol 2014;5:129.
56 Turan TN, Chimowitz MI: Yet again no benefit of stenting over medical therapy. Lancet Neurol 2015;14:565–566.
57 Derdeyn CP, Fiorella D, Lynn MJ, et al; SAMMPRIS Trial Investigators. Impact of operator and site experience on outcomes after angioplasty and stenting in the SAMMPRIS trial. J Neurointerv Surg 2013;5:528–533.
58 Holmstedt CA, Turan TN, Chimowitz MI: Atherosclerotic intracranial arterial stenosis: risk factors, diagnosis, and treatment. Lancet Neurol 2013;12:1106–1114.
59 Chaudhry SA, Watanabe M, Qureshi AI: The new standard for performance of intracranial angioplasty and stent placement after Stenting versus Aggressive Medical Therapy for Intracranial Arterial Stenosis (SAMMPRIS) Trial. AJNR Am J Neuroradiol 2011;32:E214.
60 Miao Z, Song L, Liebeskind DS, et al: Outcomes of tailored angioplasty and/or stenting for symptomatic intracranial atherosclerosis: a prospective cohort study after SAMMPRIS. J Neurointerv Surg 2015;7:331–335.
61 Miao Z, Zhang Y, Shuai J, et al: Study Group of Registry Study of Stenting for Symptomatic Intracranial Artery Stenosis in China: Thirty-Day Outcome of a Multicenter Registry Study of Stenting for Symptomatic Intracranial Artery Stenosis in China. Stroke 2015;46:2822–2829.
62 López-Cancio E, Matheus MG, Romano JG, et al: Infarct patterns, collaterals and likely causative mechanisms of stroke in symptomatic intracranial atherosclerosis. Cerebrovasc Dis 2014;37:417–422.
63 Abe A, Ueda T, Ueda M, et al: Symptomatic middle cerebral artery stenosis treated by percutaneous transluminal angioplasty: improvement of cerebrovascular reserves. Interv Neuroradiol 2012;18:213–220.
64 Derdeyn CP, Fiorella D, Lynn MJ, et al; Stenting and Aggressive Medical Management for Preventing Recurrent Stroke in Intracranial Stenosis Trial Investigators. Mechanisms of stroke after intracranial angioplasty and stenting in the SAMMPRIS trial. Neurosurgery 2013;72:777–795.
65 Yu SC, Leung TW, Lee KT, Wong LK: Learning curve of Wingspan stenting for intracranial atherosclerosis: single-center experience of 95 consecutive patients. J Neurointerv Surg 2014;6:212–218.
66 Kwon SU, Hong KS, Kang DW, et al: Efficacy and safety of combination antiplatelet therapies in patients with symptomatic intracranial atherosclerotic stenosis. Stroke 2011;42:2883–2890.
67 Jiang WJ, Cheng-Ching E, Abou-Chebl A, et al: Multicenter analysis of stenting in symptomatic intracranial atherosclerosis. Neurosurgery 2012;70:25–30.
68 Fiorella D, Levy EI, Turk AS, et al: US multicenter experience with the Wingspan stent system for the treatment of intracranial atheromatous disease: Periprocedural results. Stroke 2007;38:881–887.
69 Chimowitz MI, Lynn MJ, Turan TN, et al; SAMMPRIS Investigators: Design of the stenting and aggressive medical management for preventing recurrent stroke in intracranial stenosis trial. J Stroke Cerebrovasc Dis 2011;20:357–368.
70 Waters MF, Hoh BL, Lynn M, et al; Stenting and Aggressive Medical Management for Preventing Recurrent Stroke in Intracranial Stenosis (SAMMPRIS) Trial Investigators: Factors associated with recurrent ischemic stroke in the medical group of the SAMMPRIS trial. JAMA Neurol 2016;73:308–315.
71 Fiorella D, Derdeyn CP, Lynn MJ, et al, SAMMPRIS Trial Investigators. Detailed analysis of periprocedural strokes in patients undergoing intracranial stenting in stenting and aggressive medical management for preventing recurrent stroke in intracranial stenosis (sammpris). Stroke 2012;43:2682–2688.
72 Chimowitz MI, Derdeyn CP: Endovascular therapy for atherosclerotic intracranial arterial stenosis: back to the drawing board. JAMA 2015;313:1219–1220.
73 Meng R, Asmaro K, Meng L, et al: Upper limb ischemic preconditioning prevents recurrent stroke in intracranial arterial stenosis. Neurology 2012;79:1853–1861.
74 Meng R, Ding Y, Asmaro K, et al: Ischemic conditioning is safe and effective for octo- and nonagenarians in stroke prevention and treatment. Neurotherapeutics 2015;12:667–677.
75 Dusick JR, Liebeskind DS, Saver JL, Martin NA, Gonzalez NR: Indirect revascularization for nonmoyamoya intracranial arterial stenoses: clinical and angiographic outcomes. J Neurosurg 2012;117:94–102.

Prof. Thomas W. Leung, MD
Department of Medicine and Therapeutics, The Prince of Wales Hospital
The Chinese University of Hong Kong
Hong Kong, SAR (China)
E-Mail drtleung@cuhk.edu.hk

Kim JS, Caplan LR, Wong KS (eds): Intracranial Atherosclerosis: Pathophysiology, Diagnosis and Treatment.
Front Neurol Neurosci. Basel, Karger, 2016, vol 40, pp 164–178 (DOI: 10.1159/000448312)

Surgical Therapy

Chang Wan Oh[a] · Gary K. Steinberg[b]

[a]Department of Neurosurgery, Seoul National University Bundang Hospital, Seongnam, Korea; [b]Department of Neurosurgery, Stanford University School of Medicine, Stanford, Calif., USA

Abstract

Many prior investigations have indicated the important role of medical treatment to prevent stroke in patients with intracranial atherosclerosis, with angioplasty and stenting occasionally being performed. In a subgroup of patients with severe hemodynamic impairment, extracranial-intracranial (EC-IC) bypass surgery may be considered. Additionally, in patients with massive infarctions due to middle cerebral artery (MCA) occlusion, the use of decompressive craniectomy may lower mortality rates and improve long-term quality of life. However, the benefit of these surgical procedures in patients with intracranial atherosclerosis has long been controversial. In this chapter, we review the surgical therapies for patients with intracranial atherosclerosis. This review does not include EC-IC bypass surgery for moyamoya disease, which is discussed in another chapter.

Intracranial Revascularization Surgery

Surgical Procedures

Revascularization of the ischemic brain distal to intracranial or extracranial steno-occlusive lesions can be achieved through various EC-IC bypass surgeries using different donors, recipient arteries and conduit vessels [1, 2]. There are two types of bypass surgeries, which are defined by the amount of blood flow through the bypass: high-flow and low-flow (fig. 1). The high-flow bypass uses a free venous or arterial graft (saphenous vein or radial artery) to connect the cervical carotid artery to the proximal MCA (M1 or M2 branches in the Sylvian fissure). Extracranial internal, external, or common carotid arteries can be used as donor arteries depending on the situation, including anatomy and size of the donor arteries, and surgeon preference.

This type of bypass surgery is often used in the planned occlusion of the internal carotid artery (ICA) for the treatment of giant aneurysms or skull-base tumors, and is less commonly used to treat intracranial atherosclerotic disease because of the high risk of complications, including post-operative hemorrhage associated with hyperperfusion injury. Hemorrhagic complications occur more frequently in patients with a history of previous, multiple ischemic symptoms [3]. High-flow bypasses have relatively low short- and long-

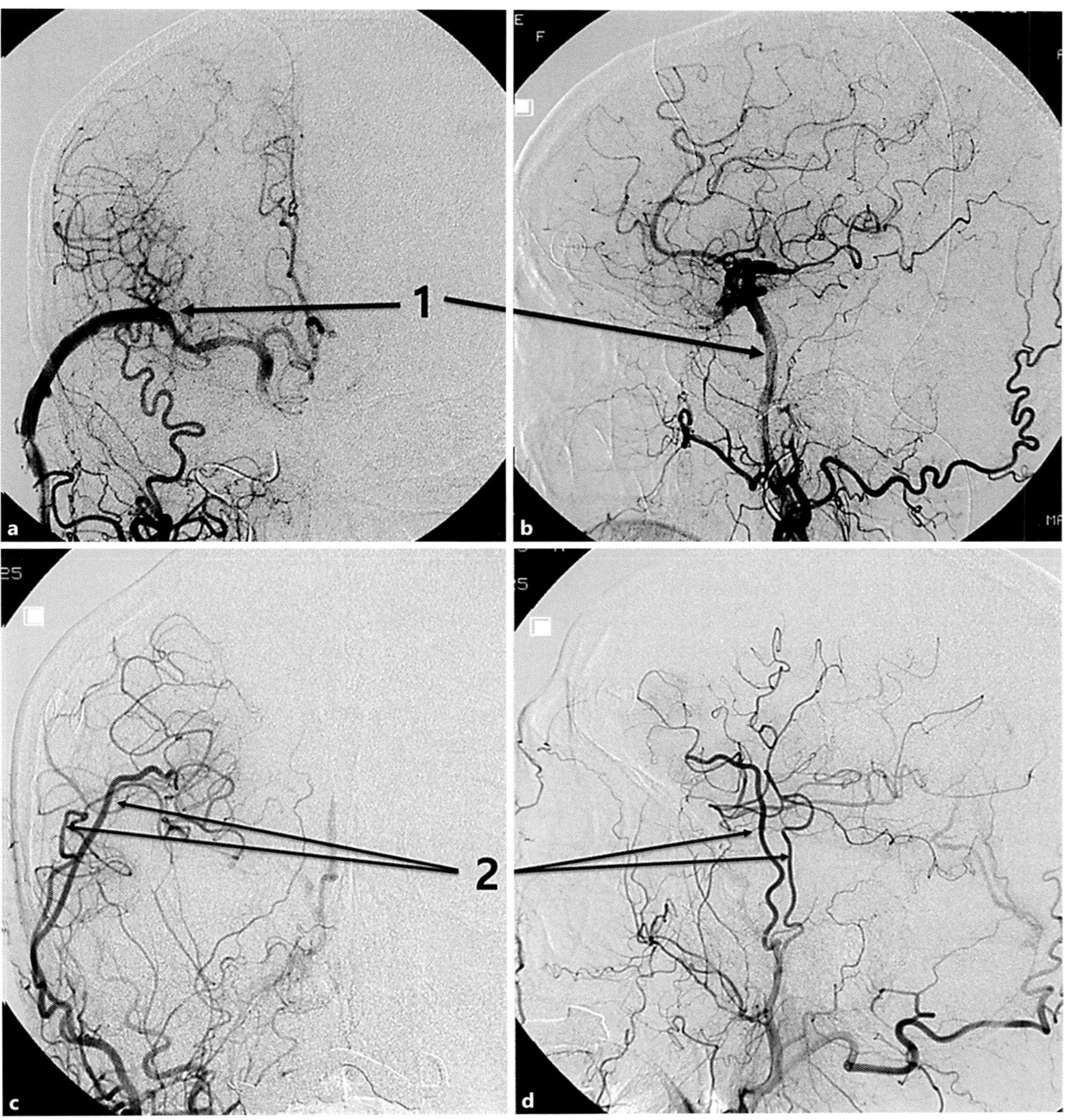

Fig. 1. a and **b**, high-flow bypass using saphenous vein graft supplies the entire territory of the internal carotid artery (arrow 1, saphenous vein graft). **c** and **d**, double-barrel bypass with two branches of the superficial temporal artery (STA) can irrigate the territory of the middle cerebral artery (arrow 2, two branches of the STA).

term patency rates, with 42% of all graft failures occurring within the first 24 hours after surgery and an occlusion rate of 14% at 1 year [4].

The low-flow bypass usually uses an arterial pedicle, a mobilized extracranial artery such as the superficial temporal artery (STA) or occipital artery (OA), and its distal cut end is directly connected to the branches of the MCA without vessel graft interposition [1, 2, 5, 6]. Compared with the high-flow bypass with vessel graft, this type of direct bypass has fewer complications and better long-term durability with a 5-year patency rate >95%. The most commonly used recipient artery is the cortical (M4) branch of the MCA, but more proximal branches (M2 or M3) can be used to increase the blood flow through the bypass [7] (fig. 2). Double-barrel anastomoses using the frontal and parietal branches of the STA can also be performed to increase flow through the anastomosis [8] (fig. 1c, d). The most popular cortical recipient arteries are those from around the temporo-occipital area, especially the angular artery. The prefrontal or anterior temporal cortical branches are also used, although they have a smaller diameter than the angular artery. The arteries supplying the eloquent area around the central sulcus are rarely used as the recipient artery because of concerns about potential complications. For posterior circulation revascularization, the donor arteries can be connected to the posterior cerebral (PCA), superior cerebellar (SCA), anterior inferior cerebellar (AICA), and posterior inferior cerebellar (PICA) arteries. Bypass surgery for posterior circulation disorders has a higher risk of complications than that for anterior circulation diseases.

History of EC-IC Bypass Surgery

In 1967, Yasargil [9] and Donaghy [10] first used STA-MCA anastomosis [11]. Since then, this procedure has been employed to revascularize the brain distal to steno-occlusive lesions that are not accessible by carotid endarterectomy. This procedure improves cerebral perfusion [12, 13] and decreases the occurrence of secondary strokes in several non-randomized, retrospective reports [13–15]. In a large series, the technical success rate was reported to be extremely high with a patency rate of 99% [16]; operative morbidity (2–4%) and mortality (1–2.5%) were also acceptable [16, 17]. The incidence of secondary stroke ipsilateral to the side of successful bypass surgery was reportedly to be 0.9% per year [17].

However, a randomized International Cooperative Study of Extracranial-Intracranial Arterial Anastomosis (EC-IC Bypass Study) performed in 1977 demonstrated that cerebral revascularization using STA-MCA anastomosis provided no benefits over medical treatment [18, 19] in reducing the subsequent risk of stroke. This study randomized 1,377 patients with minor stroke or transient ischemic attack (TIA), including retinal ischemia due to atherosclerotic steno-occlusive disease of the ICA or MCA, with an average follow-up period of 55.8 months. The analysis revealed that a single stroke occurred in 18% of patients in the medication group and 20% of patients in the surgery group. Multiple strokes occurred in 10% of patients in the medication group and in 11% of patients in the surgery group.

The result of subgroup analysis in 268 patients with MCA lesions did not show differences between the medication and surgery groups. Moreover, after bypass surgery, patients with MCA stenosis experienced worse outcomes than those with vascular lesions in other areas. This result may be due to an occlusion of the stenotic lesions after the surgery, which was observed on a postoperative angiogram in 14% of the patients [18].

The overall surgery-related morbidity and mortality rates were similar to those of the previous reports [16, 17]. During the perioperative period (<30 days after surgery), 12.2% of the patients had cerebral and retinal ischemic events ranging from trivial to fatal. The major stroke morbidity rate was 4.5%, while the mortality rate was 1.1%. During surgery and in the 30 days after surgery, however, the major stroke morbidity rate was 3%, including a 0.6% mortality rate. The

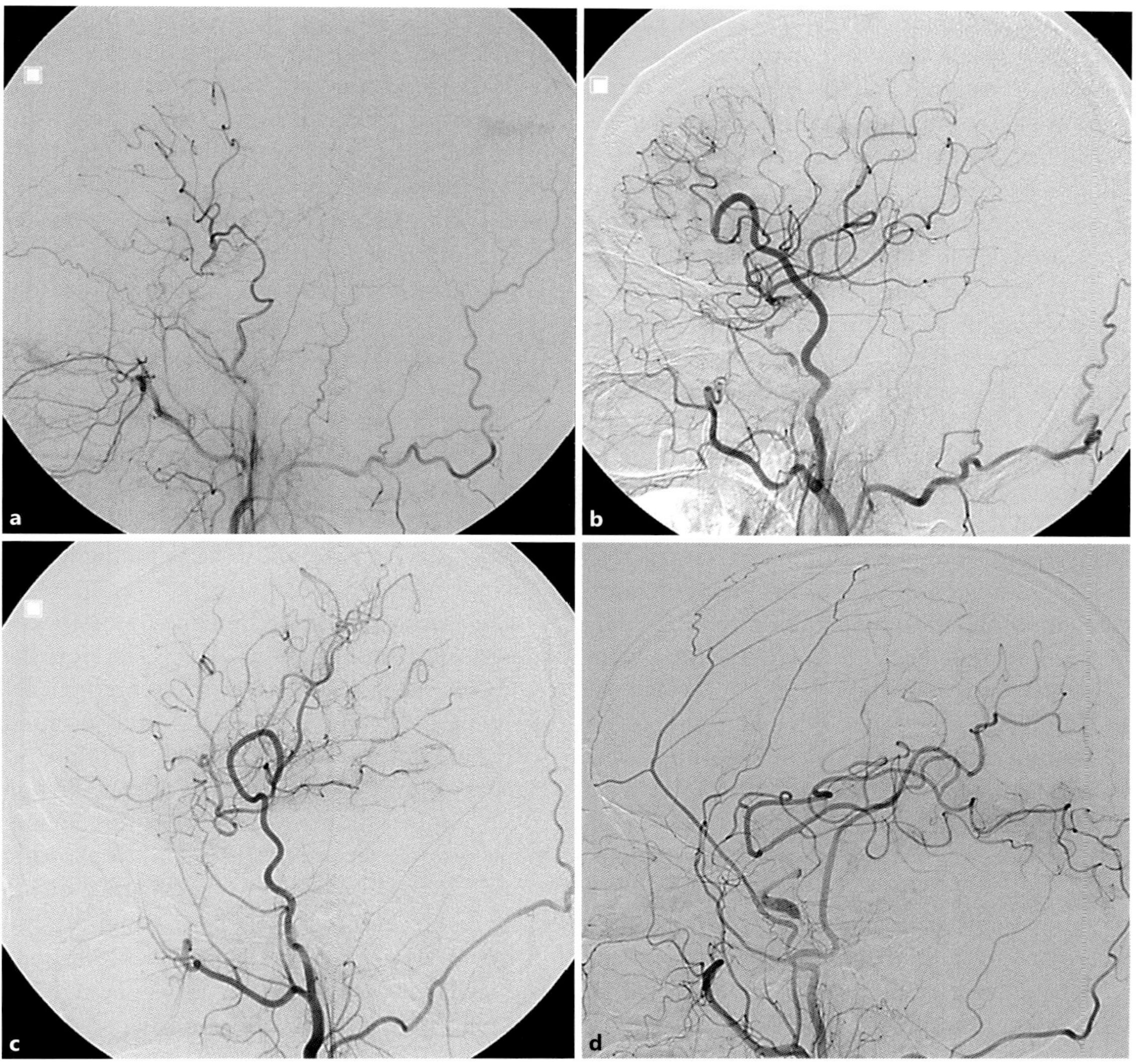

Fig. 2. Variations in the superficial temporal artery – middle cerebral artery (STA-MCA) anastomosis. The recipient artery may be the M2 branch (**a**), prefrontal artery (**b**), anterior temporal artery (**c**), or angular artery (**d**). The single STA-MCA anastomosis can resupply most of the territory of the MCA if it is ≥1 mm diameter and the recipient MCA branch is also ≥1 mm diameter.

average interval between randomization and EC-IC bypass surgery was 9 days, during which 10 cases of major stroke occurred. Many of these cases were considered to be related to the surgical preparation, such as repeated angiography or stress imposed on the patient prior to surgery [18]. This result emphasizes the importance of careful perioperative management in patients at high risk of stroke. The bypass patency rate was as high as 96%, demonstrating a high technical success rate of this procedure, which was compatible with the findings of a previous report [16].

Several criticisms have been raised against this study result, including concerns about internal and external validity [20–27]. Two important shortcomings of this trial deserve mention. The first is that a large number of patients, perhaps as many as 3,000, based on the data obtained by Sundt [21], were operated on outside of the trial, while only 663 were assigned to surgery within the trial [22]. Many of those patients who underwent surgery outside of the trial could have been eligible for and included in the trial. The omission of those patients might have diluted the efficacy of surgery. However, without detailed information on those patients undergoing surgery outside of the trial, further investigation of this question was not possible. The second and more important criticism is that this study enrolled patients based on clinical symptoms and angiographic findings only [19] and included no information about hemodynamic status [20, 25, 27]. In 1977, when the EC/IC Bypass Study was initiated, technologies assessing cerebrovascular hemodynamics were not available in many centers. With the advent of cerebral perfusion measurements, it has been shown that only a small proportion of patients with steno-occlusive lesions have decreased blood flow distal to the vascular lesions [28]. Therefore, the failure of the EC-IC Bypass Study may have been related to the inclusion of patients who did not need cerebral revascularization. Thus, it was suggested that studies should be performed that pay attention to each patient's cerebral hemodynamic status and subsequent stroke risk [20, 29].

Hemodynamic Impairment and the Risk of Subsequent Stroke

The Warfarin versus Aspirin in Symptomatic Intracranial Disease (WASID) study [30, 31], which provided a data set regarding the risk of stroke from intracranial atherosclerotic disease, found that the risk of stroke increased in proportion to the severity of stenosis [32]. This result correlated well with the findings of the North American Symptomatic Carotid Endarterectomy Trial (NASCET) [33] that showed an increased risk of stroke in patients with severe stenotic lesions of the extracranial carotid artery. These proportionately increased risks of stroke suggest that the hemodynamic problems associated with severe stenosis contribute to an increased risk of stroke. The severity of stenosis alone, however, does not correlate well with the degree of hemodynamic compromise [28]. The cerebral vasculature has a high potential for developing collateral channels, including the circle of Willis, ophthalmic artery, and leptomeningeal vessels. Accordingly, the pattern of collateral pathways, especially the development of ophthalmic and leptomeningeal collaterals, is also important in determining hemodynamic status [34–36].

The pattern of infarction may suggest the presence of hemodynamic failure. Data from the NASCET study demonstrated that internal border zone infarction (IBI) occurs in association with a high degree of ICA stenosis [37]. The incidence of pure IBI is relatively rare (3.4%) in stroke patients, but the presence of this finding along with the lesions occurring in the centrum semiovale may provide strong evidence of hemodynamic failure [38–40]. Although embolism can also result in IBI, especially in cases with isolated cortical border-zone infarcts [39], this may still be the footprint of hemodynamic impairment.

The correlation between cerebral hemodynamic impairment and the risk of subsequent stroke has been investigated via measurements of various cerebral perfusion parameters. Grubb and Powers categorized cerebral hemodynamic impairment into three stages according to changes measured by positron emission tomography (PET): from normal (stage 0) to stages 1 and 2 hemodynamic failure with a progressive decrease in cerebral perfusion pressure (CPP) [41]. In stage 1, vasodilatation of the arterioles maintains normal cerebral blood flow (CBF) associated with an increased cerebral blood volume (CBV). With a further decrease in CPP, autoregulation fails to maintain CBF, so the oxygen extraction fraction (OEF) begins to increase (stage 2) to maintain normal brain oxygen metabolism and function. This stage is termed 'misery perfusion' [42].

Stage 1 hemodynamic failure can be detected by the measurement of increased CBV or CBV/CBF ratio by PET and by computed tomography (CT)/magnetic resonance imaging (MRI) quantitatively and qualitatively, respectively. However, the clinical implications of these results have yet to be elucidated [43]. Autoregulatory vasodilatation can be evaluated by comparing the CBF before and after a variety of vasodilatory stimuli, such as hypercapnia, intravenous challenge with acetazolamide, or physiological tasks, such as hand movements [28, 44]. If the increase in CBF is impaired following the stimulus compared to the normal condition, the presence of autoregulatory vasodilatory failure is confirmed. This reduced responsiveness to stimuli is also known as reduced cerebrovascular reserve capacity (CVRC). Information about an impaired reserve capacity can be obtained by transcranial Doppler (TCD), single-photon emission CT (SPECT), xenon CT, MRI, and CT perfusion studies [44]. Such qualitative studies provide valuable information about unilateral hemodynamic impairments. However, the correlation between stage 1 hemodynamic failure and the subsequent risk of stroke is inconsistent; although many studies have demonstrated an increased risk of stroke associated with a decreased reserve capacity [45–50], other well-designed studies failed to show this correlation [51, 52].

Only PET can accurately detect the stage 2 hemodynamic impairment (misery perfusion) by measuring the increase in OEF. A well-designed prospective and blind trial demonstrated that stage 2 hemodynamic impairment correlated significantly with an increased risk of subsequent stroke [41]. This longitudinal cohort study demonstrated that the occurrence of stroke ipsilateral to the occlusive lesion in the stage 2 group was 26.5% in 2 years, whereas it was 5.3% in the patients with a normal OEF. The age-adjusted relative risk by stage 2 hemodynamic failure was 7.3 for ipsilateral stroke. Similar results were reported by another prospective study in patients with symptomatic ICA- or MCA-occlusive lesions. Over 5 years, the relative risk of ipsilateral stroke was 6.4 for patients with an increased OEF compared with those with a normal OEF [53]. Accordingly, the presence of misery perfusion has been considered a potential indication for revascularization procedures, including bypass surgery and endovascular intervention. OEF measurements using PET, however, are not widely available in clinical practice. Although a close correlation between OEF and other more commonly available hemodynamic measurements has been reported [54–56], controversy persists concerning the validity of these techniques for predicting subsequent stroke.

Indications for Revascularization Based on Hemodynamic Impairment

PET studies have demonstrated that EC-IC bypass can restore the impaired cerebral hemodynamics, including impaired cerebral vasoreactivity and increased OEF [42, 57]. Iwama and Hashimoto also showed that STA-MCA anastomosis improved neurological dysfunction in a subgroup of patients with significantly elevated OEF. They analyzed the results of pre- and postoperative PET studies in 16 patients with stable neurological dysfunction of grades 1–3 on a modified Rankin Scale (mRS). The EC-IC bypass surgery decreased the average OEF of the affected side, but only six patients showed neurological improvement after surgery. Their preoperative OEF and cerebral metabolic rate of oxygen ($CMRO_2$) values were significantly higher than those of the patients without improvement [58]. The improvement in cerebrovascular reserve capacity measured by other imaging methods has also been reported [59, 60], and several studies have confirmed the efficacy of EC-IC bypass surgery for improving anterior circulation hemodynamic impairments in selected patients [58, 61, 62].

There have been a few large bypass surgery trials based on hemodynamic impairment. The Carotid Occlusion Surgery Study trial uses PET to identify participants in stage 2 hemodynamic failure among those with symptomatic carotid occlusion [63]. To test the hypothesis that STA-MCA anastomosis can reduce the occurrence of ipsilateral stroke, the authors investigated 195 patients (97 in the surgery group, 98 in the medical group) in 49 clinical centers for 2 years. Two-year rates for the primary endpoint were 21.0% for the surgical group and 22.7% for the nonsurgical group. The difference in rates was only 1.7% (95% confidence interval [CI], –10.4% to 13.8%, p = 0.78, Z test). Thirty-day rates for ipsilateral ischemic stroke were 14.4% in the surgical group and 2.0% in the nonsurgical group with a difference of 12.4% (95% CI, 4.9–19.9%) [64].

On the other hand, the Japanese EC-IC Bypass Trial (JET) study enrolled 206 patients (103 each in the medical and surgical groups) between November 1998 and March 2002 at 28 centers in Japan [65, 66]. Participants were selected using ^{123}I-IMP SPECT among those with TIA or minor strokes within 3 months before entry. Randomized patients were to have ICA or MCA steno-occlusive lesions. In the JET study, patients were included when there was misery perfusion defined by a decreased CBF of <80% of the normal control value and a concomitant decrease of CVRC of <10%. An interim analysis of this trial of 196 patients (98 each in the medical and surgical groups) enrolled until January 31, 2002 reported that STA-MCA anastomosis reduced the ipsilateral stroke rate compared with the medically treated patients at 2 years (3.1% versus 11.2%, p = 0.045) [65]. However, the final report that includes the pre- and postoperative cognitive function test results is pending [65, 66].

Indeed, the proportion of hemodynamic stroke is relatively rare among all stroke patients [67], and impaired cerebral perfusion often improves spontaneously with time [49, 68, 69]. Therefore, a revascularization procedure should be considered carefully for those selected patients with sustained hemodynamic failure following cerebral ischemic events. The hemodynamic parameters should be measured for several weeks following the acute ischemic attack to assess the need for revascularization [58]. The potential benefit provided by EC-IC bypass should always be weighed against the morbidity that might result from the surgery, and patients with major medical problems should be excluded to avoid complications. Evidence also suggests that the best medical treatment should always be provided regardless of the need for revascularization procedures.

Because the risk of secondary stroke is highest in the early period following the first attack [31], emergency EC-IC bypass surgery may be considered, especially when the patient's neurological symptoms fluctuate or progress. Early revascularization procedure results to date have been inconsistent: some showed poor outcomes with a high risk of intracranial hemorrhage [14, 70], while others described favorable results with acceptable complication rates [71–75]. Patients with mild to moderate deficits associated with crescendo TIA or progressing stroke benefit the most from early revascularization, while those with severe fixed neurological deficits do not. The number of reported cases, however, is too small to draw definite conclusions, so further studies are needed.

Revascularization Surgery for Posterior Circulation Ischemia

Stroke patients with intracranial vertebrobasilar stenosis have a relatively poor prognosis with an annual rate of stroke recurrence or death of 24.2% [76]. Similar results were obtained in the subgroup analysis of the WASID study for intracranial posterior circulation disease, which showed an annual rate of ischemic stroke, brain hemorrhage, and non-stroke vascular death of 25% in the aspirin treated group and 24% in the warfarin treated group [31].

When the risk of stroke was evaluated using quantitative magnetic resonance angiography, patients with low-flow distal to steno-occlusive lesions demonstrated a higher risk of subsequent stroke compared to those with a normal flow [77]. Hemodynamic mechanisms may also play a role in the pathogenesis of cerebellar infarction [78]. Thus, these patients at increased risk of stroke through hemodynamic impairment may be potential candidates for revascularization procedures.

EC-IC bypass of the posterior circulation can be performed by connecting the STA or OA to the PCA or cerebellar arteries (SCA, AICA, or PICA). Free vein or arterial grafts may also be used. Ausman and Diaz reported their experience with 85 cases of EC-IC bypass surgery in the posterior circulation [79]. All of their patients had TIAs that were presumably related to severe bilateral distal vertebral artery or basilar artery disease. In their series, 69% of patients had complete symptom resolution, but the morbidity (13.3%) and mortality (8.4%) rates were high compared to those with anterior circulation disease. Recurrence of the vertebrobasilar insufficiency was observed in 11.8% of cases, and clinically stable patients showed better results than unstable patients.

A review of the literature by Hopkins also showed significant complications of EC-IC bypass in the posterior circulation [80]. In their review of 86 cases of STA-PCA or STA-SCA bypass, the patency rate was 79%, the mortality rate was 12%, and the complication rate was as high as 55%, with at least 20% of the patients having serious morbidities. A review of 76 cases of OA-to-PICA bypass demonstrated somewhat better results. The overall patency rate was 91%, mortality rate was 3%, and complication rate was 22% with a 10% rate of serious morbidities. The blood flow volume through this bypass, however, was less satisfactory than that through the STA-PCA or STA-SCA bypass. These reports suggest that further studies are needed to elucidate the possible benefit of bypass surgery in patients with intracranial diseases in the posterior circulation. Conservative approaches should be taken before considering intracranial bypass surgery in these patients [80].

Decompressive Craniectomy for Massive MCA Infarction

Intracranial atherosclerosis usually produces subcortical infarction often associated with small and scattered cortical infarcts [81]. Thus, in contrast to embolic infarction, massive infarction involving the entire MCA territory is unusual in patients with intrinsic MCA atherosclerosis. However, decompressive surgery must be considered in occasional patients with extensive MCA territory infarction associated with inadequately developed collateral circulation.

Very large infarction following MCA occlusion leads to a mortality rate as high as 80%, and the survivors suffer from serious morbidities [82–84]. The elevated intracranial pressure induced by significant edema reduces cerebral perfusion, further increasing the infarct volume, and finally leads to brain death by transtentorial herniation. For these patients, Ivamoto and Donaghy [85] proposed surgical decompression therapy in 1974. In 1981, Rengachary [86] reported on three patients who had been successfully treated by hemicraniectomy. In the 1990s, several studies reported that the surgical procedure decreased the mortality rate in these patients and sometimes improved the long term quality of life, especially in young patients with nondominant hemispheric infarcts [87–91]. A large hemicraniectomy extending to the temporal base accompanied by durotomy is currently recommended to provide appropriate reduction of the intracranial pressure (fig. 3).

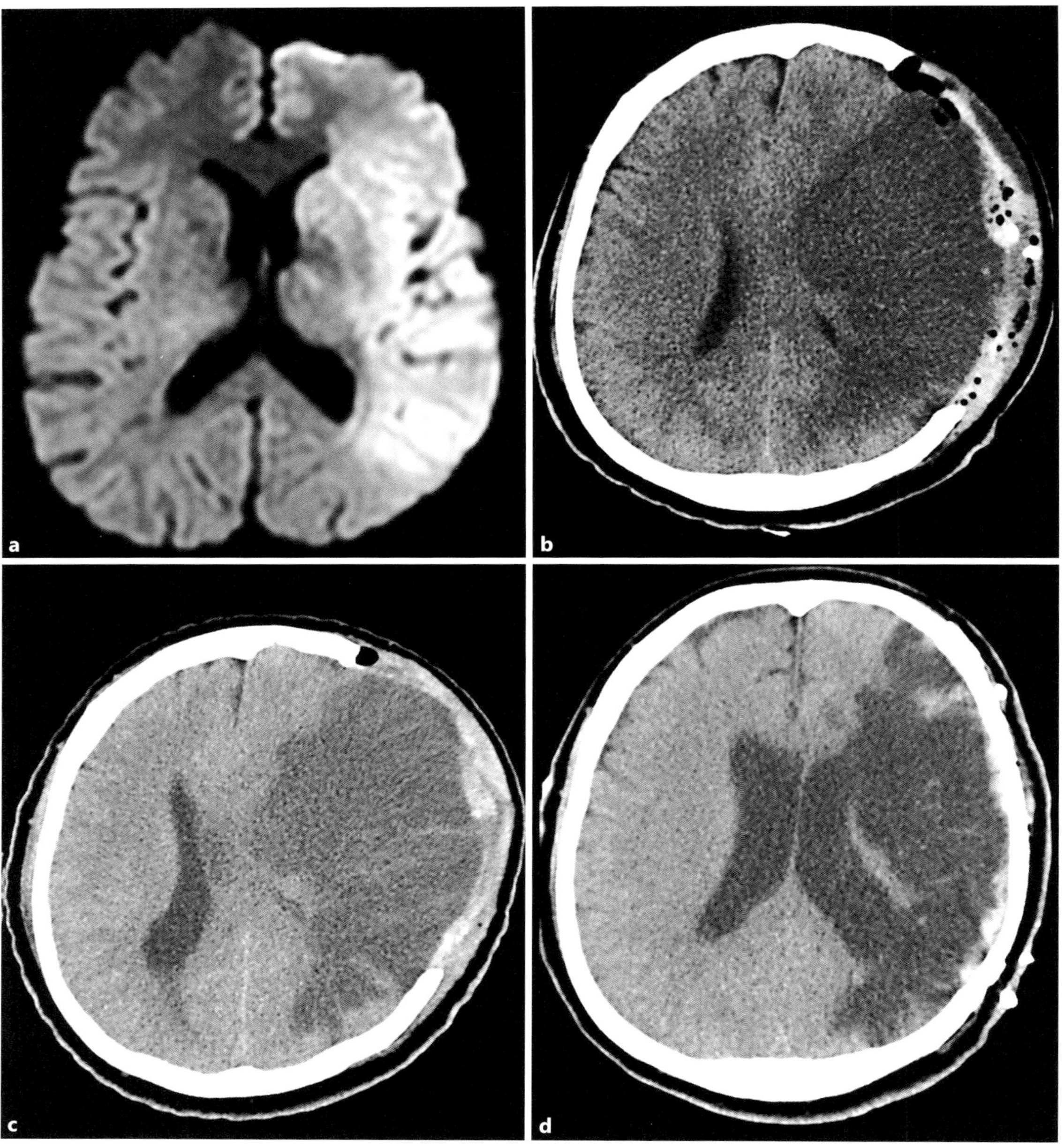

Fig. 3. Hemicraniectomy for massive infarction by the occlusion of the middle cerebral artery (MCA). **a** Diffusion-weighted image showing the left MCA territory infarction. **b** Immediately after surgery. **c** Brain swelling at 1 week of follow-up. **d** After cranioplasty.

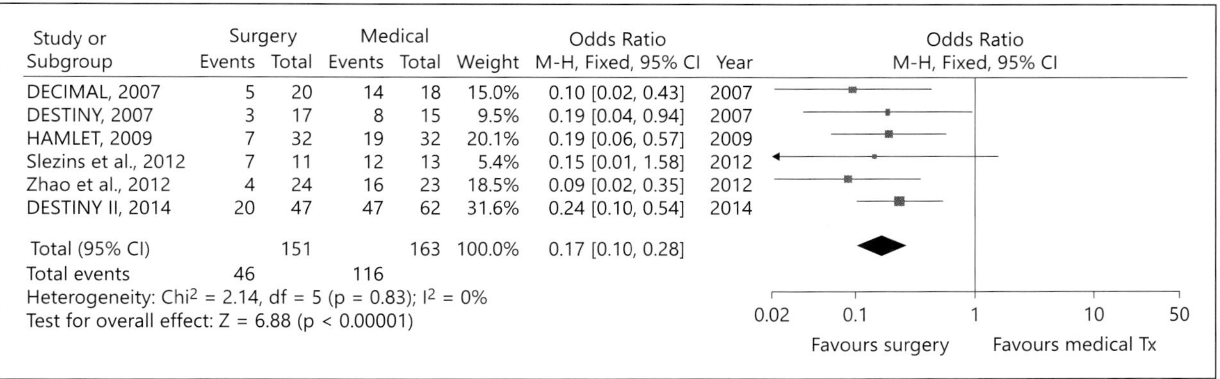

Study or Subgroup	Surgery Events	Surgery Total	Medical Events	Medical Total	Weight	Odds Ratio M-H, Fixed, 95% CI	Year
DECIMAL, 2007	5	20	14	18	15.0%	0.10 [0.02, 0.43]	2007
DESTINY, 2007	3	17	8	15	9.5%	0.19 [0.04, 0.94]	2007
HAMLET, 2009	7	32	19	32	20.1%	0.19 [0.06, 0.57]	2009
Slezins et al., 2012	7	11	12	13	5.4%	0.15 [0.01, 1.58]	2012
Zhao et al., 2012	4	24	16	23	18.5%	0.09 [0.02, 0.35]	2012
DESTINY II, 2014	20	47	47	62	31.6%	0.24 [0.10, 0.54]	2014
Total (95% CI)		151		163	100.0%	0.17 [0.10, 0.28]	
Total events	46		116				

Heterogeneity: $Chi^2 = 2.14$, df = 5 (p = 0.83); $I^2 = 0\%$
Test for overall effect: Z = 6.88 (p < 0.00001)

Fig. 4. One-year mortality reported by randomized prospective clinical trials.

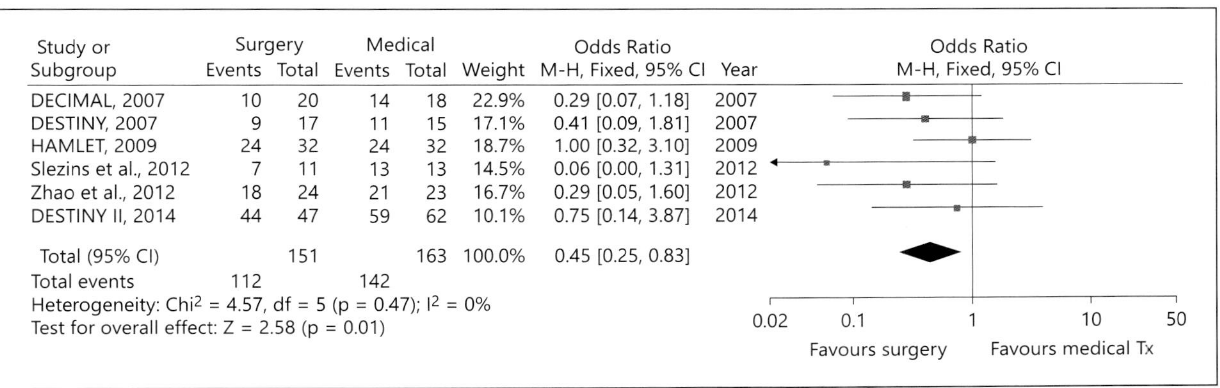

Study or Subgroup	Surgery Events	Surgery Total	Medical Events	Medical Total	Weight	Odds Ratio M-H, Fixed, 95% CI	Year
DECIMAL, 2007	10	20	14	18	22.9%	0.29 [0.07, 1.18]	2007
DESTINY, 2007	9	17	11	15	17.1%	0.41 [0.09, 1.81]	2007
HAMLET, 2009	24	32	24	32	18.7%	1.00 [0.32, 3.10]	2009
Slezins et al., 2012	7	11	13	13	14.5%	0.06 [0.00, 1.31]	2012
Zhao et al., 2012	18	24	21	23	16.7%	0.29 [0.05, 1.60]	2012
DESTINY II, 2014	44	47	59	62	10.1%	0.75 [0.14, 3.87]	2014
Total (95% CI)		151		163	100.0%	0.45 [0.25, 0.83]	
Total events	112		142				

Heterogeneity: $Chi^2 = 4.57$, df = 5 (p = 0.47); $I^2 = 0\%$
Test for overall effect: Z = 2.58 (p = 0.01)

Fig. 5. One-year disability (modified Rankin scale score of 4 or 5) including mortality from randomized prospective clinical trials.

There have been seven prospective multi-center randomized trials to date:

(1) Hemicraniectomy and Durotomy upon Deterioration from Infarction Related Swelling Trial (HeADDFIRST [American trial]) [92];

(2) Decompressive Surgery for the Treatment of Malignant Infarction of the Middle Cerebral Artery (DESTINY [German trial]) [93];

(3) Decompressive Surgery for the Treatment of Malignant Infarction of the Middle Cerebral Artery II (DESTINY II [German trial]) [94];

(4) Early Decompressive Craniectomy in Malignant Middle Cerebral Artery Infarction (DECIMAL [French trial]) [95];

(5) Hemicraniectomy after Middle Cerebral Artery Infarction with Life-threatening Edema Trial (HAMLET [Dutch trial]) [96, 97];

(6) Decompressive hemicraniectomy in malignant middle cerebral artery infarct: a randomized controlled trial enrolling patients up to 80 years old (Chinese trial) [98];

(7) Preliminary results of randomized controlled study on decompressive craniectomy in

treatment of malignant middle cerebral artery stroke ([Latvian trial]) [99].

The HeADDFIRST study demonstrated similar mortality rates at 6 months in the surgical and medical group (40 vs. 36%) [92]. However, the DESTINY trial, in which patients in the surgical group underwent surgery within 36 hours of symptom onset, showed that hemicraniectomy improved survival at 1 year compared with conservative management (82 vs. 47%, respectively). With 32 patients enrolled, this trial failed to demonstrate that hemicraniectomy had any significant benefits in improving the mRS score (0–3 vs. 4–6) at 6 and 12 months. The trial was terminated early because of the result of the pooled analysis from the three European trials [93]. In the DECIMAL trial, surgery was performed within 30 h of symptom onset. Patients with an infarct volume >145 cm^3 from diffusion-weighted MRI were enrolled. There was a 52.8% absolute reduction in death following hemicraniectomy compared with medical therapy alone ($p < 0.0001$). Study results on 38 patients showed that surgery increased the number of patients showing mild to moderate disability (mRS ≤3; 25 vs. 5.6% at 6 months); however, the difference was not statistically significant. This trial was also terminated soon after the pooled analysis results were reported [95].

Before the termination of the DESTINY and DECIMAL trials, investigators from the DESTINY, DECIMAL, and HAMLET studies decided to pool their data prospectively. Ninety-three patients were included in this pooled analysis. The surgery group showed a significantly better survival rate than the conservatively treated group (78 vs. 29%; 50% reduction in absolute risk). The patients in the decompressive surgery group showed a better clinical outcome than the patients managed conservatively (75 vs. 24% with mRS ≤4; 43 vs. 21% with mRS ≤3) [100]. Furthermore, randomized controlled studies conducted in China and Latvia also showed lower mortality and disability rates at 1 year of follow-up after randomization [98, 99]. The superiority of hemicraniectomy in older (≥60 years old) patients with MCA territory infarction was described by the DESTINY II trial. The proportion of patients without severe disability was 38% in the hemicraniectomy group and 18% in the control group ($p = 0.04$). A lower mortality rate was reported in the surgery group (33 vs. 70%) [94].

Regarding 1-year mortality, a pooled analysis using the results of six random controlled trials (not including HeADDFIRST) showed that decompressive craniectomy is effective (fig. 4). Moreover, hemicraniectomy can prevent severe disability (fig. 5). In short, decompressive surgery undertaken for massive infarction reduces mortality and increases the number of patients with a favorable functional outcome.

Surgical therapy is sometimes helpful in improving clinical outcomes for patients with intracranial atherosclerotic disease. This includes extracranial to intracranial bypass procedures to revascularize the brain in cases of hemodynamic ischemia that is not responsive to maximal medical therapy, and decompressive hemicraniectomy for extensive ICA or MCA infarcts.

References

1 Kawashima M, Rhoton AL Jr, Tanriover N, Ulm AJ, Yasuda A, Fujii K: Microsurgical anatomy of cerebral revascularization. Part I: anterior circulation. J Neurosurg 2005;102:116–131.

2 Kawashima M, Rhoton AL Jr, Tanriover N, Ulm AJ, Yasuda A, Fujii K: Microsurgical anatomy of cerebral revascularization. Part II: posterior circulation. J Neurosurg 2005;102:132–147.

3 Sundt TM Jr, Piepgras DG, Marsh WR, Fode NC: Saphenous vein bypass grafts for giant aneurysms and intracranial occlusive disease. J Neurosurg 1986;65:439–450.

4 Regli L, Piepgras DG, Hansen KK: Late patency of long saphenous vein bypass grafts to the anterior and posterior cerebral circulation. J Neurosurg 1995;83: 806–811.
5 Newell DW, Vilela MD: Superficial temporal artery to middle cerebral artery bypass. Neurosurgery 2004;54:1441–1448; discussion 1448–1449.
6 Wanebo JE, Zabramski JM, Spetzler RF: Superficial temporal artery-to-middle cerebral artery bypass grafting for cerebral revascularization. Neurosurgery 2004;55:395–398; discussion 398–399.
7 Diaz FG, Umansky F, Mehta B, Montoya S, Dujovny M, Ausman JI, Cabezudo J: Cerebral revascularization to a main limb of the middle cerebral artery in the Sylvian fissure. An alternative approach to conventional anastomosis. J Neurosurg 1985;63:21–29.
8 Lawton MT, Hamilton MG, Morcos JJ, Spetzler RF: Revascularization and aneurysm surgery: current techniques, indications, and outcome. Neurosurgery 1996;38:83–92; discussion 92–84.
9 MG Y: Microsurgery applied to neurosurgery. Stuttgart, George Thieme Verlag, 1969.
10 Donaghy RM: Neurologic surgery. Surg Gynecol Obstet 1972;134:269–270.
11 MG Y: Microvascular surgery. Stuttgart, George Thieme Verlag, 1967.
12 Heilbrun MP, Reichman OH, Anderson RE, Roberts TS: Regional cerebral blood flow studies following superficial temporal-middle cerebral artery anastomosis. J Neurosurg 1975;43:706–716.
13 Popp AJ, Chater N: Extracranial to intracranial vascular anastomosis for occlusive cerebrovascular disease: experience in 110 patients. Surgery 1977;82:648–654.
14 Gratzl O, Schmiedek P, Spetzler R, Steinhoff H, Marguth F: Clinical experience with extra-intracranial arterial anastomosis in 65 cases. J Neurosurg 1976;44:313–324.
15 Yasargil MG, Yonekawa Y: Results of microsurgical extra-intracranial arterial bypass in the treatment of cerebral ischemia. Neurosurgery 1977;1:22–24.
16 Sundt TM Jr, Whisnant JP, Fode NC, Piepgras DG, Houser OW: Results, complications, and follow-up of 415 bypass operations for occlusive disease of the carotid system. Mayo Clin Proc 1985;60: 230–240.
17 Chater N: Neurosurgical extracranial-intracranial bypass for stroke: with 400 cases. Neurol Res 1983;5:1–9.
18 Failure of extracranial-intracranial arterial bypass to reduce the risk of ischemic stroke. Results of an international randomized trial. The EC/IC bypass study group. N Engl J Med 1985;313:1191–1200.
19 The international cooperative study of extracranial/intracranial arterial anastomosis (EC/IC bypass study): methodology and entry characteristics. The EC/IC bypass study group. Stroke 1985;16: 397–406.
20 Awad IA, Spetzler RF: Extracranial-intracranial bypass surgery: a critical analysis in light of the international cooperative study. Neurosurgery 1986;19: 655–664.
21 Sundt TM Jr: Was the international randomized trial of extracranial-intracranial arterial bypass representative of the population at risk? N Engl J Med 1987; 316:814–816.
22 Goldring S, Zervas N, Langfitt T: The extracranial-intracranial bypass study. A report of the committee appointed by the American association of neurological surgeons to examine the study. N Engl J Med 1987;316:817–820.
23 Barnett HJ, Sackett D, Taylor DW, Haynes B, Peerless SJ, Meissner I, Hachinski V, Fox A: Are the results of the extracranial-intracranial bypass trial generalizable? N Engl J Med 1987;316:820–824.
24 Plum F: Extracranial-intracranial arterial bypass and cerebral vascular disease. N Engl J Med 1985;313:1221–1223.
25 Ausman JI, Diaz FG: Critique of the extracranial-intracranial bypass study. Surg Neurol 1986;26:218–221.
26 Barnett HJ, Fox A, Hachinski V, Haynes B, Peerless SJ, Sackett D, Taylor DW: Further conclusions from the extracranial-intracranial bypass trial. Surg Neurol 1986;26:227–235.
27 Day AL, Rhoton AL Jr, Little JR: The extracranial-intracranial bypass study. Surg Neurol 1986;26:222–226.
28 Powers WJ: Cerebral hemodynamics in ischemic cerebrovascular disease. Ann Neurol 1991;29:231–240.
29 Barnett HJ: Hemodynamic cerebral ischemia. An appeal for systematic data gathering prior to a new EC/IC trial. Stroke 1997;28:1857–1860.
30 Chimowitz MI, Lynn MJ, Howlett-Smith H, Stern BJ, Hertzberg VS, Frankel MR, Levine SR, Chaturvedi S, Kasner SE, Benesch CG, Sila CA, Jovin TG, Romano JG; Warfarin-Aspirin Symptomatic Intracranial Disease Trial Investigators: Comparison of warfarin and aspirin for symptomatic intracranial arterial stenosis. N Engl J Med 2005;352:1305–1316.
31 Kasner SE, Lynn MJ, Chimowitz MI, Frankel MR, Howlett-Smith H, Hertzberg VS, Chaturvedi S, Levine SR, Stern BJ, Benesch CG, Jovin TG, Sila CA, Romano JG; Warfarin Aspirin Symptomatic Intracranial Disease Trial Investigators: Warfarin vs aspirin for symptomatic intracranial stenosis: subgroup analyses from wasid. Neurology 2006;67:1275–1278.
32 Kasner SE, Chimowitz MI, Lynn MJ, Howlett-Smith H, Stern BJ, Hertzberg VS, Frankel MR, Levine SR, Chaturvedi S, Benesch CG, Sila CA, Jovin TG, Romano JG, Cloft HJ; Warfarin Aspirin Symptomatic Intracranial Disease Trial Investigators: Predictors of ischemic stroke in the territory of a symptomatic intracranial arterial stenosis. Circulation 2006;113:555–563.
33 Morgenstern LB, Fox AJ, Sharpe BL, Eliasziw M, Barnett HJ, Grotta JC: The risks and benefits of carotid endarterectomy in patients with near occlusion of the carotid artery. North American Symptomatic Carotid Endarterectomy Trial (NASCET) Group. Neurology 1997; 48:911–915.
34 Brozici M, van der Zwan A, Hillen B: Anatomy and functionality of leptomeningeal anastomoses: a review. Stroke 2003;34:2750–2762.
35 Hofmeijer J, Klijn CJ, Kappelle LJ, Van Huffelen AC, Van Gijn J: Collateral circulation via the ophthalmic artery or leptomeningeal vessels is associated with impaired cerebral vasoreactivity in patients with symptomatic carotid artery occlusion. Cerebrovasc Dis 2002;14: 22–26.
36 Yamauchi H, Kudoh T, Sugimoto K, Takahashi M, Kishibe Y, Okazawa H: Pattern of collaterals, type of infarcts, and haemodynamic impairment in carotid artery occlusion. J Neurol Neurosurg Psychiatry 2004;75:1697–1701.

37 Del Sette M, Eliasziw M, Streifler JY, Hachinski VC, Fox AJ, Barnett HJ: Internal borderzone infarction: a marker for severe stenosis in patients with symptomatic internal carotid artery disease. For the North American Symptomatic Carotid Endarterectomy (NASCET) Group. Stroke 2000;31:631–636.

38 Gandolfo C, Del Sette M, Finocchi C, Calautti C, Loeb C: Internal borderzone infarction in patients with ischemic stroke. Cerebrovasc Dis 1998;8:255–258.

39 Momjian-Mayor I, Baron JC: The pathophysiology of watershed infarction in internal carotid artery disease: review of cerebral perfusion studies. Stroke 2005; 36:567–577.

40 Yamauchi H, Fukuyama H, Nagahama Y, Nabatame H, Nakamura K, Yamamoto Y, Yonekura Y, Konishi J, Kimura J: Evidence of misery perfusion and risk for recurrent stroke in major cerebral arterial occlusive diseases from pet. J Neurol Neurosurg Psychiatry 1996;61: 18–25.

41 Grubb RL Jr, Derdeyn CP, Fritsch SM, Carpenter DA, Yundt KD, Videen TO, Spitznagel EL, Powers WJ: Importance of hemodynamic factors in the prognosis of symptomatic carotid occlusion. JAMA 1998;280:1055–1060.

42 Baron JC, Bousser MG, Rey A, Guillard A, Comar D, Castaigne P: Reversal of focal 'misery-perfusion syndrome' by extra-intracranial arterial bypass in hemodynamic cerebral ischemia. A case study with 15O positron emission tomography. Stroke 1981;12:454–459.

43 Grubb RL Jr: Extracranial-intracranial arterial bypass for treatment of occlusion of the internal carotid artery. Curr Neurol Neurosci Rep 2004;4:23–30.

44 Derdeyn CP, Grubb RL Jr, Powers WJ: Cerebral hemodynamic impairment: methods of measurement and association with stroke risk. Neurology 1999; 53:251–259.

45 Kuroda S, Houkin K, Kamiyama H, Mitsumori K, Iwasaki Y, Abe H: Long-term prognosis of medically treated patients with internal carotid or middle cerebral artery occlusion: can acetazolamide test predict it? Stroke 2001;32: 2110–2116.

46 Ogasawara K, Ogawa A, Terasaki K, Shimizu H, Tominaga T, Yoshimoto T: Use of cerebrovascular reactivity in patients with symptomatic major cerebral artery occlusion to predict 5-year outcome: comparison of xenon-133 and iodine-123-imp single-photon emission computed tomography. J Cereb Blood Flow Metab 2002;22:1142–1148.

47 Vernieri F, Pasqualetti P, Passarelli F, Rossini PM, Silvestrini M: Outcome of carotid artery occlusion is predicted by cerebrovascular reactivity. Stroke 1999; 30:593–598.

48 Webster MW, Makaroun MS, Steed DL, Smith HA, Johnson DW, Yonas H: Compromised cerebral blood flow reactivity is a predictor of stroke in patients with symptomatic carotid artery occlusive disease. J Vasc Surg 1995;21:338–344; discussion 344–335.

49 Widder B, Kleiser B, Krapf H: Course of cerebrovascular reactivity in patients with carotid artery occlusions. Stroke 1994;25:1963–1967.

50 Yonas H, Smith HA, Durham SR, Pentheny SL, Johnson DW: Increased stroke risk predicted by compromised cerebral blood flow reactivity. J Neurosurg 1993; 79:483–489.

51 Powers WJ, Tempel LW, Grubb RL Jr: Influence of cerebral hemodynamics on stroke risk: one-year follow-up of 30 medically treated patients. Ann Neurol 1989;25:325–330.

52 Yokota C, Hasegawa Y, Minematsu K, Yamaguchi T: Effect of acetazolamide reactivity on [corrected] long-term outcome in patients with major cerebral artery occlusive diseases. Stroke 1998; 29:640–644.

53 Yamauchi H, Fukuyama H, Nagahama Y, Nabatame H, Ueno M, Nishizawa S, Konishi J, Shio H: Significance of increased oxygen extraction fraction in five-year prognosis of major cerebral arterial occlusive diseases. J Nucl Med 1999;40:1992–1998.

54 Herold S, Brown MM, Frackowiak RS, Mansfield AO, Thomas DJ, Marshall J: Assessment of cerebral haemodynamic reserve: correlation between PET parameters and CO2 reactivity measured by the intravenous 133 xenon injection technique. J Neurol Neurosurg Psychiatry 1988;51:1045–1050.

55 Hirano T, Minematsu K, Hasegawa Y, Tanaka Y, Hayashida K, Yamaguchi T: Acetazolamide reactivity on 123I-IMP single photon emission computed tomography in patients with major cerebral artery occlusive disease: correlation with positron emission tomography parameters. J Cereb Blood Flow Metab 1994;14:763–770.

56 Kanno I, Uemura K, Higano S, Murakami M, Iida H, Miura S, Shishido F, Inugami A, Sayama I: Oxygen extraction fraction at maximally vasodilated tissue in the ischemic brain estimated from the regional CO2 responsiveness measured by positron emission tomography. J Cereb Blood Flow Metab 1988;8:227–235.

57 Grubb RL Jr, Powers WJ: Risks of stroke and current indications for cerebral revascularization in patients with carotid occlusion. Neurosurg Clin N Am 2001; 12:473–487, vii.

58 Iwama T, Hashimoto N, Hayashida K: Cerebral hemodynamic parameters for patients with neurological improvements after extracranial-intracranial arterial bypass surgery: evaluation using positron emission tomography. Neurosurgery 2001;48:504–510; discussion 510–512.

59 Anderson DE, McLane MP, Reichman OH, Origitano TC: Improved cerebral blood flow and CO2 reactivity after microvascular anastomosis in patients at high risk for recurrent stroke. Neurosurgery 1992;31:26–33; discussion 33–34.

60 Schmiedek P, Piepgras A, Leinsinger G, Kirsch CM, Einhupl K: Improvement of cerebrovascular reserve capacity by EC-IC arterial bypass surgery in patients with ICA occlusion and hemodynamic cerebral ischemia. J Neurosurg 1994;81: 236–244.

61 Amin-Hanjani S, Butler WE, Ogilvy CS, Carter BS, Barker FG 2nd: Extracranial-intracranial bypass in the treatment of occlusive cerebrovascular disease and intracranial aneurysms in the United States between 1992 and 2001: a population-based study. J Neurosurg 2005;103: 794–804.

62 Nussbaum ES, Erickson DL: Extracranial-intracranial bypass for ischemic cerebrovascular disease refractory to maximal medical therapy. Neurosurgery 2000;46:37–42; discussion 42–43.

63 Grubb RL Jr, Powers WJ, Derdeyn CP, Adams HP Jr, Clarke WR: The carotid occlusion surgery study. Neurosurg Focus 2003;14:e9.
64 Powers WJ, Clarke WR, Grubb RL Jr, Videen TO, Adams HP Jr, Derdeyn CP, Investigators C: Extracranial-intracranial bypass surgery for stroke prevention in hemodynamic cerebral ischemia: the carotid occlusion surgery study randomized trial. JAMA 2011;306:1983–1992.
65 Group JS: Japanese EC-IC bypass trial (JET study). 脳卒中の外科 2002;30: 434–437.
66 Ogasawara K, Ogawa A: [JET study (Japanese EC-IC bypass trial)]. Nihon Rinsho 2006;64(suppl 7):524–527.
67 Bladin CF, Chambers BR: Frequency and pathogenesis of hemodynamic stroke. Stroke 1994;25:2179–2182.
68 Hasegawa Y, Yamaguchi T, Tsuchiya T, Minematsu K, Nishimura T: Sequential change of hemodynamic reserve in patients with major cerebral artery occlusion or severe stenosis. Neuroradiology 1992;34:15–21.
69 Kleiser B, Widder B: Course of carotid artery occlusions with impaired cerebrovascular reactivity. Stroke 1992;23: 171–174.
70 Crowell R: STA-MCA bypass for acute focal cerebral ischemia; Microsurgery for stroke, Springer, 1977, pp 244–250.
71 Diaz FG, Ausman JI, Mehta B, Dujovny M, de los Reyes RA, Pearce J, Patel S: Acute cerebral revascularization. J Neurosurg 1985;63:200–209.
72 Sakai K, Nitta J, Horiuchi T, Ogiwara T, Kobayashi S, Tanaka Y, Hongo K: Emergency revascularization for acute main-trunk occlusion in the anterior circulation. Neurosurg Rev 2008;31:69–76; discussion 76.
73 Yoshimoto Y, Kwak S: Superficial temporal artery – middle cerebral artery anastomosis for acute cerebral ischemia: the effect of small augmentation of blood flow. Acta Neurochir (Wien) 1995;137:128–137; discussion 137.
74 Hwang G, Oh CW, Bang JS, Jung CK, Kwon OK, Kim JE, Bae HJ, Han MK: Superficial temporal artery to middle cerebral artery bypass in acute ischemic stroke and stroke in progress. Neurosurgery 2011;68:723–729; discussion 729–730.
75 Horiuchi T, Nitta J, Ishizaka S, Kanaya K, Yanagawa T, Hongo K: Emergency EC-IC bypass for symptomatic atherosclerotic ischemic stroke. Neurosurg Rev 2013;36:559–564; discussion 564–565.
76 Qureshi AI, Suri MFK, Ziai WC, Yahia AM, Mohammad Y, Sen S, Agarwal P, Zaidat OO, Suarez JI, Wityk RJ: Stroke-free survival and its determinants in patients with symptomatic vertebrobasilar stenosis: a multicenter study. Neurosurgery 2003;52:1033–1040.
77 Amin-Hanjani S, Du X, Zhao M, Walsh K, Malisch TW, Charbel FT: Use of quantitative magnetic resonance angiography to stratify stroke risk in symptomatic vertebrobasilar disease. Stroke 2005;36:1140–1145.
78 Chaves CJ, Caplan LR, Chung CS, Tapia J, Amarenco P, Teal P, Wityk R, Estol C, Tettenborn B, Rosengart A, et al: Cerebellar infarcts in the New England medical center posterior circulation stroke registry. Neurology 1994;44: 1385–1390.
79 Ausman JI, Diaz FG, Vacca DF, Sadasivan B: Superficial temporal and occipital artery bypass pedicles to superior, anterior inferior, and posterior inferior cerebellar arteries for vertebrobasilar insufficiency. J Neurosurg 1990;72:554–558.
80 Hopkins LN, Budny JL: Complications of intracranial bypass for vertebrobasilar insufficiency. J Neurosurg 1989;70: 207–211.
81 Lee DK, Kim JS, Kwon SU, Yoo SH, Kang DW: Lesion patterns and stroke mechanism in atherosclerotic middle cerebral artery disease: early diffusion-weighted imaging study. Stroke 2005;36: 2583–2588.
82 Berrouschot J, Sterker M, Bettin S, Koster J, Schneider D: Mortality of space-occupying ('malignant') middle cerebral artery infarction under conservative intensive care. Intensive Care Med 1998;24:620–623.
83 Hacke W, Schwab S, Horn M, Spranger M, De Georgia M, von Kummer R: 'Malignant' middle cerebral artery territory infarction: clinical course and prognostic signs. Arch Neurol 1996;53:309–315.
84 Wijdicks EF, Diringer MN: Middle cerebral artery territory infarction and early brain swelling: progression and effect of age on outcome. Mayo Clin Proc 1998; 73:829–836.
85 Ivamoto HS, Numoto M, Donaghy RM: Surgical decompression for cerebral and cerebellar infarcts. Stroke 1974;5:365–370.
86 Rengachary SS, Batnitzky S, Morantz RA, Arjunan K, Jeffries B: Hemicraniectomy for acute massive cerebral infarction. Neurosurgery 1981;8:321–328.
87 Carter BS, Ogilvy CS, Candia GJ, Rosas HD, Buonanno F: One-year outcome after decompressive surgery for massive nondominant hemispheric infarction. Neurosurgery 1997;40:1168–1175; discussion 1175–1166.
88 Delashaw JB, Broaddus WC, Kassell NF, Haley EC, Pendleton GA, Vollmer DG, Maggio WW, Grady MS: Treatment of right hemispheric cerebral infarction by hemicraniectomy. Stroke 1990;21:874–881.
89 Mori K, Nakao Y, Yamamoto T, Maeda M: Early external decompressive craniectomy with duroplasty improves functional recovery in patients with massive hemispheric embolic infarction: timing and indication of decompressive surgery for malignant cerebral infarction. Surg Neurol 2004;62:420–429; discussion 429–430.
90 Rieke K, Schwab S, Krieger D, von Kummer R, Aschoff A, Schuchardt V, Hacke W: Decompressive surgery in space-occupying hemispheric infarction: results of an open, prospective trial. Crit Care Med 1995;23:1576–1587.
91 Sakai K, Iwahashi K, Terada K, Gohda Y, Sakurai M, Matsumoto Y: Outcome after external decompression for massive cerebral infarction. Neurol Med Chir (Tokyo) 1998;38:131–135; discussion 135–136.
92 Frank JI, Schumm LP, Wroblewski K, Chyatte D, Rosengart AJ, Kordeck C, Thisted RA; HeADDFIRST Trialists: Hemicraniectomy and durotomy upon deterioration from infarction-related swelling trial: randomized pilot clinical trial. Stroke 2014;45:781–787.
93 Juttler E, Schwab S, Schmiedek P, Unterberg A, Hennerici M, Woitzik J, Witte S, Jenetzky E, Hacke W; DESTINY Study Group: Decompressive surgery for the treatment of malignant infarction of the middle cerebral artery (DESTINY): a randomized, controlled trial. Stroke 2007;38:2518–2525.

94 Juttler E, Unterberg A, Woitzik J, Bosel J, Amiri H, Sakowitz OW, Gondan M, Schiller P, Limprecht R, Luntz S, Schneider H, Pinzer T, Hobohm C, Meixensberger J, Hacke W; DESTINY II Investigators: Hemicraniectomy in older patients with extensive middle-cerebral-artery stroke. N Engl J Med 2014;370: 1091–1100.
95 Vahedi K, Vicaut E, Mateo J, Kurtz A, Orabi M, Guichard JP, Boutron C, Couvreur G, Rouanet F, Touze E, Guillon B, Carpentier A, Yelnik A, George B, Payen D, Bousser MG; DECIMAL Investigators: Sequential-design, multicenter, randomized, controlled trial of early decompressive craniectomy in malignant middle cerebral artery infarction (DECIMAL Trial). Stroke 2007;38:2506–2517.
96 Hofmeijer J, Amelink GJ, Algra A, van Gijn J, Macleod MR, Kappelle LJ, van der Worp HB; HAMLET Investigators: Hemicraniectomy after middle cerebral artery infarction with life-threatening edema trial (HAMLET). Protocol for a randomised controlled trial of decompressive surgery in space-occupying hemispheric infarction. Trials 2006;7: 29.
97 Geurts M, van der Worp HB, Kappelle LJ, Amelink GJ, Algra A, Hofmeijer J; HAMLET Streeing Committee : Surgical decompression for space-occupying cerebral infarction: Outcomes at 3 years in the randomized HAMLET trial. Stroke 2013;44:2506–2508.
98 Zhao J, Su YY, Zhang Y, Zhang YZ, Zhao R, Wang L, Gao R, Chen W, Gao D: Decompressive hemicraniectomy in malignant middle cerebral artery infarct: a randomized controlled trial enrolling patients up to 80 years old. Neurocrit Care 2012;17:161–171.
99 Slezins J, Keris V, Bricis R, Millers A, Valeinis E, Stukens J, Minibajeva O: Preliminary results of randomized controlled study on decompressive craniectomy in treatment of malignant middle cerebral artery stroke. Medicina (Kaunas) 2012;48:521–524.
100 Vahedi K, Hofmeijer J, Juettler E, Vicaut E, George B, Algra A, Amelink GJ, Schmiedeck P, Schwab S, Rothwell PM, Bousser M-G, van der Worp HB, Hacke W: Early decompressive surgery in malignant infarction of the middle cerebral artery: a pooled analysis of three randomised controlled trials. Lancet Neurol 2007;6:215–222.

Chang Wan Oh, MD, PhD
Department of Neurosurgery, Seoul National University Bundang Hospital
82 Gumri-ro 173 Beon-gil, Bundang-gu
Seongnam 13620 (Korea)
E-Mail wanoh@snu.ac.kr

Kim JS, Caplan LR, Wong KS (eds): Intracranial Atherosclerosis: Pathophysiology, Diagnosis and Treatment.
Front Neurol Neurosci. Basel, Karger, 2016, vol 40, pp 179–203 (DOI: 10.1159/000448313)

Non-Atherosclerotic Intracranial Arterial Diseases

Jong S. Kim[a] · Louis R. Caplan[b]

[a]Department of Neurology, Asan Medical Center, University of Ulsan, Seoul, Republic of Korea; [b]Department of Neurology, Beth Israel Deaconess Medical Center, Boston, Mass., USA

Abstract

Atherosclerosis is not the only cause of intracranial arterial disease. Arterial dissection, moyamoya disease, vascular inflammatory disease, vasospasm and immunologic disorders are important non-atherosclerotic intracranial arterial diseases. Identification of the correct etiology is important in establishing treatment strategies and assessing prognosis. Careful history taking and appropriate laboratory testing are essential. Although catheter angiography is the most important diagnostic tool to examine various intracranial arterial diseases, other diagnostic modalities such as CT angiography and MR angiography are nowadays widely used. High resolution vessel wall MRI also can assist in making the correct diagnosis as this can yield information regarding vessel wall pathology. Certain diseases such as infectious vasculopathies and moyamoya disease are more prevalent in certain parts of the world, and physicians practicing in these regions should be mindful of these disorders. In this chapter, these non-atherosclerotic intracranial arterial diseases are discussed. Moyamoya disease will be described in another chapter.

Arterial Dissection

Cervicocerebral artery dissections account for 1–2% of all ischemic strokes [1–3], and 10–25% of ischemic strokes in young and middle-aged patients [4, 5]. According to population-based studies, the incidence of spontaneous arterial dissections was 1.7–3.0/100,000 in the internal carotid arteries (ICAs) and was 1.0–1.5/100,000 in the vertebral arteries (VAs) [1, 6, 7]. The prevalence is higher in men than in women [8, 9], and females are younger and more often have migraine and multiple dissections [8].

Cervicocerebral artery dissections can result from either primary intimal tear with secondary dissection into the media layer or primary intramedial hemorrhage. The intramural hematoma is located within the medial layer or near the intimal or adventitial layer. A subintimal dissection leads to luminal stenosis and obstruction, resulting in an ischemic event. A subadventitial dissection may cause aneurysmal formation (dissecting aneurysm) and, when intracranial, may cause subarachnoid hemorrhage (SAH).

Dissections are categorized as traumatic or spontaneous (non-traumatic). In patients with spontaneous dissections, minor trauma in the form of stretching of the neck still plays a causative role. Inherent conditions predisposing to spontaneous arterial dissections include fibromuscular dysplasia, cystic medial necrosis, α1 antitrypsin deficiency, Ehlers-Danlos syndrome type IV, Loeys-Dietz syndrome, Marfan's syndrome, autosomal dominant polycystic kidney disease, tuberous sclerosis, migraine, and hyperhomocysteinemia [3, 10]. Ultrastructural morphological aberrations of dermal connective tissue were found in more than half of patients with spontaneous cervical artery dissections [11].

Intracranial Arterial Dissection

Intracranial arterial dissections are known to be less frequent than extracranial dissections. In a retrospective analysis of 263 patients with spontaneous cervicocerebral artery dissections at the Mayo Clinic between 1970 and 1991, 33 (12.5%) had intracranial dissections [3]. Another study showed that among 67 patients with cervicocerebral artery dissections, 9 (13.4%) had intracranial dissections [12]. In a study including a series of 169 patients with 195 VA dissections, 21 dissections (11%) occurred intracranially [8].

The frequency of intracranial dissections may have been underestimated because the diagnosis of intracranial dissection is more difficult than that of the extracranial counterpart. Extensive evaluation, such as repeated MRA in suspected patients [13], and utilization of high resolution vessel wall MRI, that can identify dissection, flap, or mural hematoma more easily [14], will increase the likelihood of diagnosis of intracranial dissection [15]. With advanced imaging, a recent study on dissections causing ischemic stroke or transient ischemic attack (TIA) reported that intracranial arterial dissection is two times more common than extracranial arterial dissection [15]. The most frequent site was the intracranial VA (ICVA).

In contrast to the cervical arteries, the intracranial arteries lack external elastic lamina and have only a thin adventitial layer. Intracranial dissections more readily lead to the development of subadventitial dissections and dissecting aneurysm formation and SAH [16, 17]. Pathological studies have shown that subadventitial dissections are more frequent in the ICVA than in the middle cerebral artery (MCA) [18, 19]. This could explain the relatively high frequency of SAH in ICVA dissections as compared to dissections occurring in the MCA. Trauma, either serious or minor is more closely associated with extracranial dissections than intracranial dissections [3, 15, 17]. Extracranial vessels may be more susceptible to compression against bony structures after trauma, such as that caused by neck rotation. As in atherothrombotic infarction, extracranial dissection usually cause stroke or TIA via artery to artery embolism, whereas branch occlusion is an important stroke mechanism in intracranial dissections. Intracranial dissection frequently causes deep (subcortical and brainstem) infarction [20].

Clinical Manifestations

Dissection in the Anterior Circulation

In the anterior circulation, dissections most often occur in the supraclinoid ICA or the proximal MCA. Distal ICA dissection occasionally extends to the MCA (fig. 1). In a recent series, MCA dissection (19%) was the more prevalent than distal ICA dissection (12%) as a cause of ischemic stroke. In a review of 54 patients with MCA dissections who had 59, most presented with cerebral infarction (91%), while SAH was uncommon (9%) [21]. Most patients showed vascular luminal stenosis (87%), and a small number of patients had aneurysmal dilatation (11%) or a double

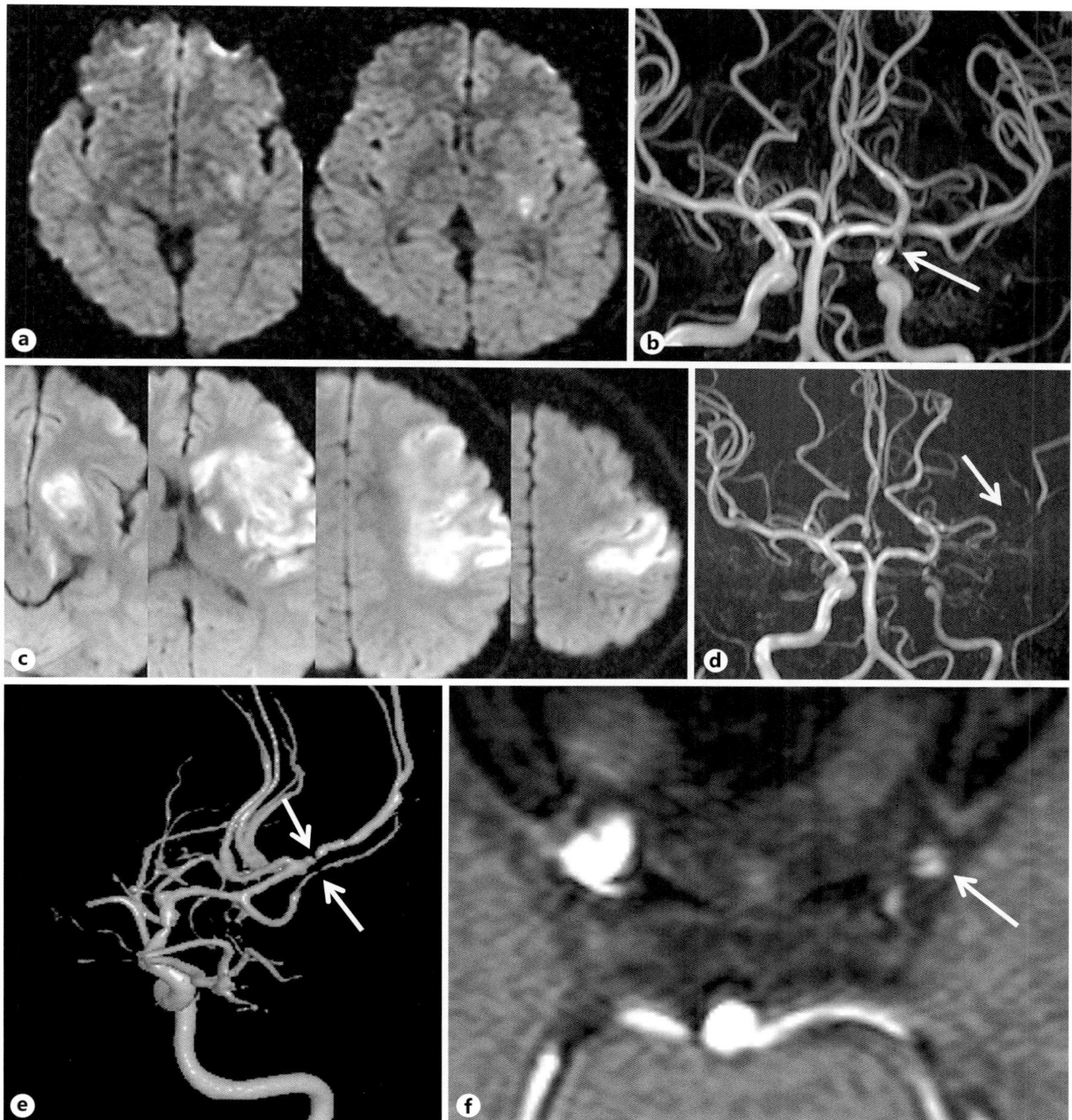

Fig. 1. A 26-year-old woman developed mild (IV/V) right limb weakness. Diffusion weighted MRI (DWI) showed an acute, focal, left basal ganglia infarction (**a**). MR angiogram showed focal stenosis in the left terminal internal carotid artery (ICA) (**b**, arrow). Three days later, she developed aphasia and her limb weakness progressed to grade I/V. Follow-up DWI showed extension of the infarction that involved most of the left middle cerebral artery (MCA) territory (**c**). MR angiogram showed more severe ICA stenosis and poor visualization of the left MCA (**d**, arrow). 3D reconstruction of conventional angiography showed severe stenosis in the left distal ICA, and diffuse narrowing of the M1 portion of the MCA, which suggests extension of the dissection. Multiple stenoses of the M2 portion of the MCA suggest embolic occlusion (**e**, arrows). Source image of three-dimensional time-of-flight (TOF) MR angiography showed a flap like structure inside the distal ICA and proximal MCA (**f**, arrow).

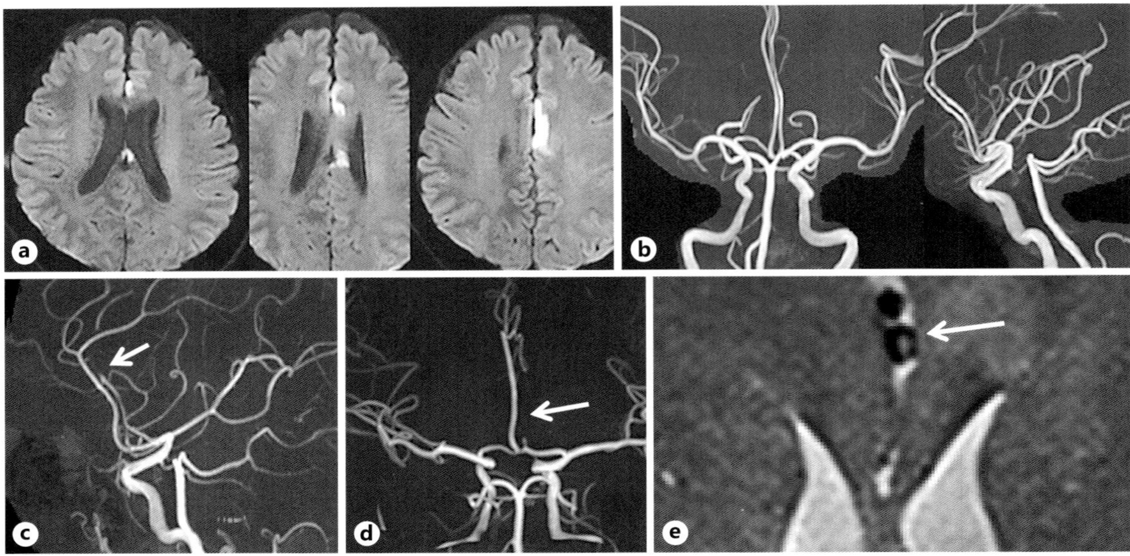

Fig. 2. A 54-year-old man without vascular risk factors developed slight (IV/V) right leg weakness. Diffusion weighted MRI showed left anterior cerebral artery (ACA) territory infarction (**a**). MR angiography findings were normal (**b**). After admission, the leg weakness worsened progressively (II/V). Four days later, an MR angiogram showed stenosis in the A2-A3 junction of the ACA (**c**, arrow). Five days later, an MR angiogram showed extension of the ACA stenosis (**d**, arrow). High resolution MRI showed dissection flap in one of the two ACAs (**e**, arrow), illustrating that he had an ACA dissection.

lumen (2%). Hemiparesis was the most frequent presenting symptom (92%), followed by headache (61%) and consciousness change (44%). Preceding trauma was more often found in isolated MCA dissections than intracranial ICA-MCA dissections (35 vs. 19%). The exact mechanism of how a blunt head injury causes MCA dissection is not clear. One proffered suggestion is that the impact of the MCA against the sphenoid ridge causes an intimal tear, which results in dissection [22]. In contrast, congenital vessel wall defects were found more often in intracranial ICA-MCA dissections than in isolated MCA dissections (26 vs. 4%) [21].

Dissection may account for the majority of fusiform aneurysms arising from the MCA. In a review of 102 cases of spontaneous fusiform MCA aneurysms, the mean age was 38 years, and the male-to-female ratio was 1.4:1.22/[18]. Most MCA aneurysms originated proximal to the MCA genu (M1 segment, 69%) and presented with ischemic symptoms or were found incidentally.

Dissections involving the anterior cerebral artery (ACA) are uncommon, but now are more easily detected by high resolution vessel wall imaging (fig. 2). In a study of 18 patients with nontraumatic ACA dissections, 9 had ischemia, 5 had SAH, and 4 patients had both [23]. Dissection should be suspected when patients with ACA territory infarction progressively deteriorate. The lesion sites of ACA dissections were mainly at the A2 portion for the patients with ischemia and at the A1 portion for those having SAH.

Dissection in the Posterior Circulation

In the posterior circulation, dissection most often develop in the ICVA. Although extracranial VA dissection has been traditionally emphasized [24,

25], recent reports from Asia suggest that intracranial VA dissection may be an even more important cause of ischemic stroke [26]. Many ECVA dissections that begin in the V3 portion high in the neck extend intracranially into the ICVA. VA dissections are often attributed to trauma associated with rotating neck motion such as chiropractic procedures or other neck manipulations [27]. Some arise from very minor trauma that include heavy coughing, falling on the back, and turning the head to back-up a car. Many others, however, do not have such a history [27–31].

The most common symptom of VA dissection is pain in the head or neck. Usually, the pain is in the posterior neck with radiation to the occiput, sometimes to the shoulder. Headache and neck pain may be the only complaints. Ischemic symptoms and signs may develop at the same time as the pain or after a delay of hours to a few days. The lateral medulla and cerebellum are the regions most susceptible to ischemia from VA dissection [24, 25] (fig. 3). Intracranial VA dissections most frequently involve the VA near the origin of the PICA. The dissections occasionally extend into the BA. Dissecting aneurysms can act as a mass lesion compressing the brainstem, cranial nerves or vessels [32]. In a study of 31 patients with ICVA dissections, 55% had headache, 48% had infarction involving the brainstem or cerebellum, and 10% presented with SAH [33].

Basilar artery (BA) dissections are uncommon and usually carry a more grave prognosis than VA dissections. They often produce extensive, bilateral pontine infarction clinically manifested as sudden altered consciousness and quadriparesis [34]. In a review of 38 patents with BA dissections, 27 had brainstem ischemia, 5 had SAH, and 6 patients had both ischemia and SAH. Thirty patients (79%) died [35]. A more recent study showed that unilateral pontine infarction with a favorable outcome is actually more common [36]. In another study of 10 patients with BA dissections, 5 had impaired consciousness, 4 SAH and one had mass effect on the brainstem, while the remaining 5 patients had brainstem ischemia [37].

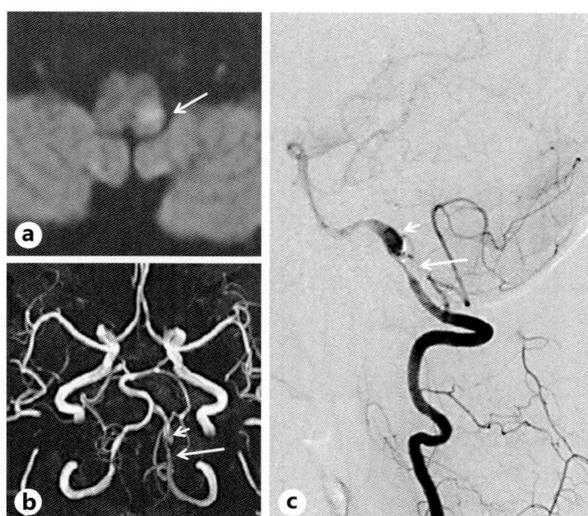

Fig. 3. A 36-year-old woman without vascular risk factors suddenly developed posterior neck/occipital headache followed by vertigo, nausea, and gait instability. Examination showed right-beating nystagmus, left Horner syndrome, decreased sensory perception on the left face and right arm, and gait ataxia. Diffusion weighted MRI showed left lateral medullary infarction (**a**, arrow). An MR angiogram showed severe stenosis in the left distal vertebral artery (**b**, long arrow) and a fusiform aneurysmal dilatation (**b**, short arrow), which was more clearly documented by catheter angiography (**c**). These findings are consistent with dissection that probably caused branch (perforator) occlusion leading to lateral medullary infarction. The Posterior inferior cerebellar artery remained intact.

Dissections occurring in the posterior cerebral artery (PCA) are rare [38]. In a review of 40 patients with PCA dissections, 15 had ischemia, 15 had SAH, and 6 had aneurysmal mass effect. Precipitating factors were found in nearly half of patients, including trauma, migraine, substance abuse, migraine, and the postpartum status [39].

Isolated dissections of the posterior inferior cerebellar artery (PICA) without involvement of

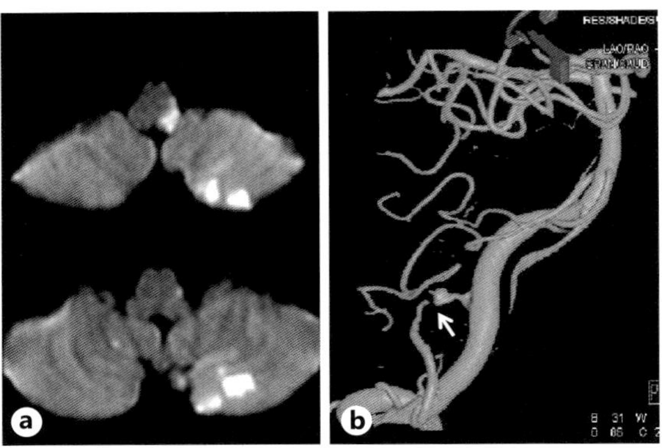

Fig. 4. A 52-year-old man without vascular risk factors developed sudden headache and interscapular pain followed by whirling vertigo, gait ataxia and dysphagia. Examination showed right beating nystagmus, skew deviation, left Horner sign, pinprick and temperature sensation loss in the left face and right hemibody. He also felt tingling sensation in the left forearm and hand. He had dysphagia, hoarseness and felt to the left on standing. Diffusion weighted MRI showed infarcts involving the left lateral medulla and medial cerebellum (**a**). MR angiogram did not reveal any abnormalities (not shown). An angiogram (3D reconstruction image) showed aneurysmal dilation and stenosis (**b**, arrow) consistent with posterior inferior cerebellar artery dissection.

the VA are rare and present either SAH or ischemic symptoms [40, 41]. PICA dissection presenting with ischemic symptoms may have been underdiagnosed, since cerebral angiography is often omitted in these patients (fig. 4). One report suggested that dissections occurring in the proximal PICA tend to produce ischemic symptoms, while those in the distal portion tend to cause SAH [42]. A recent study reported that among 167 patients with isolated PICA territory infarction, PICA dissection was the cause of stroke in 10 patients (6%) [13]. In 6 of these 10 patients PICA dissections had not been suspected on initial MRA, and were confirmed by follow-up MRA or digital subtraction angiography. Thus, more extensive work ups will find more cases of PICA dissection.

Fibromuscular Dysplasia

Fibromuscular dysplasia (FMD) is an idiopathic, segmental, noninflammatory, nonatherosclerotic vascular disease that most commonly affects the renal and carotid arteries. Bilateral ICA involvement is common (86%); abnormalities most often involve the pharyngeal portion of the artery, with sparing of the carotid bifurcation and the intracranial ICA. About 1/5th of these individuals have coexistent FMD in the VA.

The most common form of FMD affects the media. Constricting bands made up of fibrous dysplastic tissue and proliferating smooth-muscle cells in the media alternate with areas of luminal dilatation with medial thinning and disruption of the elastic membrane. These abnormalities are imaged as the characteristic string-of-beads appearance on arteriography. Hypertrophy of fibrous tissues in the adventitia or intima can cause segmental regions of stenosis. Superimposed thrombi sometimes develop in these dilated regions and outpouchings. FMD may not be a single disease, but a variety of different conditions that affect the arterial walls [43].

Most FMD lesions are asymptomatic and found incidentally, but patients may develop ischemic stroke or TIAs. Some patients also develop complications such as arterial dissection [44], aneurysms [45], and carotid-cavernous fistulas [46]. SAH may result from intracranial aneurysm rupture [45]. Although extracranial FMD occasionally extends to intracranial arteries [47], isolated intracranial FMD is rare. FMDs occurring in the BA [48], PCA [49], distal ICA and the MCA [50, 51] have been reported. FMD may also be associated with the Moyamoya syndrome [52].

Dolichoectasia

With the advent of vascular imaging, fusiform, tortuous, and ectatic arteries (dolichoectasia) are increasingly recognized. They may be found in the distal ICA or the MCA, but are most often observed in the BA [53]. The etiologies of fusiform arterial dilatations remains unclear, but may involve degenerative process under genetic influences that lead to structural arterial defects characterized by fibrous dysplasia, internal elastic lamina degeneration, and fibrous and collagen replacement of the media [54]. Dilative arteriopathy has been found in children and young adults with AIDS, Marfan syndrome, Ehlers-Danlos syndrome, sickle cell disease, and Fabry disease. A genetic deficiency in α-glucosidase was found in some patients with fusiform BA aneurysms [55].

Unlike atherosclerosis, a condition that primarily involves the intima and endothelia of large- and medium-size arteries, dilatative arteriopathy involves mainly the media of intracranial arteries. Dolichoectatic arteries have an abnormally large external diameter and a thin arterial wall; intraluminal thrombi may also be present. Histological studies show degeneration of the internal elastic lamina, multiple gaps in the internal elastica, thinning of the media secondary to reticular fiber deficiency and smooth muscle atrophy. At times, the intima is thickened, and there is severe elastic tissue degeneration and an increase in the vasa vasorum.

In adults, atherosclerotic changes in the vessels may interact with congenital structural defects to augment fusiform dilatation. In the ectatic vessel, slowed blood flow predisposes atherothrombus formation, which may lead to infarction via artery to artery embolism or perforator occlusion [56–58]. Symptoms may occur due to compression and traction on posterior fossa structures [57, 59] that include occipital headache and cranial nerve palsies [60–62].

Infectious Diseases

Bacterial Infection

Autopsy [63, 64], clinical [63, 65, 66], and angiographic studies [67–69], have documented the involvement of cerebral vessels in bacterial meningitis. Vascular events typically occur within the first 2 weeks of disease and are most commonly seen with *Streptococcus pneumonia* infections in adults and *Haemophilus influenza* infections in children. The vascular involvement is attributed to endothelial or smooth muscle damage by direct invasion of organisms or generation of immune reaction in the course of extensive inflammation. Hypercoagulation, vasospasm, and resultant thrombus formation play additional roles in the development of cerebral ischemia. The vascular event is usually a sentinel event; however, it may be persistent and produce recurrent infarctions [70, 71], suggesting the role of the ongoing immunologic process.

Vascular involvement after bacterial meningitis is one of the most feared complications. According to Pfister et al. [66, 72], the cerebrovascular complications comprised 37% of all the central nervous system complications in patients with bacterial meningitis. Cerebral angiography showed abnormalities in about half of the patients, which included irregularities, narrowing, obstruction or ectatic changes of the intracranial large arteries, focal abnormal parenchymal blush suggesting small vessel involvement, and thrombosis of the superior sagittal sinus or cortical veins. The prognosis in the patients with involvement of intracranial arteries is unfavorable. Ries et al. [73] prospectively investigated the changes of intracranial cerebral blood flow velocities in 22 patients with bacterial meningitis, by means of transcranial doppler (TCD). Elevated blood flow velocity in the MCA was documented in 18 patients. Seven patients with markedly increased systolic peak velocities (>210 cm/s) had low Glasgow Coma Scales on admission, focal cerebral ischemic deficits, and seizures. Although corticosteroids are often used in patients with meningitis complicated by cerebrovascular disease, it remains unclear whether this improves or prevents ischemic symptoms.

Tuberculosis

It has been shown that 6 to 47% of patients with tuberculous meningitis develop brain infarction [74–76]. The agent may involve small, medium, or large arteries or veins, characterized pathologically by mononuclear infiltrates, caseating necrosis, and fibrinoid changes. Vasculitis involving vessels in the base of the brain is a common histopathologic feature. The vascular involvement can be silent or manifest either as a stroke or diffuse symptoms such as obtundation, delirium, or cognitive dysfunction.

In a study of 25 young patients with tuberculous meningitis with brain infarction, most patients (23 patients) had anterior circulation involvement. The territories involved were lenticulostriate in 16, MCA in 3, and multiple in 3 patients. A majority (23 patients) had a concomitant hydrocephalus. The outcomes were poor, and none recovered completely [75]. In another study [77], 5 out of 12 patients (42%) with cerebral infarction associated with tuberculosis had large artery territory infarction only, while the remaining 7 (58%) patients had small deep infarcts with or without coexisting large artery infarction. Intracranial artery involvement is frequent in tuberculous meningitis [78] (fig. 5). Once patients have vascular involvement, the outcome is poor and full recovery is uncommon [75, 77].

Viral Infection

Herpes Zoster

Herpes zoster infection is caused by varicella zoster virus, a DNA virus of the herpes family. The skin vesicles characteristically appear in a peripheral nerve or root dermatome. The virus occasionally affects cerebral vessels. Pathologically, necrotizing granulomatous angiitis of small- and medium-sized cerebral arteries are shown [79–81]. Viral particles are detected in the outer walls or within the media of affected vessels [82, 83]. The most plausible mechanism is intraneuronal migration of the virus from the trigeminal ganglion to the cerebral arteries [84]; the distribution of vascular lesions (MCA, ACA, and BA) matches the density of trigeminal innervation at the circle of Willis [85, 86].

Neurologic signs typically develop one week to months after the skin involvement. The symptoms are usually focal but diffuse symptoms such as stupor, somnolence, and confusion are present in approximately half of the patients [85]. The infarcts are either subcortical or cortical. Angiographic studies show irregular, beaded, or segmental narrowing or occlusion of the ipsilateral MCA, intracranial ICA, or ACA [87]. The PCA or BA can be involved, albeit uncommonly, and deep-seated infarcts in the thalamus, brainstem, and spinal cord may be shown [88]. CSF studies reveal abnormal findings in 70% of the patients [85]. The prognosis is poor in patients with a vascular complication, with the mortality ranging from 20–28% [81, 85]. Although post-varicella cerebral arteriopathy usually follows a monophasic course with a gradual regression [89], the vascular lesion may progress in some patients [90] which may be related to the continuing immunologic process.

Human Immunodeficiency Virus

Vascular complications are relatively common in patients affected with human immuondeficiency virus (HIV). However, autopsy findings of cerebrovascular disease were generally not correlated with clinical stroke before death [91]. After a review of the literature, Pinto [91] reported that only 1.3% of patients had a clinically overt stroke syndrome.

The cause of vascular involvement in HIV infection is complex, especially in adult patients. Cerebral infarcts are usually caused by nonbacterial thrombotic endocarditis or concomitant opportunistic central nervous system infection [91]. In a recent review of 82 patients with stroke (77 with ischemic stroke and 5 with intracerebral

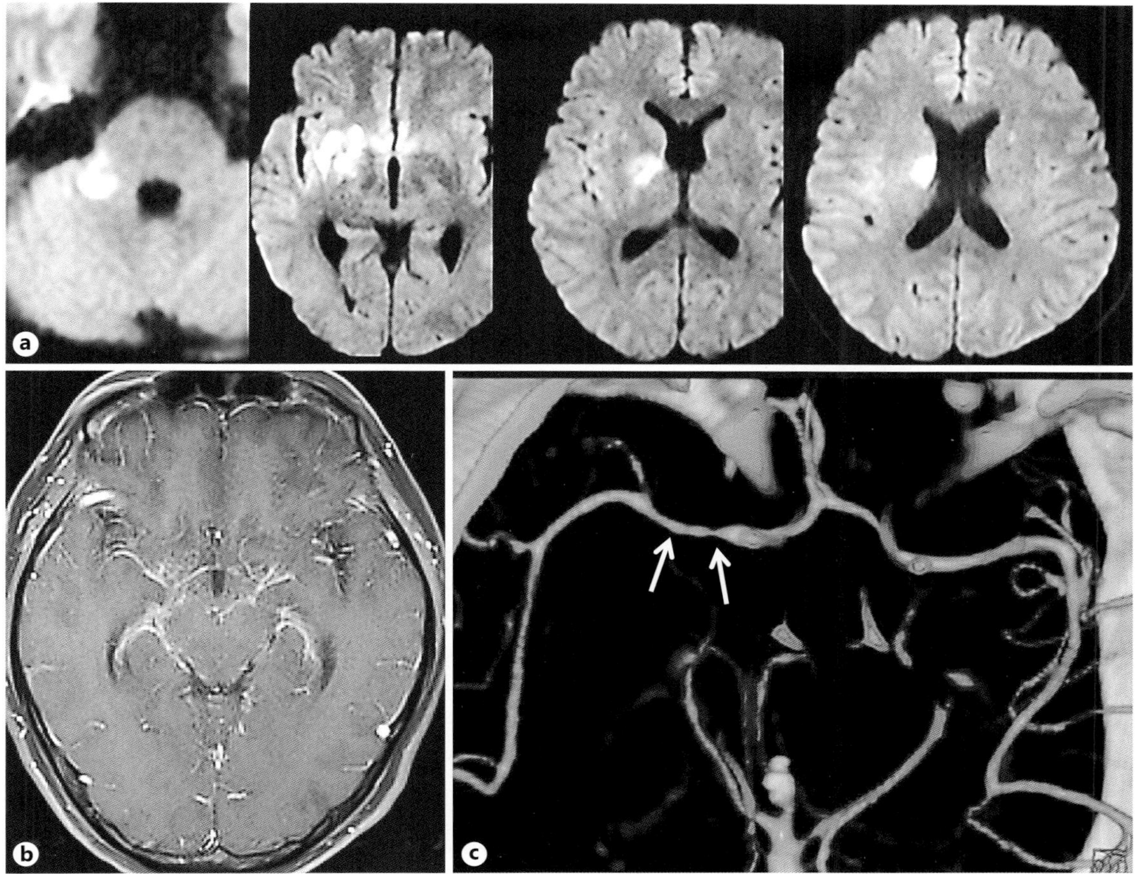

Fig. 5. A 43-year-old man developed headache, nausea and fever. A few days later he had difficulty in speaking and visual hallucinations. Neurologic examination showed that he was confused, disoriented, and had neck stiffness but without any focal signs. CSF study results showed increased white blood cell count (132) and protein (143 mg/dl) with dominant neutrophils. Blood T-spot and CSF AFB culture were positive. With anti-Tb medication and steroids he gradually improved. Diffusion weighted MRI showed acute infarcts in the right corona radiata, basal ganglia, and right cerebellar peduncle (**a**). Gadolinium enhanced MRI showed leptomeningeal enhancement in the basal and suprasellar cisterns (**b**). A CT angiogram showed segmental narrowing of the right middle cerebral artery trunk, consistent with vasculitis due to tuberculous infection (**c**, arrows).

hemorrhage), the mechanism of ischemic stroke was large artery atherosclerosis in 12%, cardiac embolism in 18%, small vessel occlusion in 18%, other determined etiology in 23%, and undetermined in 29%. Protein S deficiency was noted in 45% and anticardiolipin antibodies were present in 29% of the patients tested. Vasculitis was considered responsible for the stroke only in 10 patients (13%) [92]. Intracranial vasculitis, usually in association with concomitant opportunistic infection such as syphilis, varicella zoster, tuberculosis or cryptococcal meningitis is an important mechanism in some patients with HIV infection [92]. The direct role of HIV on the development of cerebrovascular disease remains uncertain.

In children and adolescence, the incidence of cerebrovascular disease in HIV-positive patients is 1.3–2.6% [93, 94], while autopsy shows evidence of cerebrovascular disease in as high as 24% of patients [93]. In this age group, strokes appear to be more directly related to HIV. Cerebral arteriopathy with or without fusiform aneurysm formation is often observed even without concomitant opportunistic infection [93, 94]. The vasculopathy frequently involves intracranial arteries such as the MCA or ACA. The arterial lesions can be transient and reversible [95, 96]. Autopsies show panarteritis involving vasa vasorum and multiple fusiform aneurysms in the major cerebral vessels. Microscopically, thickened vascular wall are observed, due primarily to subintimal fibrosis [97].

Parasitic Infections

Among parasites affecting central nervous system, cysticercosis is the most important agent that causes vascular involvement. Cysticercosis is prevalent in Southern Asia, sub-Saharan Africa, or Latin America. Patients with neurocysticerosis are nowadays occasionally observed in developed countries, due to increasing international travel and the high incidence of HIV infection.

Cerebral cysticercosis can be divided into parenchymal and subarachoid (or cisternal) cysticercosis. The parenchymal form produces seizures and focal neurologic deficits [98] whereas subarachoid cysticercosis results in arachnoiditis, hydrocephalus, and vasculitis. Occlusive arteritis of small perforating artery is more common than large artery involvement [99, 100]. Pathologically, the involved vessels show advanced endarteritic changes with luminal narrowing, adventitial fibrosis, and chronic panarteritis [101].

In some patients, especially in those with cysticercosis involving the Sylvian cisterns, occlusion of the main MCA trunk is observed [102–104], which causes significant hemiparesis, aphasia, apraxia, and seizures. Hydrocephalus is commonly accompanied, and the prognosis of these patients is usually poor. Barinagarrementeria and Cantú [105], studied 28 patients with subarachnoid cysticercosis using cerebral arteriography and brain MRI. Among them, 15 patients had angiographic evidence of cerebral arteritis (53%), in whom 12 had clinical stroke syndromes, and 8 had evidence of cerebral infarction on MRI. The vessels most commonly involved were the MCA and the PCA. Subarachnoid cysticercosis should be considered one of the causes of non-atherosclerotic intracranial vascular disease in endemic areas.

The treatment of cysticercosis with vascular involvement is not well established. Albendazol or praziquantel should not be used, or should be cautiously used in conjunction with a high dose of corticosteroid because degenerated parasites may induce extensive inflammation and immunologic reactions, further augmenting vascular damage and ischemic symptoms [106].

Spirochetal Infection

Syphilis

Syphilis used to be the most common causes of strokes occurring in young adults. The incidence has dramatically decreased with the advent of penicillin. However, recent increase in syphilitic infection has been noted due to the increased incidence of HIV infection. The importance meningovascular syphilis has become greater as compared to other subtypes of neurosyphilis such as general paresis or tabes dorsalis.

Meningovascular syphilis develops 1–12 years (mostly 6–7 years) after the original infection. The CSF studies show increased cells, protein and positive serologic tests. The infarcts may develop anywhere in the brain but most often occur in the subcortical area of the anterior circulation such as the internal capsule and basal ganglia, which produce hemiparesis, speech disturbances, hemisensory changes and cognitive impairment.

Pathologically, wide-spread arteritis is noted, characterized by lymphocytes and plasma cell infiltration in the vasa vasorum, the adventitia and eventually the media of medium-sized and large arteries. Occlusion of vasa vasorum destroys the smooth muscle and elastic tissue of the media, which are replaced by fibrous tissue, producing progressive narrowing and eventual occlusion of the vessel along with superimposed thrombosis [107]. In many autopsied patients, atherosclerosis or embolic occlusion was observed without active inflammation, in whom chronic inflammatory environments may have accelerated the progression of atherosclerosis. The presence of central nervous system (CNS) syphilis should be suspected in patients with rapidly progressive intracranial artery stenosis (fig. 6). Antibiotics may arrest the active inflammation but cannot reverse the existing vascular and brain damage.

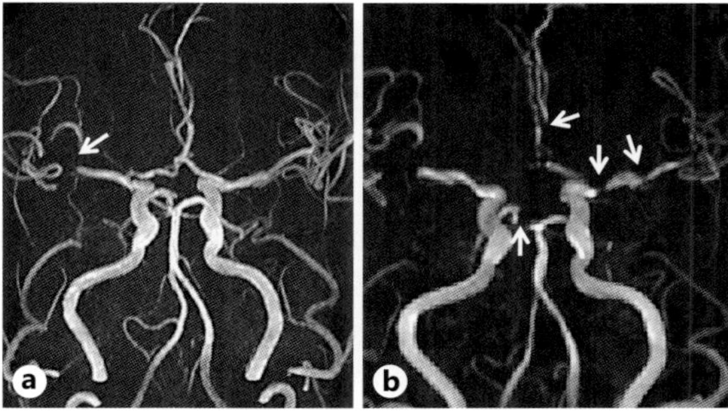

Fig. 6. A 64-year-old woman who had a history of myelitis developed transient left hemparesis. She had no vascular risk factors. MRI findings were normal (not shown). An MR angiogram showed severe stenosis in the distal M1 portion of the right middle cerebral artery (MCA) (**a**, arrow). Despite antiplatelets and statin therapy, she developed recurrent transient right hemparesis 6 months later. A follow-up MR angiogram showed newly developed multiple stenoses in the left MCA, left anterior cerebral artery and right P1 portion of the posterior cerebral artery (**b**, arrows). CSF study showed 113 cells (Lymphocyte 81%) and increased protein (148.0 mg/dl). Serum and CSF VDRL were positive and she was treated with penicillin, under the diagnosis of meningovascular syphilis.

Leptospirosis

Leptospirosis is a sprochetal infection characterized by hepatitis, conjunctival suffusion and photophobia. Aseptic meningitis, sometimes severe in degree, may develop as a second phase illness. Leptospiral meningitis is an important cause of cerebral arteritis of children or young adults in the rural area of China [108]. Among 12 pathologically verified cases of cerebrovascular leptospirosis, there were multiple occlusive vascular disorders in 9, intracranial hemorrhage in 2, and intracranial hypertension in one patient. Cerebral panarteritis involving the main trunks of large arteries at the base of the brain was a common pathologic finding. Narrowing of the intracranial portions of ICA was common, and infarcts usually developed in the MCA territory often at the watershed areas. Leptospirosis seems to be one of the important causes of moyamoya syndrome in this region [109].

Fungal Infections

Fungal infection is a rare cause of intracranial arterial disease. The affected patients are usually immuno-compromised; they have transplatation surgery, HIV infection or uncontrolled diabetes mellitus. In patients with mucormycosis, thrombotic occlusion of the distal ICA is occasionally observed because the agent frequently invades the orbit or the cavernous sinus. In these patients, numerous hyphae are present within the thrombi and vessel wall, often invading the surrounding parenchyma. Pontine infarction due to arteritis involving the BA was reported in a patient with mucormycosis [110]. Hyphae invasion of brain arteries is also observed in patients with aspergillosis, resulting in thrombotic occlusion and hemorrhages [111–113]. Patients usually develop infarcts in the perforating artery territory [112, 113], but large cortical infarction may occur [114].

Kawasaki Disease

Kawasaki disease (KD) is an acute, systemic vasculitis affecting mainly children. Although infectious etiology is suspected, the cause of KD remains still unknown. Diagnosis of KD requires persistent fever for at least 5 days and at least four of the following symptoms/signs: extremity edema or erythema, polymorphous exanthema, bilateral conjunctival injection, strawberry tongue or cracking lips, and cervical lymphadenopathy [115]. Neurological complications, such as aseptic meningitis and facial palsy are occasionally present. The disease is more prevalent in East Asia, but may affect children of all races [116]. Although KD is one of the most common causes of acquired heart disease in children, stroke is rare in this condition. Cardioembolism, vasculitic arterial occlusion or acquired thrombophilia may be considered as stroke mechanisms. Steno-occlusions of the intracranial arteries has been described, most often MCA occlusion [117].

Reversible Cerebral Vasoconstriction Syndrome

In 1988, Call, Fleming and colleagues described four patients who had vasoconstriction of intracranial arteries and presented with acute headache, with or without focal neurologic deficits and seizures, and called this syndrome as 'reversible cerebral arterial segmental vasoconstriction' [118]. Later, Calabrese et al proposed the term 'reversible cerebral vasoconstriction syndromes (RCVS)'. It was defined as a group of disorders characterized by prolonged but reversible vasoconstriction of the cerebral arteries, usually associated with acute-onset, severe headaches, with or without additional neurologic signs and symptoms [119]. The syndrome most often affects women during the puerperium or menopause, but can occur in any sex and any age.

Stroke in Patients with Vasoconstriction

In brain regions perfused by an artery that is severely constricted, ischemic stroke can develop while some develop parenchymal hemorrhages or SAH overlying the cortical surface [120–123]. Hemorrhage is most likely related to reperfusion injury and leakage or rupture of cortical surface vessels in the setting of impaired auto-regulation. In a prospective series of 67 patients, hemorrhages were found to be an early complications, occurring within the first week, while ischemic events occurred later mainly during the second week [124].

Small areas of infarction, hemorrhage and brain edema can be found on brain CT and more clearly on MRI (fig. 7), the most frequent finding being bi-hemispheric infarcts in the parieto-occipital lobes and 'borderzone' territories. Ischemic lesions are often crescentic or horseshoe-shaped, but may appear wedge-shaped. FLAIR imaging often shows dot-shaped or linear hyperintensities along the cortical surfaces, which may reflect slow flow within dilated vessels. Cortical SAH, a frequent complication of RCVS (22%), consisted of small localized bleedings at the surface of the brain [124]. Up to one third of patients with RCVS show no abnormality on brain imaging despite multifocal arterial narrowing on angiograms [122].

Vasoconstriction may begin distally and progresses towards medium sized and larger arteries [124]. The most frequently involved intracranial vessels are medium-sized cerebral arteries, including the MCA, ACA, ICVA, BA, PCA and cerebellar arteries. Angiography typically shows diffuse, multifocal, segmental vascular narrowing, with focal regions of vasodilatation, called 'sausage string' or 'string of beads' [125] (fig. 7). Repeated angiography after a few weeks or months shows normalization of cerebral arteries. TCD can be used as a useful diagnostic tool in assessing the reversal of vasoconstriction [126].

A transient abnormality in the control of cerebral vascular tone appears to be the main cause

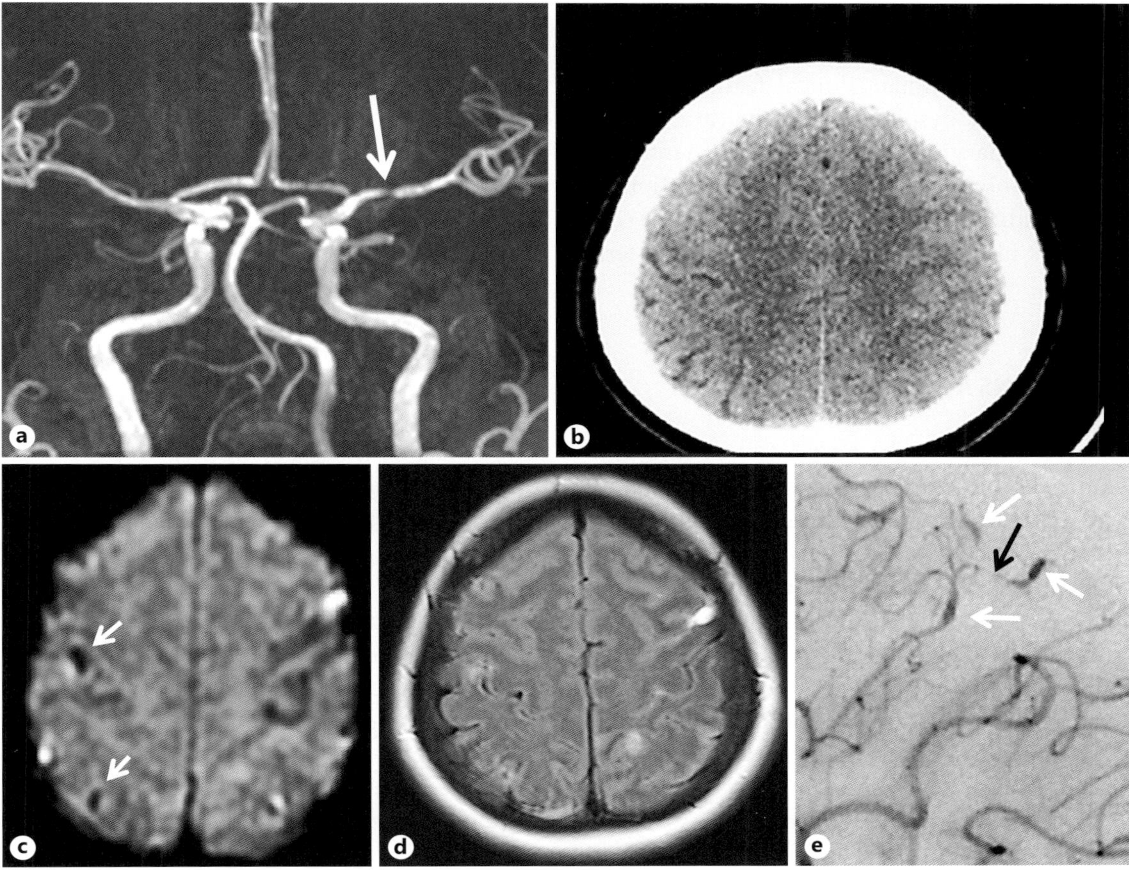

Fig. 7. A 52-year-old, hypertensive woman suddenly developed severe, generalized headache. The next day, an MR angiogram showed left middle cerebral artery narrowing (**a**, arrow) that resembled intracranial atherosclerosis. CT showed grossly normal brain, but sulci effacement was suspected in the left hemisphere (**b**). Diffusion weighted MRI showed acute convexal cortical subarachnoid hemorrhages (**c**, arrows) and FLAIR showed high signals in sulcal areas (**d**). Angiography showed diffuse, multifocal, segmental vascular narrowing (**e**, dark arrow), with focal, sausage arterial vasodilatation (**e**, white arrows).

of RCVS. Many patients who develop RCVS have a history of migraine, implying that there is a genetic susceptibility to develop vascular constriction after a vasoactive stimulus. Chemical factors, such as circulating catecholamines, serotonin, endothelin-1, calcium, nitric oxide, prostaglandins may be involved in the pathophysiology of vascular constriction associated with sympathomimetic or serotonergic drugs, hypercalcemia, intravenous immunoglobulin, carotid endarterectomy, neurosurgical trauma, uncontrolled hypertension and tumors [127–130]. The frequent occurrence in women, soon after menarche, and menopause, suggests a role of hormonal effect.

Vasospasm after aneurysmal SAH should be differentiated from RCVS. In patients with SAH, vasospasm usually correlates with the location and amount of bleeding and is not multifocal, and most often occurs between 7 and 14 days after the onset of SAH [131]. It is also important to distinguish stroke caused by RCVS from other disorders with similar clinical feature, such as fibromuscular dysplasia, inflammatory vasculitis, and primary angiitis of the CNS, and intracranial atherosclerosis because consideration of these conditions may expose patients to the risks of brain biopsy or to unnecessary, long-term therapy.

Isolated CNS Angiitis

Isolated angiitis of the CNS is a very rare idiopathic vasculitis restricted to small leptomeningeal and parenchymal arteries and veins, without apparent systemic involvement [132]. It is now regarded as an immunological, non-specific T cell-mediated inflammatory reaction rather than a specific entity [133]. It is a rare condition with an estimated incidence of less than 1:2,000,000 [134]. Symptoms may develop acutely within a few weeks, or evolve for a period of months to years. Any age can be affected and there is a male predominance (nearly 2 to 1) [135]. Diffuse or multifocal encephalopathy associated with cognitive or behavioral changes and high CSF protein are the main clinical findings. Due to the protean, yet nonspecific clinical manifestations, it is often difficult to make this diagnosis. Definitive diagnosis depends on brain/leptomeningeal biopsy findings, which include a segmental, necrotizing granulomatous vasculitis affecting mostly the leptomeningeal, cortical, and spinal vessels. The intima and adventitia of arteries are infiltrated with lymphocytes, giant cells, and granulomas, with preservation of the media. Granulomas can extend into the adjacent brain parenchyma. Isolated CNS angiitis is a rare cause of stroke. Although angiitis can produce brain infarction, the lesions are usually small and do not present as clinical strokes. All types of strokes have been observed in isolated CNS angiitis, including definite cerebral infarcts, TIA, intraparenchymal hemorrhage or SAH. A multi-infarct state has also been reported [136–138].

Intracranial Arterial Disease in Isolated CNS Angiitis

Intracranial vessels of any size may be involved although there is a predilection for small arteries and arterioles [132, 139]. Angiography may show sausage-like, multiple segmental intracranial arterial narrowing. These findings are not specific, and may be observed in patients with drug abuse or those having RCVS. RCVS is a much more common condition. Conventional angiography shows arterial abnormalities in less than 50% of the cases or shows abnormalities only after repeated tests [140]. Involved small arterioles and venules are often less than 300 μm in diameter [141], which are below the resolution of conventional angiography [142, 143].

Systemic Lupus Erythematosus

Systemic lupus erythematosus (SLE) is a chronic inflammatory connective tissue disorder characterized by multisystem autoimmunity. The clinical picture can be complex, with an array of different presentations. The American College of Rheumatology developed criteria for the diagnosis of SLE, which includes documentation of 4 of 11 abnormalities [144].

Strokes are reported to be present in 2.6–20% of SLE patients [145–151], and tests for SLE have been included in the evaluation of stroke in young patients. Brain Imaging shows a wide spectrum of stroke lesions in various locations, including cortical and/or white matter, the basal ganglia and the brain stem. MRI often shows discrete focal, asymptomatic lesions in SLE patients [152], which are consistent with autopsy findings showing microinfarcts and microhemorrhages in the brain [153]. Occlusions of large arteries resulting in major strokes also occurs in lupus patients [154].

Intracranial Arterial Disease in SLE
In lupus patients, cortical and cortical-subcortical infarcts are most often caused by cardiac-origin embolism and abnormalities of coagulation. One study reported that about 50% of patients who underwent cerebral angiography had intracranial lesions, and about half of them were branch occlusions, suggesting an embolic origin [155]. On echocardiography, as many as 75% of SLE patients had cardiac abnormalities, 37.5% with valvular lesions [156]. Abnormalities of the mitral valve, and infective endocarditis are frequently observed [157]. Libman-Sacks endocarditis is also common, which is a verrucous endocarditis with deposition of hyalinized blood and platelet thrombus, not covered by endothelium. All of these cardiac lesions can produce emboli. SLE patients often have a hypercoagulable state characterized by the lupus anticoagulants, anticardiolipin antibodies [158], or low functional levels of antithrombin III [159]. Immune complex–induced endothelial dysfunction and fibrinolytic defects were also reported in SLE patients [160, 161]. Atherosclerosis in lupus patients is more frequent than can be explained by conventional vascular risk factors [162]. Long term steroid therapy [163], and anticardiolipin antibodies may increase atherogenic potential [164].

Although cerebral vasculitis has been described, there are only a few case reports in the literature of what appears to be a true vasculitis. The most common pathology is a vasculopathy, with perivascular inflammatory infiltrates, perivascular hemorrhages and proliferation of blood vessels, including vascular occlusion with multiple channels of recanalization [165, 166]. Cytokine abnormalities in patients with SLE may contribute to unusually severe white matter damage [167, 168].

Polyarteritis Nodosa

Polyarteritis nodosa (PAN) is a focal, segmental, necrotizing vasculitis of small and medium-sized arteries, characterized by skin, muscle, kidney, gastrointestinal tract and peripheral nervous system involvement [169]. PAN affects middle-aged patients (average age 40 to 60 years) with the annual incidence of approximately 6.3 per 100,000 habitants [170]. One of the most common neurological manifestations is mononeuritis multiplex, which is usually a part of the initial presentation. On the other hand, symptoms related to CNS involvement typically occur 2–3 years after the onset. Strokes, ischemic or hemorrhagic, occurs in 11–14% of PAN patients [171].

Intracranial Arterial Disease in PAN
Small branches of the major cerebral arteries are most often affected [172]. Infiltration of polymorphonuclear leukocytes and monocytes is followed by intimal proliferation, fibrinoid necrosis, and thrombosis of arteries. In some cases, marked loss of the muscular coatings of small intracranial arteries has been reported, with replacement by collagenous tissue, resulting in severe luminal narrowing [173]. Reports of the cerebral angiographic findings in PAN have shown alternating segments of narrowing and widening of small and medium-sized intracranial arteries [174–176]. Occasionally, arteries as large as the MCA or ACA are involved [177]. Small deep infarcts are the most frequent (73%) stroke pattern associated with PAN [178], affecting internal capsule, striatum, corona radiate and the pons. This preponderance of lacunar stroke may be partially explained by associated hypertension [179].

Recreational Drug Use

Drug abuse is a major social and medical problem and has become a significant cause of stroke, especially in adolescents and young adults. A case-control study reported an estimated relative risk of stroke of 6.5 in recreational drug users [180]. Intracranial hemorrhage caused by drugs is most often caused by cocaine and amphetamines [181] while ischemic strokes are usually related to the use of cocaine and heroin [182]. Associated infection, such as hepatitis, AIDS, endocarditis and fungal infections also contribute to ischemic stroke [183, 184]. In some patients who take cocaine and amphetamine, segmental changes in intracerebral vessels with prominent beading are observed on cerebral angiograms suggesting vasocontriction, while necrotizing angiitis has been demonstrated pathologically [185, 186].

Radiation Injury

Cerebral arteriopathy may result from therapeutic irradiation of neck or intracranial malignancies such as lymphoma, thyroid cancer, or glioma. Similarly, autopsy findings of human cases showed vacuolization and thickening of the intima, degeneration of endothelial cells, and accumulation of fat-laden macrophages in the media [187]. Proliferation and calcification of the intima are also observed [188]. The vascular complications usually develop 6 months to 10 years after irradiation.

According to a study that reviewed 12 patients with radiation-induced arteriopathy who presented with stroke syndromes, vascular lesions generally correlated with the irradiation sites [189]. The mean interval from the time of irradiation to the development of stroke was 13.4 years (ranging from 4 to 30 years) for extracranial lesions and 5.1 years (ranging from 2 to 9 years) for intracranial lesions. The interval between the irradiation and the onset of stroke appears to correlate with the diameter of arteries. Extensive arterial lesions may produce vasculopathy mimicking moyamoya disease [190, 191].

Sarcoidosis

Sarcoidosis affects the central nervous system in about 5% of patients usually in the form of cranial neuropathies, basilar meningitis, intracranial masses, diabetes insipidus, encephalopathies, and seizures [192]. Despite the frequent observation of vasculitis and cerebral infarcts on autopsy, clinical stroke events are rare [193, 194]. Veins and venules are more often involved than arteries. Characteristic postmortem findings of these patients include the invasion of the arterial wall by epithelioid cell granulomas that disrupt the media and the internal elastica causing vascular stenosis or occlusion. Small perforating and medium-sized arteries are primarily affected [192, 195], and the involvement of large intracranial arteries is rare although segmental narrowing and dilatation of large cerebral arteries [196], and moyamoya-like vasculopathy [194, 197] have been reported.

Thromboangiitis Obliterans

Thromboangiitis obliterans (TAO) or Buerger's disease is a vasoocclusive disease of unknown cause affecting mainly the peripheral vessels of the upper and lower extremities. Nearl all reported patients were very heavy tobacco smokers. Ischemic stroke and TIAs have been occasionally described to complicate TAO [198–204]. The incidence of cerebral TAO has been shown to range from 0.5 to 18% [202, 204]. Angiography studies describe thrombotic stenosis/occlusion of ICAs, proximal MCAs, ACA, or PCA [199]. These findings were not clearly distinguishable from usual atherosclerosis in these patients who had a long standing history of heavy smoking. Controversies remain regarding whether there are specific pathologic or angiographic findings in patients with cerebral TAO [205].

In occasional reported patients, the vascular occlusion described as worm-like white strings was limited to distal small arteries, while the proximal vessels remained intact [202]. This finding was distinguishable from usual atherosclerosis. A few studies [206] have reported interesting angiographic findings, which included multiple alternative areas of arterial occlusions in the distal segments of both MCAs and extensive pathological collateral vessels around the occluded segment, resembling the 'tree root' or 'corkscrew' vessels described in the peripheral arteries in patients with TAO [207]. Although uncommon, at least some of the patients present with characteristic intracranial vascular diseases that resemble pathologic changes shown in limb arteries of TAO patients.

Takayasu's Arteritis

Takayasu's arteritis is an idiopathic granulomatous vasculitis that affects the aortic arch and its main branches [208]. Although certain genetic predisposition, chronic inflammation, and immunologic process have been considered [209], the etiology still remains elusive. Most patients present between the ages of 11 and 30 years with systemic symptoms such as fever, malaise, weight loss, night sweats and arthralgia. Symptoms associated with vascular involvement follow that include diminished or absent pulses, bruits, extremity claudication, angina, hypertension and congestive heart failure. Pathologically, lymphoplasmacytic inflammation affects primarily the tunica media causing destruction of the elastic lamina. As the disease process continues, fibrous thickening and loss of compliance of the vessel walls develop, and occlusion of the vessel due to superimposed thrombosis may ensue. Approximately 10–15% of patients with Takayasu's arteritis present with ischemic stroke or TIAs [210, 211]. Hemodynamic insufficiency and embolism from the stenosed extracranial arteries, aorta, or diseased heart are the main mechanisms of stroke. Takayasu's arteritis is essentially an extracranial arterial disease. There is a report that described autopsy finding of intracranial arteritis in a patient with Takayasu's arteritis [212]. More recently, two patients who showed angiographic evidence of extensive intracranial arterial involvement were described [213].

CADASIL

CADASIL (cerebral autosomal dominant arteriopathy with subcortical infarcts and leukoencephalopathy) is a hereditary disorder characterized clinically by recurrent migraine, stroke episodes, and dementia. Various mutations in the Notch 3 gene in chromosome 19 are responsible for this disease [214]. In these patients stroke manifests usually with lacunar syndromes. As strokes recur, depression and subcortical dementia develop. The symptoms worsen gradually or step-wise, and the patients become significantly disabled before they die at the mean age of 65. Autopsy findings show that the involved vessels are cerebral and leptomeningeal arterioles. The media is thickened and smooth muscle cells are swollen and degenerated. On electron microscopy, dense, granular osmiophilic materials (GOM) are characteristically observed [215]. MRI shows multifocal or diffuse white matter changes especially in the anterior temporal lobes, subcortical lacunar infarcts, dilated Virchow-Robin spaces, and microbleeds [216].

Since the involved vessels are mainly small arterioles, angiographic findings are usually negative. However, a patient with multifocal segmental stenosis of cerebral arteries similar to primary angiitis of the central nervous system was reported [217]. The presence of occlusive changes in the intracranial arteries was described in Japanese patients with CADASIL who did not have vascular risk factors [218]. Recent series of patients from East Asia found that ischemic stroke can be attributed to intracranial ar-

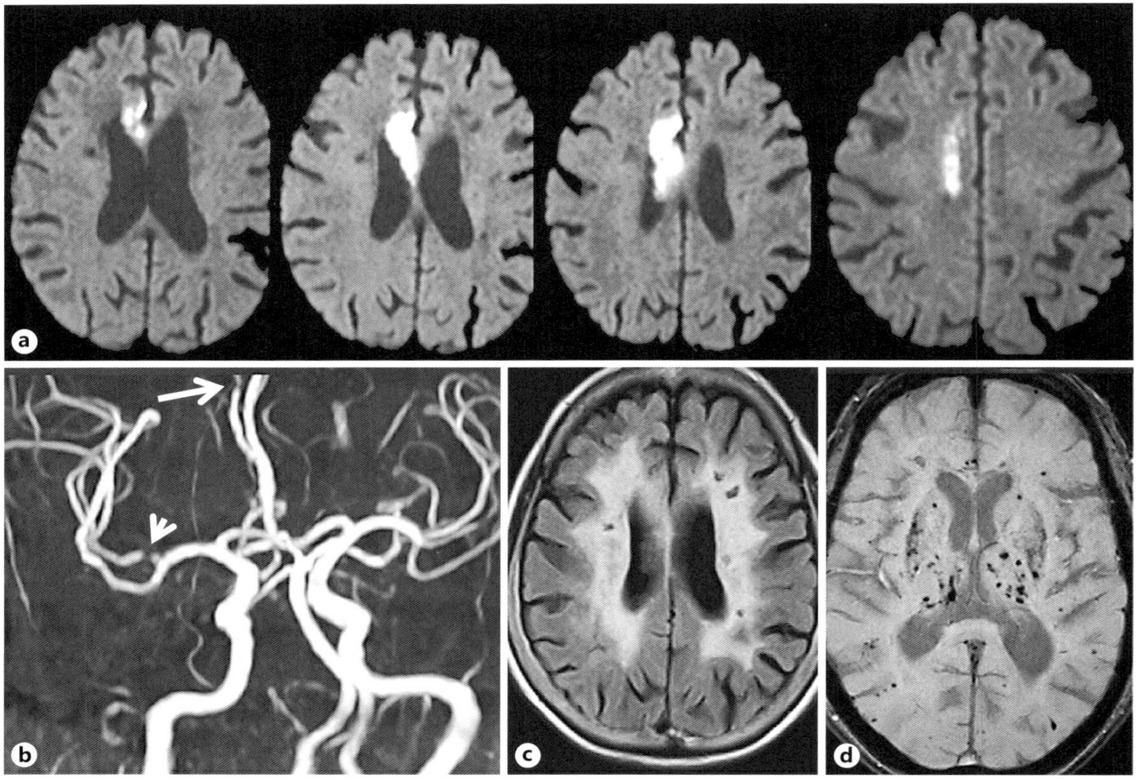

Fig. 8. A 66-year-old woman suddenly developed abulia and left hemiparesis worse in the leg than in the arm. She had no vascular risk factors, and had been diagnosed as having dementia and depression. Genetic studies revealed that she had CADASIL. Diffusion weighted MRI showed right anterior cerebral artery territory infarction (**a**). MR angiogram showed left A3 stenosis (**b**, long arrow). Asymptomatic M2 stenosis was also observed (**b**, short arrow). FLAIR showed diffuse white matter ischemic abnormalitiess and multiple old lacunes (**c**). A SWI image showed multiple microbleeds in the brain (**d**). Holter and echocardiogram findings were normal, and follow-up MRA two months later revealed that the stenoses remained unchanged.

terial disease in 7–26% of the CADASIL patients [219–221]. Kang and Kim [221] stressed that arterial stenosis was generally located in relatively small vessels (e.g., ACA, anterior inferior cerebellar artery, or M2 portion of MCA) compared to the usual locations for intracranial atherosclerosis (e.g., proximal MCA) They posited that this may represent an accelerated atherosclerosis in the presence of endothelial cell damage associated with GOM deposition. Intracranial arterial disease may be a manifestation of CADASIL at least in East Asian countries (fig. 8).

References

1 Giroud M, Fayolle H, Andre N, Dumas R, Becker F, Martin D, Baudoin N, Krause D: Incidence of internal carotid artery dissection in the community of dijon. J Neurol Neurosurg Psychiatry 1994;57:1443.

2 Bogousslavsky J, Van Melle G, Regli F: The Lausanne stroke registry: analysis of 1,000 consecutive patients with first stroke. Stroke 1988;19:1083–1092.

3 Schievink WI, Mokri B, O'Fallon WM: Recurrent spontaneous cervical-artery dissection. N Eng J Med 1994;330:393–397.

4 Bogousslavsky J, Pierre P: Ischemic stroke in patients under age 45. Neurol Clin 1992;10:113–124.

5 Lee TH, Hsu WC, Chen CJ, Chen ST: Etiologic study of young ischemic stroke in Taiwan. Stroke 2002;33:1950–1955.

6 Schievink WI, Mokri B, Whisnant JP: Internal carotid artery dissection in a community. Rochester, Minnesota, 1987–1992. Stroke 1993;24:1678–1680.

7 Lee VH, Brown RD, Jr., Mandrekar JN, Mokri B: Incidence and outcome of cervical artery dissection: a population-based study. Neurology 2006;67:1809–1812.

8 Arnold M, Kappeler L, Georgiadis D, Berthet K, Keserue B, Bousser MG, Baumgartner RW: Gender differences in spontaneous cervical artery dissection. Neurology 2006;67:1050–1052.

9 Metso TM, Metso AJ, Helenius J, Haapaniemi E, Salonen O, Porras M, Hernesniemi J, Kaste M, Tatlisumak T: Prognosis and safety of anticoagulation in intracranial artery dissections in adults. Stroke 2007;38:1837–1842.

10 Rubinstein SM, Peerdeman SM, van Tulder MW, Riphagen I, Haldeman S: A systematic review of the risk factors for cervical artery dissection. Stroke 2005;36:1575–1580.

11 Hausser I, Muller U, Engelter S, Lyrer P, Pezzini A, Padovani A, Moormann B, Busse O, Weber R, Brandt T, Grond-Ginsbach C: Different types of connective tissue alterations associated with cervical artery dissections. Acta Neuropathol 2004;107:509–514.

12 Pelkonen O, Tikkakoski T, Leinonen S, Pyhtinen J, Sotaniemi K: Intracranial arterial dissection. Neuroradiology 1998;40:442–447.

13 Kobayashi J, Ohara T, Shiozawa M, Minematsu K, Nagatsuka K, Toyoda K: Isolated posterior inferior cerebellar artery dissection as a cause of ischemic stroke: clinical features and prognosis. Cerebrovasc Dis 2015;40:215–221.

14 Choi YJ, Jung SC, Lee DH: Vessel wall imaging of the intracranial and cervical carotid arteries. J Stroke 2015;17:238–255.

15 Kwon JY, Kim NY, Suh DC, Kang DW, Kwon SU, Kim JS: Intracranial and extracranial arterial dissection presenting with ischemic stroke: lesion location and stroke mechanism. J Neurol Sci 2015;358:371–376.

16 Wilkinson IM: The vertebral artery. Extracranial and intracranial structure. Arch Neurol 1972;27:392–396.

17 Yonas H, Agamanolis D, Takaoka Y, White RJ: Dissecting intracranial aneurysms. Surg Neurol 1977;8:407–415.

18 Day AL, Gaposchkin CG, Yu CJ, Rivet DJ, Dacey RG Jr: Spontaneous fusiform middle cerebral artery aneurysms: characteristics and a proposed mechanism of formation. J Neurosurg 2003;99:228–240.

19 Endo S, Nishijima M, Nomura H, Takaku A, Okada E: A pathological study of intracranial posterior circulation dissecting aneurysms with subarachnoid hemorrhage: report of three autopsied cases and review of the literature. Neurosurgery 1993;33:732–738.

20 Kim JS: Pure lateral medullary infarction: clinical-radiological correlation of 130 acute, consecutive patients. Brain 2003;126:1864–1872.

21 Lin CH, Jeng JS, Yip PK: Middle cerebral artery dissections: differences between isolated and extended dissections of internal carotid artery. J Neurol Sci 2005;235:37–44.

22 Piepgras DG, Mcgrail KM, Tazelaar HD: Intracranial dissection of the distal middle cerebral-artery as an uncommon cause of distal cerebral-artery aneurysm. J Neurosurg 1994;80:909–913.

23 Ohkuma H, Suzuki S, Kikkawa T, Shimamura N: Neuroradiologic and clinical features of arterial dissection of the anterior cerebral artery. AJNR Am J Neuroradiol 2003;24:691–699.

24 Chiras J, Marciano S, Vega Molina J, Touboul J, Poirier B, Bories J: Spontaneous dissecting aneurysm of the extracranial vertebral artery (20 cases). Neuroradiology 1985;27:327–333.

25 Mokri B, Houser OW, Sandok BA, Piepgras DG: Spontaneous dissections of the vertebral arteries. Neurology 1988;38:880–885.

26 Huang YC, Chen YF, Wang YH, Tu YK, Jeng JS, Liu HM: Cervicocranial arterial dissection: experience of 73 patients in a single center. Surg Neurol 2009;72(suppl 2):S20–S27; discussion S27.

27 Frumkin LR, Baloh RW: Wallenberg's syndrome following neck manipulation. Neurology 1990;40:611–615.

28 Easton JD, Sherman DG: Cervical manipulation and stroke. Stroke 1977;8:594–597.

29 Goldstein SJ: Dissecting hematoma of the cervical vertebral artery. Case report. J Neurosurg 1982;56:451–454.

30 Biousse V, Chabriat H, Amarenco P, Bousser MG: Roller-coaster-induced vertebral artery dissection. Lancet 1995;346:767.

31 Norris JW, Beletsky V, Nadareishvili ZG: Sudden neck movement and cervical artery dissection. The canadian stroke consortium. CMAJ 2000;163:38–40.

32 Caplan LR, Baquis GD, Pessin MS, D'Alton J, Adelman LS, DeWitt LD, Ho K, Izukawa D, Kwan ES: Dissection of the intracranial vertebral artery. Neurology 1988;38:868–877.

33 Hosoya T, Adachi M, Yamaguchi K, Haku T, Kayama T, Kato T: Clinical and neuroradiological features of intracranial vertebrobasilar artery dissection. Stroke 1999;30:1083–1090.

34 Alexander CB, Burger PC, Goree JA: Dissecting aneurysms of the basilar artery in 2 patients. Stroke 1979;10:294–299.

35 Masson C, Krespy Y, Masson M, Colombani JM: Magnetic resonance imaging in basilar artery dissection. Stroke 1993;24:1264–1266.

36 Ruecker M, Furtner M, Knoflach M, Werner P, Gotwald T, Chemelli A, Zangerle A, Prantl B, Matosevic B, Schmidauer C, Schmutzhard E, Willeit J, Kiechl S: Basilar artery dissection: series of 12 consecutive cases and review of the literature. Cerebrovasc Dis 2010;30:267–276.

37 Yoshimoto Y, Hoya K, Tanaka Y, Uchida T: Basilar artery dissection. J Neurosurg 2005;102:476–481.
38 Caplan LR, Estol CJ, Massaro AR: Dissection of the posterior cerebral arteries. Arch Neurol 2005;62:1138–1143.
39 Inoue T, Nishimura S, Hayashi N, Numagami Y, Takazawa H, Nishijima M: Postpartum dissecting aneurysm of the posterior cerebral artery. J Clin Neurosci 2007;14:576–581.
40 Wetjen NM, Link MJ, Reimer R, Nichols DA, Giannini C: Clinical presentation and surgical management of dissecting posterior inferior cerebellar artery aneurysms: 2 case reports. Surg Neurol 2005; 64:462–467; discussion 467.
41 Sedat J, Chau Y, Mahagne MH, Bourg V, Lonjon M, Paquis P: Dissection of the posteroinferior cerebellar artery: clinical characteristics and long-term follow-up in five cases. Cerebrovasc Dis 2007;24: 183–190.
42 Kanou Y, Arita K, Kurisu K, Ikawa F, Eguchi K, Monden S, Watanabe K: Dissecting aneurysm of the peripheral posterior inferior cerebellar artery. Acta Neurochir 2000;142:1151–1156.
43 Slovut DP, Olin JW: Fibromuscular dysplasia. N Engl J Med 2004;350:1862–1871.
44 Ringel SP, Harrison SH, Norenberg MD, Austin JH: Fibromuscular dysplasia: Multiple 'spontaneous' dissecting aneurysms of the major cervical arteries. Ann Neurol 1977;1:301–304.
45 Cloft HJ, Kallmes DF, Kallmes MH, Goldstein JH, Jensen ME, Dion JE: Prevalence of cerebral aneurysms in patients with fibromuscular dysplasia: a reassessment. J Neurosurg 1998;88:436–440.
46 Zimmerman R, Leeds NE, Naidich TP: Carotid-cavernous fistula associated with intracranial fibromuscular dysplasia. Radiology 1977;122:725–726.
47 Osborn AG, Anderson RE: Angiographic spectrum of cervical and intracranial fibromuscular dysplasia. Stroke 1977;8: 617–626.
48 Hegedus K, Nemeth G: Fibromuscular dysplasia of the basilar artery. Case report with autopsy verification. Arch Neurol 1984;41:440–442.
49 Frens DB, Petajan JH, Anderson R, Deblanc JH Jr: Fibromuscular dysplasia of the posterior cerebral artery: report of a case and review of the literature. Stroke 1974;5:161–166.
50 Rinaldi I, Harris WO Jr, Kopp JE, Legier J: Intracranial fibromuscular dysplasia: report of two cases, one with autopsy verification. Stroke 1976;7: 511–516.
51 Shea KJ, Hoang JK, Smith EC: Ischemic stroke because of intracranial fibromuscular dysplasia. Pediatr Neurol 2011;44: 214–217.
52 Pilz P, Hartjes HJ: Fibromuscular dysplasia and multiple dissecting aneurysms of intracranial arteries. A further cause of moyamoya syndrome. Stroke 1976;7:393–398.
53 Little JR, St Louis P, Weinstein M, Dohn DF: Giant fusiform aneurysm of the cerebral arteries. Stroke 1981;12:183–188.
54 Hirsch CS, Roessmann U: Arterial dysplasia with ruptured basilar artery aneurysm: report of a case. Hum Pathol 1975; 6:749–758.
55 Makos MM, McComb RD, Hart MN, Bennett DR: Alpha-glucosidase deficiency and basilar artery aneurysm: report of a sibship. Ann Neurol 1987;22:629–633.
56 Kwon HM, Kim JH, Lim JS, Park JH, Lee SH, Lee YS: Basilar artery dolichoectasia is associated with paramedian pontine infarction. Cerebrovasc Dis 2009;27: 114–118.
57 Pessin MS, Chimowitz MI, Levine SR, Kwan ES, Adelman LS, Earnest MP, Clark DM, Chason J, Ausman JI, Caplan LR: Stroke in patients with fusiform vertebrobasilar aneurysms. Neurology 1989;39:16–21.
58 Passero S, Filosomi G: Posterior circulation infarcts in patients with vertebrobasilar dolichoectasia. Stroke 1998;29: 653–659.
59 Moseley IF, Holland IM: Ectasia of the basilar artery: the breadth of the clinical spectrum and the diagnostic value of computed tomography. Neuroradiology 1979;18:83–91.
60 Kerber CW, Margolis MT, Newton TH: Tortuous vertebrobasilar system: a cause of cranial nerve signs. Neuroradiology 1972;4:74–77.
61 Nishizaki T, Tamaki N, Takeda N, Shirakuni T, Kondoh T, Matsumoto S: Dolichoectatic basilar artery: a review of 23 cases. Stroke 1986;17:1277–1281.
62 Paulson G, Nashold BS Jr, Margolis G: Aneurysms of the vertebral artery: report of 5 cases. Neurology 1959;9:590–598.
63 Adams RD, Kubik CS, Bonner FJ: The clinical and pathological aspects of influenzal meningitis. Arch Pediatr 1948; 65:408–441.
64 Dodge PR, Swartz MN: Bacterial meningitis – a review of selected aspects. II. Special neurologic problems, postmeningitic complications and clinicopathological correlations. N Engl J Med 1965; 272:1003–1010 CONCL.
65 Igarashi M, Gilmartin RC, Gerald B, Wilburn F, Jabbour JT: Cerebral arteritis and bacterial meningitis. Arch Neurol 1984;41:531–535.
66 Pfister HW, Borasio GD, Dirnagl U, Bauer M, Einhaupl KM: Cerebrovascular complications of bacterial meningitis in adults. Neurology 1992;42:1497–1504.
67 Ferris EJ, Rudikoff JC, Shapiro JH: Cerebral angiography of bacterial infection. Radiology 1968;90:727–734.
68 Davis DO, Dilenge D, Schlaepfer W: Arterial dilatation in purulent meningitis. Case report. J Neurosurg 1970;32:112–115.
69 Leeds NE, Goldberg HI: Angiographic manifestations in cerebral inflammatory disease. Radiology 1971;98:595–604.
70 Czartoski T, Hallam D, Lacy JM, Chun MR, Becker K: Postinfectious vasculopathy with evolution to moyamoya syndrome. J Neurol Neurosurg Psychiatry 2005;76:256–259.
71 Pugin D, Copin JC, Goodyear MC, Landis T, Gasche Y: Persisting vasculitis after pneumococcal meningitis. Neurocrit Care 2006;4:237–240.
72 Pfister HW, Feiden W, Einhaupl KM: Spectrum of complications during bacterial meningitis in adults. Results of a prospective clinical study. Arch neurol 1993;50:575–581.
73 Ries S, Schminke U, Fassbender K, Daffertshofer M, Steinke W, Hennerici M: Cerebrovascular involvement in the acute phase of bacterial meningitis. J Neurol 1997;244:51–55.
74 Dastur DK, Lalitha VS, Udani PM, Parekh U: The brain and meninges in tuberculous meningitis-gross pathology in 100 cases and pathogenesis. Neurol India 1970;18:86–100.
75 Leiguarda R, Berthier M, Starkstein S, Nogues M, Lylyk P: Ischemic infarction in 25 children with tuberculous meningitis. Stroke 1988;19:200–204.

76 Lan SH, Chang WN, Lu CH, Lui CC, Chang HW: Cerebral infarction in chronic meningitis: a comparison of tuberculous meningitis and cryptococcal meningitis. QJM 2001;94:247–253.
77 Chan KH, Cheung RT, Lee R, Mak W, Ho SL: Cerebral infarcts complicating tuberculous meningitis. Cerebrovasc Dis 2005;19:391–395.
78 Hsieh FY, Chia LG, Shen WC: Locations of cerebral infarctions in tuberculous meningitis. Neuroradiology 1992;34: 197–199.
79 Kolodny EH, Rebeiz JJ, Caviness VS, Jr., Richardson EP Jr: Granulomatous angiitis of the central nervous system. Arch Neurol 1968;19:510–524.
80 Ruppenthal M: Changes of the central nervous system in herpes zoster. Acta Neuropathol 1980;52:59–68.
81 Hilt DC, Buchholz D, Krumholz A, Weiss H, Wolinsky JS: Herpes zoster ophthalmicus and delayed contralateral hemiparesis caused by cerebral angiitis: diagnosis and management approaches. Ann Neurol 1983;14:543–553.
82 Linnemann CC Jr, Alvira MM: Pathogenesis of varicella-zoster angiitis in the cns. Arch Neurol 1980;37:239–240.
83 Brower MC, Rollins N, Roach ES: Basal ganglia and thalamic infarction in children. Cause and clinical features. Arch Neurol 1996;53:1252–1256.
84 Mayberg M, Langer RS, Zervas NT, Moskowitz MA: Perivascular meningeal projections from cat trigeminal ganglia: Possible pathway for vascular headaches in man. Science 1981;213:228–230.
85 Reshef E, Greenberg SB, Jankovic J: Herpes zoster ophthalmicus followed by contralateral hemiparesis: report of two cases and review of literature. J Neurol Neurosurg Psychiatry 1985;48: 122–127.
86 Askalan R, Laughlin S, Mayank S, Chan A, MacGregor D, Andrew M, Curtis R, Meaney B, deVeber G: Chickenpox and stroke in childhood: a study of frequency and causation. Stroke 2001;32:1257–1262.
87 Ueno M, Oka A, Koeda T, Okamoto R, Takeshita K: Unilateral occlusion of the middle cerebral artery after varicella-zoster virus infection. Brain 2002;24: 106–108.
88 Gilden DH, Lipton HL, Wolf JS, Akenbrandt W, Smith JE, Mahalingam R, Forghani B: Two patients with unusual forms of varicella-zoster virus vasculopathy. N Engl J Med 2002;347:1500–1503.
89 Lanthier S, Armstrong D, Domi T, deVeber G: Post-varicella arteriopathy of childhood: natural history of vascular stenosis. Neurology 2005;64:660–663.
90 Miravet E, Danchaivijitr N, Basu H, Saunders DE, Ganesan V: Clinical and radiological features of childhood cerebral infarction following varicella zoster virus infection. Dev Med Child Neurol 2007;49:417–422.
91 Pinto AN: Aids and cerebrovascular disease. Stroke 1996;27:538–543.
92 Ortiz G, Koch S, Romano JG, Forteza AM, Rabinstein AA: Mechanisms of ischemic stroke in hiv-infected patients. Neurology 2007;68:1257–1261.
93 Park YD, Belman AL, Kim TS, Kure K, Llena JF, Lantos G, Bernstein L, Dickson DW: Stroke in pediatric acquired immunodeficiency syndrome. Ann Neurol 1990;28:303–311.
94 Patsalides AD, Wood LV, Atac GK, Sandifer E, Butman JA, Patronas NJ: Cerebrovascular disease in HIV-infected pediatric patients: neuroimaging findings. AJR Am J Roentgenol 2002; 179:999–1003.
95 Sebire G: Transient cerebral arteriopathy in childhood. Lancet 2006;368: 8–10.
96 Leeuwis JW, Wolfs TF, Braun KP: A child with hiv-associated transient cerebral arteriopathy. Aids 2007;21: 1383–1384.
97 Shah SS, Zimmerman RA, Rorke LB, Vezina LG: Cerebrovascular complications of hiv in children. AJNR Am J Neuroradiol 1996;17:1913–1917.
98 Collister RE, Dire DJ: Neurocysticercosis presenting to the emergency department as a pure motor hemiparesis. J Emerg Med 1991;9:425–429.
99 Barinagarrementeria F, Delbrutto OH: Lacunar syndrome due to neurocysticercosis. Arch Neurol 1989;46:415–417.
100 Del Brutto OH: Cysticercosis and cerebrovascular disease: a review. J Neurol Neurosurg Psychiatry 1992;55:252–254.
101 Aditya GS, Mahadevan A, Santosh V, Chickabasaviah YT, Ashwathnarayanarao CB, Krishna SS: Cysticercal chronic basal arachnoiditis with infarcts, mimicking tuberculous pathology in endemic areas. Neuropathology 2004;24:320–325.
102 McCormick GF, Giannotta S, Zee C, Fisher M: Carotid occlusion in cysticercosis. Neurology 1983;33:1078–1080.
103 Rodriguezcarbajal J, Delbrutto OH, Penagos P, Huebe J, Escobar A: Occlusion of the middle cerebral-artery due to cysticercotic angiitis. Stroke 1989; 20:1095–1099.
104 Levy AS, Lillehei KO, Rubinstein D, Stears JC: Subarachnoid neurocysticercosis with occlusion of the major intracranial-arteries – case-report. Neurosurgery 1995;36:183–188.
105 Barinagarrementeria F, Cantu C: Frequency of cerebral arteritis in subarachnoid cysticercosis: an angiographic study. Stroke 1998;29: 123–125.
106 Bang OY, Heo JH, Choi SA, Kim DI: Large cerebral infarction during praziquantel therapy in neurocysticercosis. Stroke 1997;28:211–213.
107 EC T: Syphilis of the central nervous system. Lamber HP ed, B.C. Decker Inc, Philadelphia 1991.
108 Chen Y: [A clinicopathological analysis of 12 cases of cerebrovascular leptospirosis]. Zhonghua shen jing jing shen ke za zhi1990;23:226–228, 255.
109 Cheng MK: A review of cerebrovascular surgery in the people's Republic of China. Stroke 1982;13:249–255.
110 Calli C, Savas R, Parildar M, Pekindil G, Alper H, Yunten N: Isolated pontine infarction due to rhinocerebral mucormycosis. Neuroradiology 1999;41:179–181.
111 Miaux Y, Ribaud P, Williams M, Guermazi A, Gluckman E, Brocheriou C, Lavaljeantet M: MR of cerebral aspergillosis in patients who have had bone-marrow transplantation. Am J Neuroradiol 1995;16:555–562.
112 Denning DW: Invasive aspergillosis. Clin Infect dis 1998;26:781–803; quiz 804–785.

113 DeLone DR, Goldstein RA, Petermann G, Salamat MS, Miles JM, Knechtle SJ, Brown WD: Disseminated aspergillosis involving the brain: distribution and imaging characteristics. AJNR Am J Neuroradiol 1999;20:1597–1604.
114 Norlinah MI, Ngow HA, Hamidon BB: Angioinvasive cerebral aspergillosis presenting as acute ischaemic stroke in a patient with diabetes mellitus. Singapore Med J 2007;48:e1–e4.
115 Newburger JW, Takahashi M, Gerber MA, Gewitz MH, Tani LY, Burns JC, Shulman ST, Bolger AF, Ferrieri P, Baltimore RS, Wilson WR, Baddour LM, Levison ME, Pallasch TJ, Falace DA, Taubert KA; Committee on Rheumatic Fever, Endocarditis and Kawasaki Disease; Council on Cardiovascular Disease in the Young; American Heart Association; American Academy of Pediatrics: Diagnosis, treatment, and long-term management of Kawasaki disease: a statement for health professionals from the committee on rheumatic fever, endocarditis and Kawasaki disease, council on cardiovascular disease in the young, American heart association. Circulation 2004;110:2747–2771.
116 Uehara R, Belay ED: Epidemiology of Kawasaki disease in Asia, Europe, and the United States. J Epidemiol 2012;22:79–85.
117 Sabatier I, Chabrier S, Brun A, Hees L, Cheylus A, Gollub R, Hadjikhani N, Kong J, des Portes V, Floret D, Curie A: Stroke by carotid artery complete occlusion in kawasaki disease: case report and review of literature. Pediatr Neurol 2013;49:469–473.
118 Call GK, Fleming MC, Sealfon S, Levine H, Kistler JP, Fisher CM: Reversible cerebral segmental vasoconstriction. Stroke 1988;19:1159–1170.
119 Calabrese LH, Dodick DW, Schwedt TJ, Singhal AB: Narrative review: reversible cerebral vasoconstriction syndromes. Ann Intern Med 2007;146:34–44.
120 Doss-Esper CE, Singhal AB, Smith MS, Henderson GV: Reversible posterior leukoencephalopathy, cerebral vasoconstriction, and strokes after intravenous immune globulin therapy in Guillain-Barre syndrome. J Neuroimaging 2005;15:188–192.
121 Singhal AB: Cerebral vasoconstriction syndromes. Top Stroke Rehabil 2004;11:1–6.
122 Singhal AB, Topcuoglu MA, Caviness VS, Koroshetz WJ: Call-Fleming syndrome versus isolated cerebral vasculitis: MRI lesion patterns. Stroke 2003;34:264–264.
123 Ursell MR, Marras CL, Farb R, Rowed DW, Black SE, Perry JR: Recurrent intracranial hemorrhage due to postpartum cerebral angiopathy: implications for management. Stroke 1998;29:1995–1998.
124 Ducros A, Boukobza M, Porcher R, Sarov M, Valade D, Bousser MG: The clinical and radiological spectrum of reversible cerebral vasoconstriction syndrome. A prospective series of 67 patients. Brain 2007;130:3091–3101.
125 Singhal AB, Bernstein RA: Postpartum angiopathy and other cerebral vasoconstriction syndromes. Neurocrit Care 2005;3:91–97.
126 Bogousslavsky J, Despland PA, Regli F, Dubuis PY: Postpartum cerebral angiopathy: reversible vasoconstriction assessed by transcranial Doppler ultrasounds. Eur Neurol 1989;29:102–105.
127 Singhal AB, Caviness VS, Begleiter AF, Mark EJ, Rordorf G, Koroshetz WJ: Cerebral vasoconstriction and stroke after use of serotonergic drugs. Neurology 2002;58:130–133.
128 Nighoghossian N, Trouillas P, Loire R, Perrin L, Trillet V, Gamondes P: Catecholamine syndrome, carcinoid lung tumor and stroke. Eur Neurol 1994;34:288–289.
129 Yarnell PR, Caplan LR: Basilar artery narrowing and hyperparathyroidism: Illustrative case. Stroke 1986;17:1022–1024.
130 Dagher HN, Shum MK, Campellone JV: Delayed intracranial vasospasm following carotid endarterectomy. Cerebrovasc Dis 2005;20:205–206.
131 Weidauer S, Lanfermann H, Raabe A, Zanella F, Seifert V, Beck J: Impairment of cerebral perfusion and infarct patterns attributable to vasospasm after aneurysmal subarachnoid hemorrhage: a prospective MRI and DSA study. Stroke 2007;38:1831–1836.
132 Cravioto H, Feigin I: Noninfectious granulomatous angiitis with a predilection for the nervous system. Neurology 1959;9:599–609.
133 Moore PM: Central nervous system vasculitis. Curr Opin Neurol 1998;11:241–246.
134 Moore PM: The vasculitides. Curr Opin Neurol 1999;12:383–388.
135 Hankey GJ: Isolated angiitis angiopathy of the central-nervous-system. Cerebrovasc Dis 1991;1:2–15.
136 Biller J, Loftus CM, Moore SA, Schelper RL, Danks KR, Cornell SH: Isolated central nervous system angiitis first presenting as spontaneous intracranial hemorrhage. Neurosurgery 1987;20:310–315.
137 Koo EH, Massey EW: Granulomatous angiitis of the central nervous system: protean manifestations and response to treatment. J Neurol Neurosurg Psychiatry 1988;51:1126–1133.
138 Kumar R, Wijdicks EFM, Brown RD, Parisi JE, Hammond CA: Isolated angiitis of the CNS presenting as subarachnoid haemorrhage. J Neurol Neurosur Psychiatry 1997;62:649–651.
139 Budzilovich GN, Feigin I, Siegel H: Granulomatous angiitis of the nervous system. Arch Pathol 1963;76:250–256.
140 Alhalabi M, Moore PM: Serial angiography in isolated angiitis of the central nervous system. Neurology 1994;44:1221–1226.
141 Lie JT: Primary (granulomatous) angiitis of the central nervous system: a clinicopathologic analysis of 15 new cases and a review of the literature. Hum Pathol 1992;23:164–171.
142 Takahashi M, Bussaka H, Nakagawa N: Evaluation of the cerebral vasculature by intraarterial DSA–with emphasis on in vivo resolution. Neuroradiology 1984;26:253–259.
143 Harder DR, Schulte ML, Clough AV, Dawson CA: An angiographic method for in vivo study of arteries of the circle of willis in small animals. Am J Physiol 1992;263:H1616–H1622.
144 Tan EM, Cohen AS, Fries JF, Masi AT, McShane DJ, Rothfield NF, Schaller JG, Talal N, Winchester RJ: The 1982 revised criteria for the classification of systemic lupus erythematosus. Arthritis Rheum 1982;25:1271–1277.

145 Futrell N, Millikan C: Frequency, etiology, and prevention of stroke in patients with systemic lupus erythematosus. Stroke 1989;20:583–591.

146 Jonsson H, Nived O, Sturfelt G: Outcome in systemic lupus erythematosus: a prospective study of patients from a defined population. Medicine 1989;68: 141–150.

147 Roldan CA, Shively BK, Crawford MH: An echocardiographic study of valvular heart disease associated with systemic lupus erythematosus. N Eng J Med 1996;335:1424–1430.

148 Toubi E, Khamashta MA, Panarra A, Hughes GR: Association of antiphospholipid antibodies with central nervous system disease in systemic lupus erythematosus. Am J Med 1995;99: 397–401.

149 Sibley JT, Olszynski WP, Decoteau WE, Sundaram MB: The incidence and prognosis of central nervous system disease in systemic lupus erythematosus. J Rheumatol 1992;19:47–52.

150 Eustace S, Hutchinson M, Bresnihan B: Acute cerebrovascular episodes in systemic lupus erythematosus. Q J Med 1991;80:739–750.

151 Kitagawa Y, Gotoh F, Koto A, Okayasu H: Stroke in systemic lupus erythematosus. Stroke 1990;21:1533–1539.

152 Aisen AM, Gabrielsen TO, McCune WJ: MR imaging of systemic lupus erythematosus involving the brain. AJR Am J Roentgenol 1985;144:1027–1031.

153 Hanly JG, Walsh NM, Sangalang V: Brain pathology in systemic lupus erythematosus. J Rheumatol 1992;19:732–741.

154 Trevor RP, Sondheimer FK, Fessel WJ, Wolpert SM: Angiographic demonstration of major cerebral vessel occlusion in systemic lupus erythematosus. Neuroradiology 1972;4:202–207.

155 Clinical and laboratory findings in patients with antiphospholipid antibodies and cerebral ischemia. The antiphospholipid antibodies in stroke study group. Stroke 1990;21:1268–1273.

156 Ong ML, Veerapen K, Chambers JB, Lim MN, Manivasagar M, Wang F: Cardiac abnormalities in systemic lupus erythematosus: prevalence and relationship to disease activity. Int J Cardiol 1992;34:69–74.

157 Fluture A, Chaudhari S, Frishman WH: Valvular heart disease and systemic lupus erythematosus: therapeutic implications. Heart Dis 2003;5: 349–353.

158 Espinoza LR, Hartmann RC: Significance of the lupus anticoagulant. Am J Hematol 1986;22:331–337.

159 Cosgriff TM, Martin BA: Low functional and high antigenic antithrombin iii level in a patient with the lupus anticoagulant and recurrent thrombosis. Arthritis Rheum 1981;24:94–96.

160 Byron MA, Allington MJ, Chapel HM, Mowat AG, Cederholm-Williams SA: Indications of vascular endothelial cell dysfunction in systemic lupus erythematosus. Ann Rheum Dis 1987;46: 741–745.

161 Awada H, Barlowatz-Meimon G, Dougados M, Maisonneuve P, Sultan Y, Amor B: Fibrinolysis abnormalities in systemic lupus erythematosus and their relation to vasculitis. J Lab Clin Med 1988;111:229–236.

162 Esdaile JM, Abrahamowicz M, Grodzicky T, Li Y, Panaritis C, du Berger R, Cote R, Grover SA, Fortin PR, Clarke AE, Senecal JL: Traditional framingham risk factors fail to fully account for accelerated atherosclerosis in systemic lupus erythematosus. Arthritis Rheum 2001;44:2331–2337.

163 Kabakov AE, Tertov VV, Saenko VA, Poverenny AM, Orekhov AN: The atherogenic effect of lupus sera: systemic lupus erythematosus-derived immune complexes stimulate the accumulation of cholesterol in cultured smooth muscle cells from human aorta. Clini Immunol Immunopathol 1992;63:214–220.

164 MacGregor AJ, Dhillon VB, Binder A, Forte CA, Knight BC, Betteridge DJ, Isenberg DA: Fasting lipids and anticardiolipin antibodies as risk factors for vascular disease in systemic lupus erythematosus. Ann Rheuma Dis 1992; 51:152–155.

165 Smith RW, Ellison DW, Jenkins EA, Gallagher PJ, Cawley MI: Cerebellum and brainstem vasculopathy in systemic lupus erythematosus: two clinicopathological cases. Ann Rheum Dis 1994;53:327–330.

166 Futrell N, Asherson RA, Lie JT: Probable antiphospholipid syndrome with recanalization of occluded blood vessels mimicking proliferative vasculopathy. Clin Exp Rheumatol 1994;12:230–231.

167 al-Janadi M, al-Balla S, al-Dalaan A, Raziuddin S: Cytokine profile in systemic lupus erythematosus, rheumatoid arthritis, and other rheumatic diseases. J Clin Immunol 1993;13:58–67.

168 Gilad R, Lampl Y, Eshel Y, Barak V, Sarova-Pinhas I: Cerebrospinal fluid soluble interleukin-2 receptor in cerebral lupus. Br J Rheumatol 1997;36: 190–193.

169 Jennette JC, Falk RJ, Andrassy K, Bacon PA, Churg J, Gross WL, Hagen EC, Hoffman GS, Hunder GG, Kallenberg CG, et al: Nomenclature of systemic vasculitides. Proposal of an international consensus conference. Arthritis Rheum 1994;37:187–192.

170 Moore PM, Cupps TR: Neurological complications of vasculitis. Ann Neurol 1983;14:155–167.

171 Brown MM, Swash M: Polyarteritis Nodosa and Other Systemic Vasculitides. Amsterdam, Elsevier Science Publishers, 1989.

172 Provenzale JM, Allen NB: Neuroradiologic findings in polyarteritis nodosa. AJNR Am J Neuroradiol 1996;17: 1119–1126.

173 Sheehan B, Harriman DG, Bradshaw JP: Polyarteritis nodosa with ophthalmic and neurological complications. AMA Arch Ophthalmol 1958;60:537–547.

174 Kasantikul V, Suwanwela N, Pongsabutr S: Magnetic resonance images of brain stem infarct in periarteritis nodosa. Surg Neurol 1991;35: 133–136.

175 Engel DG, Gospe SM Jr, Tracy KA, Ellis WG, Lie JT: Fatal infantile polyarteritis nodosa with predominant central nervous system involvement. Stroke 1995; 26:699–701.

176 Ferris EJ, Levine HL: Cerebral arteritis: classification. Radiology 1973;109: 327–341.

177 Kernohan JW, Woltman HW: Periarteritis nodosa: a clinicopathologic study with special reference to the nervous system. Arch Neurol Psychiatry 1938; 39:655–686.

178 Reichart MD, Bogousslavsky J, Janzer RC: Early lacunar strokes complicating polyarteritis nodosa: thrombotic microangiopathy. Neurology 2000;54: 883–889.
179 Lhote F, Cohen P, Guillevin L: Polyarteritis nodosa, microscopic polyangiitis and churg-strauss syndrome. Lupus 1998;7:238–258.
180 Kaku DA, Lowenstein DH: Emergence of recreational drug abuse as a major risk factor for stroke in young adults. Ann Int Med 1990;113:821–827.
181 Caplan LR. Drugs. In CS Kase LC: Intracerebral hemorrhage. Boston, Butterworth-Heinemann, 1994.
182 Brust JC, Richter RW: Stroke associated with addiction to heroin. J Neurol Neurosurg Psychiatry 1976;39:194–199.
183 Walsh TJ, Hier DB, Caplan LR: Fungal infections of the central nervous system: comparative analysis of risk factors and clinical signs in 57 patients. Neurology 1985;35:1654–1657.
184 Walsh TJ, Hier DB, Caplan LR: Aspergillosis of the central nervous system: clinicopathological analysis of 17 patients. Ann Neurol 1985;18:574–582.
185 Rumbaugh CL, Bergeron RT, Scanlan RL, Teal JS, Segall HD, Fang HC, McCormick R: Cerebral vascular changes secondary to amphetamine abuse in the experimental animal. Radiology 1971;101:345–351.
186 Rumbaugh CL, Bergeron RT, Fang HC, McCormick R: Cerebral angiographic changes in the drug abuse patient. Radiology 1971;101:335–344.
187 Levinson SA, Close MB, Ehrenfeld WK, Stoney RJ: Carotid artery occlusive disease following external cervical irradiation. Arch Surg 1973;107:395–397.
188 Glick B: Bilateral carotid occlusive disease. Following irradiation for carcinoma of the vocal cords. Arch Pathol 1972;93:352–355.
189 Kang JH, Kwon SU, Kim JS: Radiation-induced angiopathy in acute stroke patients. J Stroke Cerebrovasc Dis 2002;11:315–319.
190 Servo A, Puranen M: Moyamoya syndrome as a complication of radiation therapy. Case report. J Neurosurg 1978;48:1026–1029.
191 Kestle JR, Hoffman HJ, Mock AR: Moyamoya phenomenon after radiation for optic glioma. J Neurosurg 1993;79:32–35.
192 Herring AB, Urich H: Sarcoidosis of the central nervous system. J Neurol Sci 1969;9:405–422.
193 Brown MM, Thompson AJ, Wedzicha JA, Swash M: Sarcoidosis presenting with stroke. Stroke 1989;20: 400–405.
194 Takenaka K, Ito M, Kumagai M, Yamakawa H, Sugimoto Y, Yamakawa H, Nishimura Y, Sakai N: Moyamoya disease associated with pulmonary sarcoidosis – case report. Neurol Med Chir 1998;38:566–568.
195 Reske-Nielsen E, Harmsen A: Periangiitis and panangiitis as a manifestation of sarcoidosis of the brain: report of a case. J Nerv Ment Dis 1962;135: 399–412.
196 Lawrence WP, el-Gammal T, Pool WH Jr, Apter L: Radiological manifestations of neurosarcoidosis: report of three cases and review of literature. Clin Radiol 1974;25:343–348.
197 Kim JS, No YJ: Moyamoya-like vascular abnormality in pulmonary sarcoidosis. Cerebrovasc Dis 2006;22: 71–73.
198 E J: Zur pathologischen anatomie der thromboangiitis obliterans bei juveniler extremitätengangrän. Virchow's Arch Pathol Anat 1932;284: 284.
199 Lippmann HI: Cerebrovascular thrombosis in patients with Buerger's disease. Circulation 1952;5:680–692.
200 Drake ME Jr: Winiwarter-Buerger disease ('thromboangiitis obliterans') with cerebral involvement. JAMA 1982;248:1870–1872.
201 Inzelberg R, Bornstein NM, Korczyn AD: Cerebrovascular symptoms in thromboangiitis obliterans. Acta Neurolog Scand 1989;80:347–350.
202 Fisher CM: Cerebral thromboangiitis obliterans. Medicine 1957;36:169–209.
203 Bernsmeier A HK: Thromboangiitis obliterans cerebri. Amsterdam, 1972.
204 Biller J, Asconape J, Challa VR, Toole JF, McLean WT: A case for cerebral thromboangiitis obliterans. Stroke 1981;12:686–689.
205 H S: Über die beteiligung des gehirns bei v. Winiwarter-buergerschen krankheit (thrombo-endangiitis obliterans). Deutsche Ztschr Nervenheilk 1935;136:86–132.
206 No YJ, Lee EM, Lee DH, Kim JS: Cerebral angiographic findings in thromboangiitis obliterans. Neuroradiology 2005;47:912–915.
207 Shionoya S: Diagnostic criteria of buerger's disease. Int J Cardiol 1998; 66(suppl 1):S243–S245; discussion S247.
208 Arend WP, Michel BA, Bloch DA, Hunder GG, Calabrese LH, Edworthy SM, Fauci AS, Leavitt RY, Lie JT, Lightfoot RW Jr, et al: The American college of rheumatology 1990 criteria for the classification of takayasu arteritis. Arthritis Rheum 1990;33:1129–1134.
209 Y S: In uncommon causes of stroke (eds). Cambridge, UK, 2001.
210 Takano K, Sadoshima S, Ibayashi S, Ichiya Y, Fujishima M: Altered cerebral hemodynamics and metabolism in takayasu's arteritis with neurological deficits. Stroke 1993;24:1501–1506.
211 Kerr GS, Hallahan CW, Giordano J, Leavitt RY, Fauci AS, Rottem M, Hoffman GS: Takayasu arteritis. Ann Int Med 1994;120:919–929.
212 Molnar P, Hegedus K: Direct involvement of intracerebral arteries in takayasu's arteritis. Acta Neuropatholog 1984;63:83–86.
213 Klos K, Flemming KD, Petty GW, Luthra HS: Takayasu's arteritis with arteriographic evidence of intracranial vessel involvement. Neurology 2003; 60:1550–1551.
214 Joutel A, Corpechot C, Ducros A, Vahedi K, Chabriat H, Mouton P, Alamowitch S, Domenga V, Cecillion M, Marechal E, Maciazek J, Vayssiere C, Cruaud C, Cabanis EA, Ruchoux MM, Weissenbach J, Bach JF, Bousser MG, Tournier-Lasserve E: Notch3 mutations in CADASIL, a hereditary adult-onset condition causing stroke and dementia. Nature 1996;383:707–710.
215 Ruchoux MM, Maurage CA: CADASIL: Cerebral autosomal dominant arteriopathy with subcortical infarcts and leukoencephalopathy. J Neuropathol Exp Neurol 1997;56:947–964.

216 Kim Y, Choi EJ, Choi CG, Kim G, Choi JH, Yoo HW, Kim JS: Characteristics of CADASIL in Korea: a novel cysteine-sparing notch3 mutation. Neurology 2006;66:1511–1516.

217 Engelter ST, Rueegg S, Kirsch EC, Fluri F, Probst A, Steck AJ, Lyrer PA: CADASIL mimicking primary angiitis of the central nervous system. Arch Neurol 2002;59:1480–1483.

218 Santa Y, Uyama E, Chui DH, Arima M, Kotorii S, Takahashi K, Tabira T: Genetic, clinical and pathological studies of CADASIL in Japan: a partial contribution of notch3 mutations and implications of smooth muscle cell degeneration for the pathogenesis. J Neurol Sci 2003;212:79–84.

219 Choi JC, Song SK, Lee JS, Kang SY, Kang JH: Diversity of stroke presentation in CADASIL: study from patients harboring the predominant notch3 mutation R544C. J Stroke Cerebrovasc Dis 2013;22:126–131.

220 Yin X, Wu D, Wan J, Yan S, Lou M, Zhao G, Zhang B: Cerebral autosomal dominant arteriopathy with subcortical infarcts and leukoencephalopathy: phenotypic and mutational spectrum in patients from mainland China. Int J Neurosci 2014.

221 Kang HG, Kim JS: Intracranial arterial disease in CADASIL patients. J Neurol Sci 2015;359:347–350.

Jong S. Kim, MD, PhD
Department of Neurology, University of Ulsan, Asan Medical Center
388–1 Pungnap-dong, Songpa-gu
Seoul 138-736 (Korea)
E-Mail jongskim@amc.seoul.kr

Kim JS, Caplan LR, Wong KS (eds): Intracranial Atherosclerosis: Pathophysiology, Diagnosis and Treatment.
Front Neurol Neurosci. Basel, Karger, 2016, vol 40, pp 204–220 (DOI: 10.1159/000448314)

Moyamoya Disease

Miki Fujimura[a] · Oh Young Bang[b] · Jong S. Kim[c]

[a]Department of Neurosurgery, Tohoku University Graduate School of Medicine, Sendai, Japan; [b]Department of Neurology, Samsung Medical Center, Sungkyunkwan University School of Medicine, and [c]Department of Neurology, Asan Medical Center, University of Ulsan, Seoul, Korea

Abstract

Moyamoya disease (MMD) is a chronic occlusive cerebrovascular disease characterized by progressive stenosis at the terminal portion of the internal carotid artery and an abnormal vascular network at the base of the brain. Although its etiology is unknown, recent genetic studies have identified *RNF213* in the 17q25-ter region as an important susceptibility gene of MMD among East Asian populations. A c.14576G>A polymorphism in *RNF213* was identified in 95% of MMD patients with a family history and in 79% of sporadic cases, and patients carrying this polymorphism exhibited significantly earlier disease onset and a more-severe form of MMD. Due possibly to genetic differences, the prevalence of MMD is higher in East Asia (e.g., Korea and Japan) than in Western countries. The MMD prevalence peaks at two ages with different clinical presentations: around 10 years and at 30–45 years. Ischemic symptoms, including transient ischemic attacks, are the most important clinical manifestation in both children and adults. Intracranial hemorrhages are more frequent in adults than in children. Catheter angiography is a diagnostic method of choice. Magnetic resonance angiography and computed tomography angiography are noninvasive diagnostic methods. High-resolution vessel-wall magnetic resonance imaging also helps in diagnosing MMD by revealing concentric vessel-wall narrowing with basal collaterals. Surgical revascularization such as extracranial-intracranial bypass is the preferred procedure for MMD patients presenting with ischemic stroke. Surgical therapy may also be effective in patients with hemorrhages, based on recent observations in the Japan Adult Moyamoya trial. Procedure-related cerebral infarction and hyperperfusion syndrome are potential complications that can lead to neurological deterioration.

Introduction

Moyamoya disease (MMD) is a chronic occlusive cerebrovascular disease with unknown etiology characterized by steno-occlusive changes at the terminal portion of the internal carotid artery (ICA) and an abnormal vascular network at the

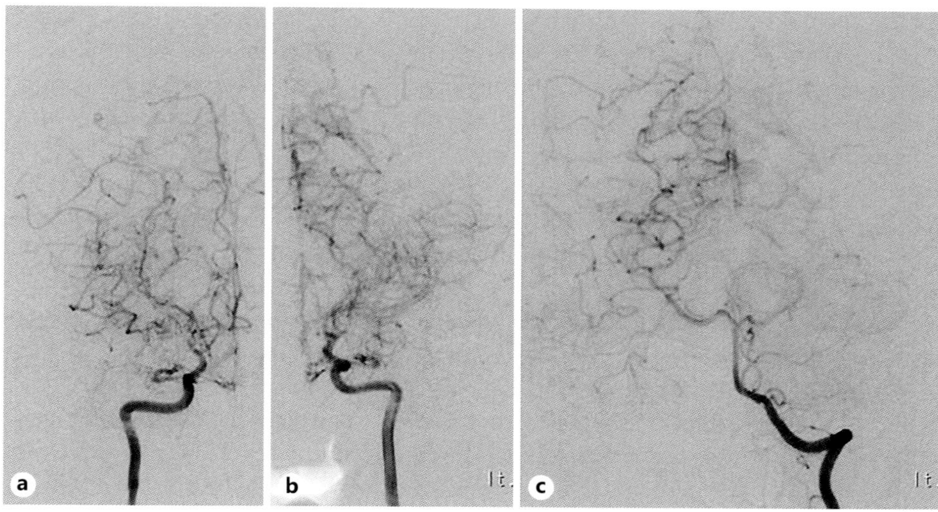

Fig. 1. Right (**a**) and left (**b**) ICA angiograms, and vertebral (**c**) angiography. Steno-occlusive changes in the bilateral ICA and the development of abnormal vascular networks are evident, making a definitive diagnosis of MMD with a Suzuki angiographic grade of stage 3.

base of the brain (fig. 1) [1]. Because of the identification of the increasing number of the patients with unilateral involvement [2] that progress overtime to a bilateral presentation [3, 4], the Research Committee of MMD of the Japanese Ministry of Health, Labour, and Welfare revised the diagnostic criteria for definitive MMD in 2015 to include patients with both bilateral and unilateral presentations of terminal ICA stenosis with an abnormal vascular network at the base of the brain. The current diagnostic criteria also state that a definitive diagnosis of MMD requires catheter angiography in unilateral cases, while bilateral cases can be promptly diagnosed using catheter angiography, magnetic resonance imaging (MRI), or magnetic resonance angiography (MRA). When there are causative diseases or associated conditions, terms such as 'moyamoya syndrome' and 'angiographic moyamoya' are often used [5]. The posterior circulation is usually spared, but may be involved in the late stage, most often the posterior cerebral artery (PCA). Although uncommon, MMD is an important cause of nonatherosclerotic intracranial arterial disease, especially in East Asian countries. Cases with isolated middle cerebral artery (MCA) stenosis are observed in young patients in this region, and they eventually evolve into MMD [6]. MMD is also the most-important cause of stroke and transient ischemic attack (TIA) in children in this region.

Epidemiology

The prevalence of MMD is relatively high in East Asian countries. The reported incidence and prevalence rate in Japan were 0.35 and 3.16 per 100,000, respectively, in 1995 [7], and they increased to 0.54 and 6.03 per 100,000 in 2003 [8]. An epidemiological study from Korea based on National Health Insurance (NHI) data [8] found that the prevalence of MMD increased from 6.3 per 100,000 in 2004 to 9.1 per 100,000 in 2008. The incidence was 1.0 per 100,000 in 2008. According to a more-recent data set obtained between 2007 and 2011 [9], the annual incidence increased from 1.7 to 2.3 per 100,000 persons. The male-to-female ratio was approximately 1:2 in both Japan and Korea, and 10–15% of the patients had a family history of MMD. The incidence peaked in two age ranges: 10–20 and 35–50 years.

The inpatient databases of the Taiwan NHI program contain information on MMD patients from 2000 to 2011 [10]. During this 12-year period, 422 patients were identified, representing an incidence of 0.15 per 100,000 person. An epidemiology study conducted in Nanjing, China showed a prevalence of 3.92 per 100,000 during 2000–2007 [11]. Although hemorrhages were found to be more common there than in Korean and Japanese studies, a more-recent Chinese study of 802 MMD patients [12] showed that the clinical presentations are similar to those from Korea and Japan. There was also a bimodal occurrence, at age ranges of 5–9 and 35–39 years. The difference in the sex distribution of MMD is less marked among Chinese patients than in Japanese and Koreans [11, 12]. A family history of MMD is less common in China (1.5% [11] or 5.2% [12]). However, definitive conclusions require caution since national data for the whole of mainland China are not available.

Studies involving non-Asian populations are rare. In the states of Washington and California in the USA, the annual incidence of MMD was 0.086 per 100,000 based on there being 298 patients. The incidence was the highest among Asians, followed by Blacks, Whites, and Hispanics [13]. However, a recent study based on the Nationwide Inpatient Sample found that MMD was distributed among racial/ethnic groups based on their corresponding proportions in the total US population [14]. There was a bimodal age distribution with peaks in the first and fourth decades, and the female-to-male ratio was 2.2. Thus, MMD in the USA might not differ from MMD in East Asia, although a family history (approximately 2%) appears to be less common.

Both the incidence and prevalence of MMD are increasing worldwide, which may indicate an increase in the actual number of MMD cases. A more-plausible explanation could be that increasing numbers of patients are being newly diagnosed following recent applications of noninvasive diagnostic tools such as MRA or computed tomography angiography (CTA). Another reason could be an increasing number of survivors due to improved management.

Pathology and Pathogenesis

Pathology

The main pathological changes induced by MMD in the stenotic segment are fibrocellular thickening of the intima, irregular undulation of the internal elastic laminae, medial thinness (weakening of the media), and a decrease in the outer diameter [15, 16]. Recent applications of neuroimaging techniques such as high-resolution MRI in MMD patients have demonstrated narrowing of the arterial outer diameter of affected segments and concentric enhancement in symptomatic segments [17, 18]. High-resolution MRI data obtained from a large adult-onset MMD cohort revealed that most patients (90.6%) showed constrictive remodeling and long-segment concentric enhancement of the distal ICA and/or MCA [19], findings that are consistent with previous pathological reports of intimal hyperplasia and medial thinness [20, 21].

There is growing evidence that MMD is primarily a proliferative disease of the intima. Histopathological findings in the distal ICA have shown proliferation of smooth-muscle cells or endothelium [22, 23], and stenosis or occlusion associated with fibrocellular thickening of the intima [15]. The proliferation of smooth-muscle tissue associated with *ACTA2* mutations has been postulated as the key mechanism of arterial occlusion in familial MMD [24].

Moyamoya vessels are dilated perforating arteries that exhibit various histopathological changes, including fibrin deposits in the wall, fragmented elastic laminae, weakened media, and the formation of microaneurysms [15]. Besides moyamoya vessels, cortical microvascularization, which is characterized by substantially increased microvascular density and microvascular diameter, is suggested as a specific finding of MMD [25]. These basal and cortical vessels may represent compensatory mechanisms for the reduced cerebral blood flow (CBF) or aberrant active neovascularization prior to vascular occlusion. An angiographic study of a large cohort of pediatric MMD patients showed that cortical neovascularization may occur before significant hemodynamic impairment, suggesting that neovascularization is an active process rather than a passive compensation for the vascular occlusion [26].

Genetic Factors Underlying MMD

Recent studies have suggested the importance of genetic factors in the pathogenesis of MMD [27–30]. A recent genome-wide association study identified the *ring finger protein (RNF)* 213 gene *(RNF213)* in the 17q25.3 region as a susceptibility gene for MMD in an East Asian population [31]. Those authors reported that the c14576G>A single-nucleotide polymorphism (SNP) was detected in *RNF213* in 95% of familial MMD cases and 79% of sporadic cases among Japanese patients [33]. The c.14576G>A homozygous variant of *RNF213* predicted an early-onset and severe form of MMD in both Japanese [32] and Korean [33] patients with MMD.

However, the exact function of *RNF213* and the mechanism underlying SNPs in this gene in MMD patients have not yet been determined. Recent in vivo experiments using genetically engineered mice (*RNF213*-deficient mice and *RNF213*-knock-in mice expressing a missense mutation in mouse *RNF213*, p.R4828K) failed to show histological and angiographic findings for MMD under normal conditions [34, 35]. In contrast, postischemic angiogenesis was significantly enhanced in mice lacking *RNF213* after inducing chronic hind-limb ischemia [36]. The results from these animal studies seem to be consistent with the low penetrance rate of *RNF213* polymorphisms in patients with MMD, and suggest the importance of environmental factors in addition to genetic factors [37]. *RNF213* genetic variants may also be associated with vascular risk factors, such as hypertension [38], or could lead to vascular fragility (including medial thinness), which may make vessels more vulnerable to hemodynamic stress after secondary insults [37].

Further genetic studies of MMD are needed in populations outside East Asia; Novel non-c14576G>A *RNF213* variants were recently found in Caucasian and Chinese patients with MMD [39], in Chinese hemorrhagic-type MMD [40], and in the USA [41].

Environmental Factors Underlying MMD

Considering that *RNF213* polymorphisms characteristic of MMD are evident in 1.4% of the normal control population [31], and only a small portion of them develop MMD, environmental factors or secondary insults may also be important in the pathogenesis of MMD. The proposed candidate secondary insults have included infection, autoimmunity, other inflammatory conditions, and cranial irradiation [42]. Among them, an autoimmune response may be the strongest secondary insult given the high prevalence of autoimmune thyroid disease among East Asia patients with MMD [43]. Autoimmune thyroid disease and type 1 diabetes are also associated with MMD patients in the USA [44]. Alternatively, *RNF213* polymorphisms could affect autoimmunity and thus contribute to the development of MMD, because this gene is predominantly expressed in white blood cells and the spleen [31].

Moyamoya Syndrome with Associated Conditions

Moyamoya-disease-like vasculopathy associated with other disease conditions is called moyamoya syndrome. Numerous conditions have been reported to be associated with moyamoya vasculopathy, and they may be categorized as follows:

(1) Genetic, hereditary disorders: Neurofibromatosis [45, 46], Down syndrome [47], Noonan syndrome [48], and trisomy 12p syndrome [49].

(2) Hematological disorders: Sickle-cell disease [52, 53], essential thrombocythemia [50], hereditary spherocytosis [51], protein C deficiency [52], and protein S deficiency [53].

(3) Connective-tissue diseases: Systemic lupus erythematosus [54], antiphospholipid antibody [55], and livedo reticularis [56].

(4) Infectious or chronic inflammatory conditions: Pneumococcal meningitis [57], tuberculous meningitis [58], HIV infection [59], leptospirosis [60], pulmonary sarcoidosis [61], and Behcet's disease [62].

(5) Metabolic diseases: Diabetes mellitus, thyrotoxicosis [63], and hyperhomocysteinemia [64].

(6) Vascular injury: Radiation therapy [65].

(7) Others: Renovascular hypertension [66] and oral contraceptive use, especially in cigarette smokers [67].

Whether these disease conditions are causally related to moyamoya vasculopathy remains unclear. They may be mere bystander conditions or simply play a role as triggering factors for symptom development. However, it is also possible that these conditions play a role in the as-yet-unknown cascades of the disease process. Czartoski et al. [57] described a 20-year-old woman who developed cerebral infarction due to vasculitis caused by pneumococcal meningitis. Approximately 4 months later she developed new infarcts, at which time her anti-b2-glycoprotein titers were elevated. Another 4 months later she developed an additional infarct, and an angiogram showed lenticulostriate artery collaterals reminiscent of moyamoya vessels. An autopsy confirmed severe narrowing of the vessels without evidence of inflammation or atherosclerosis, mimicking moyamoya pathology. This observation seems to be consistent with the hypothesis that the development of moyamoya vessels is related to a long-standing immunological process that is initially triggered by a vascular injury, possibly in a genetically susceptible subject.

Biomarkers Underlying Vascular Stenosis and Aberrant Angiogenesis

Besides genetic biomarkers, circulating factors that may also be involved in the pathogenesis of MMD are circulating endothelial/smooth-muscle progenitor cells (SPCs), cytokines, and growth factors.

(1) Circulating Vascular Progenitor Cells

In patients with acute myocardial infarcts or ischemic stroke, there is increasing evidence that circulating endothelial progenitor cells (EPCs) originating from the bone marrow play a role in maintaining the vasculature and blood flow in the infarcted area [68]. EPCs potentially contribute to neovascularization at the site of ischemic brain injury in MMD patients [69]. Although an increased level of circulating EPCs was reported in patients with MMD [70], defective angiogenic function of EPCs has been reported in pediatric [71] and adult [72] MMD patients, suggesting that abnormal angiogenesis forms part of the pathogenesis of MMD. Besides endothelial cells, smooth-muscle cells are also involved in this disease process. Kang and colleagues recently cultured and isolated SPCs from the peripheral blood of MMD patients, and found that these cells tended to make more irregularly arranged and thickened tubules compared with healthy controls [73]. These findings suggest that the maturation process of SPCs from MMD patients is defective. Genetic factors may be associated with defective functions of EPCs and SPCs in MMD patients, such as the down-regulated retinaldehyde dehydrogenase 2 (RALDH2) gene of EPCs [74] and mutations of smooth-muscle alpha-actin (encoded by *ACTA2*) [24]. Aberrant angiogenesis is an active angiogenetic process and may cause both stenosis (by the proliferation of endothelial and/or smooth-muscle cells) and abnormal collateral formation [23].

(2) Cytokines and Their Polymorphisms
The levels of various cytokines and their polymorphisms have also been reported to be associated with MMD, including (a) growth factors, such as vascular endothelial growth factor, fibroblast growth factor, platelet-derived growth factor, and hepatocyte growth factor, (b) cytokines related to vascular remodeling and angiogenesis, such as matrix metalloproteinases and their inhibitors, hypoxia-inducible factor-1α, and cellular retinoic binding protein-1, and (c) cytokines related to inflammation [70, 75, 76]. These study results, however, have not been always consistent; [77] therefore, further studies are needed to confirm the findings. In addition, changes in the levels of these factors may be secondary to the cerebral infarct rather than the primary pathology of MMD [78].

Clinical Features

The clinical presentations of MMD include TIA, ischemic stroke, hemorrhagic stroke, seizures, headache, and cognitive impairment. The incidence of each symptom varies with the age of the patients [42]. Ischemic symptoms, especially TIAs, predominate in children (70%) [79], and intellectual decline, seizures, and involuntary movements are also common in this age group. On the other hand, adult patients present with intracranial hemorrhages more often than pediatric patients do.

An ischemic event is the most-important clinical manifestation of MMD. Cerebral hypoperfusion due to progressive major-vessel occlusion results in repeated hemodynamic TIAs or ischemic strokes in children and young adults. Repeated TIAs may be associated with episodes of hyperventilation, such as when crying or eating hot noodles. Less commonly, patients develop a territorial infarction due to embolism or thrombotic occlusion in the distribution of the MCA, anterior cerebral artery (ACA), or PCA [80]. Ischemic symptoms were attributed to the MCA, ACA, and PCA territories in 92, 52, and 10 of 410 pediatric cases of MMD, respectively [79].

Stroke in the posterior circulation has been considered uncommon, developing usually in the late stages of MMD [81] (fig. 2). However, a more-recent study found PCA involvement in 29% of the patients, with 17% demonstrating an infarction in the PCA territory [82]. Unexpectedly, the prevalence of PCA involvement did not differ markedly between pediatric (26%) and adult (33%) patients. PCA involvement may be one of the factors related to a poor prognosis [79]. The infarct topography in MMD often extends beyond the classical vascular territories (fig. 2). This is probably due to the vascular territories being altered secondarily to the long-standing major vessel occlusion, along with the development of diverse collateral channels [83].

Approximately 30% of MMD patients presented with intracerebral hemorrhage (ICH) or, less commonly, subarachnoid hemorrhage (SAH) secondary to friable collateral vessels harboring microaneurysms or false aneurysms [84]. One case-control study showed that the location of hemorrhage differed between primary ICH and ICH associated with MMD [85]. The locations of primary ICH were the putamen (46.2%), thalamus (19.4%), and pons (14%), whereas those of ICH associated with MMD were intraventricular (37.6%), lobar (23.7%), and in the putamen (22.6%), in the order of frequency. Rupture of a focal microaneurysm in abnormally dilated anterior choroidal artery branches may explain the high prevalence of intraventricular hemorrhages in MMD patients. In addition, gradient-echo, T2*-weighted, and susceptibility-weighted MRI has identified cere-

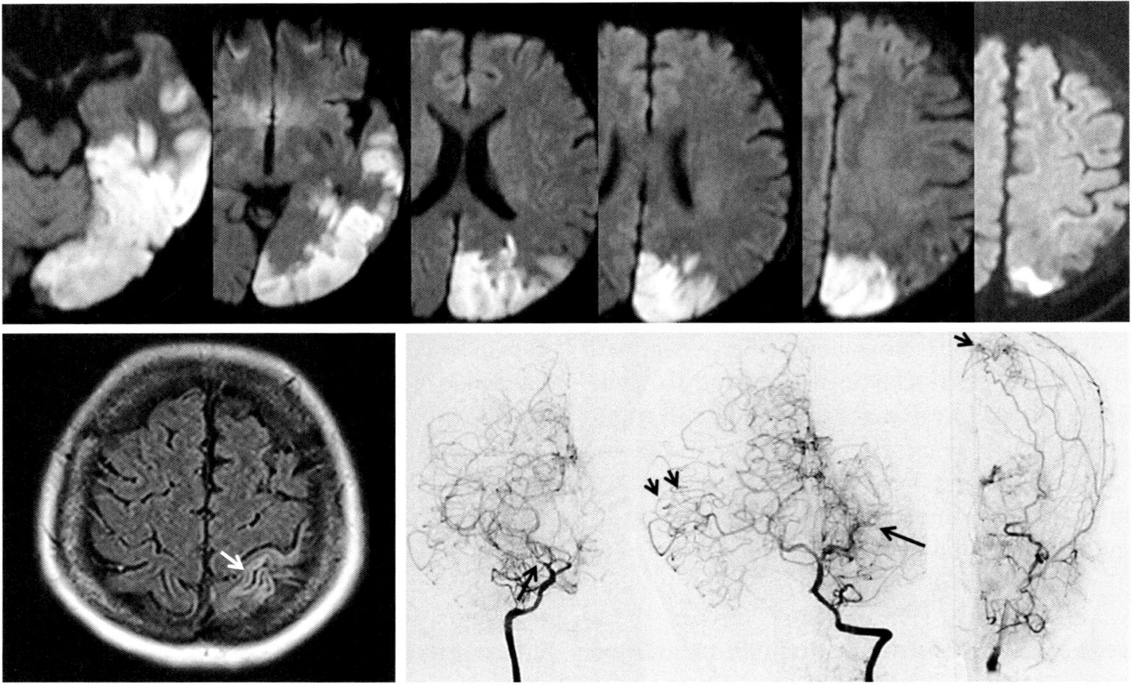

Fig. 2. A 44-year-old woman developed transient right limb weakness. Six months later, she developed headache and right homonymous hemianopia. Diffusion weighted MRI showed an infarction in the left posterior cerebral artery (PCA) territory that somewhat extended upward to the middle cerebral artery (MCA) territory (upper row). Flair MRI (lower row, first image) showed an old infarction in the left parietal area (white arrow) explaining previous hemiparesis. Transfemoral angiography showed an occlusion of the right middle cerebral artery (MCA) (dark arrow, the first angiogram image in the lower row) with basal collaterals. Left PCA was occluded with development of fine collaterals (long dark arrow). Right PCA was intact and supplies right MCA territory (short dark arrows, lower row, the second image). There was an occlusion of left distal internal carotid artery (not shown) and a part of left MCA territory was supplied by prominent external carotid artery system (dark arrow, lower row, the last image). (From Kim JS, Moyamoya Disease: Epidemiology, Clinical Features and Diagnosis, J Stroke 2016;18:2–11.)

bral microbleeds in 28–46% of MMD patients [86–88].

Significant brain hypoperfusion may lead to cognitive impairment or intellectual disability (intellectual developmental disorder) [89–91], which is a serious problem for school-age children. Seizures occur in approximately 5% of patients secondary to ischemic lesions or hypoperfusion, and they usually develop early in childhood. Headache either presents as a symptom of MMD or develops following bypass surgery. Seol et al. [92] reported that 44 of 204 MMD children (21.6%) suffered from headache. The cause of headache in MMD remains unclear, but it is possible that cerebral hypoperfusion decreases the threshold for migraine development and increases the risk of spreading cortical depression [93].

An uncommon manifestation of MMD is involuntary movements, usually among children [15]. In one study, 17 of 410 pediatric MMD patients (4%) developed involuntary movements [79], which include chorea, dystonia, and dyskinesia [94], presumably due to a cerebral perfusion defect in the basal ganglia or cerebral cortical areas.

Diagnosis of MMD

The definitive diagnosis of MMD previously required the bilateral presentation of steno-occlusive changes in the ICA. However, after a recent revision of diagnostic guidelines, the diagnostic criteria of definitive MMD now also include patients with unilateral terminal ICA steno-occlusion. A definitive MMD diagnosis requires catheter cerebral angiography in unilateral cases, while bilateral cases can be promptly diagnosed by either catheter cerebral angiography or MRA.

Based on various angiographic findings, Suzuki and Takaku [1] proposed the following six stages of angiographic evolution:

Stage 1: Segmental narrowing of the distal portion of the ICA.

Stage 2: Initial appearance of basal moyamoya, and segmental narrowing of the proximal portions of the ACA and MCA.

Stage 3: Basal moyamoya becomes very prominent. The proximal portions of the ACA and MCA are no longer visualized, and their distal branches may appear as collaterals from branches of the PCA.

Stage 4: Basal moyamoya begins to disappear. The proximal portion of the PCA becomes narrowed.

Stage 5: Basal moyamoya becomes less apparent. All of the major intracranial arteries are no longer visualized.

Stage 6: Basal moyamoya is absent. Only meningeal-pial collaterals arising from branches of the external carotid arteries supply the cerebral hemispheres.

However, the stepwise progression from stage 1 through stage 6 has been observed only in a small number of patients [95], and the practical value of this classification remains questionable.

MRI is the method of choice for detecting symptomatic or asymptomatic ischemic brain lesions. Moreover, MRI can reveal the following features that should lead clinicians to suspect MMD: the absence of flow voids in the distal ICA and MCA, multiple signal voids in the basal ganglia, and dilated leptomeningeal and cortical collateral vessels. However, for a definite diagnosis, MRA or CTA should additionally be used for the noninvasive detection of steno-occlusion of the distal ICA, MCA, and ACA. Note that MRA and CTA are less sensitive than catheter angiography in demonstrating basal moyamoya vessels [96] and small saccular aneurysms, and for assessing the status of the external carotid artery circulation. Thus, catheter cerebral angiography is generally required before considering bypass surgery.

It is often challenging to diagnose MMD in patients at the early stage of the angiographic grading of Suzuki and Takaku [1], when the abnormal vascular network is not yet evident. High-resolution vessel-wall MRI has been used recently to improve the diagnostic capability. Kaku et al. [17] proposed the constrictive remodeling theory, whereby outer diameter narrowing of the affected intracranial vessels was the early characteristic change of MMD, as demonstrated by the presence of three-dimensional (3D) constructive interference in steady-state (CIISS) MRI images. Yuan et al. [18] also reported that thinning of the vascular wall and narrowing of the arterial outer diameter evident in high-resolution MRI could be early morphological changes characteristic of MMD. Recent high-resolution MRI data obtained from a large cohort of adult-onset MMD revealed that most patients (90.6%) showed constrictive remodeling and long-segment concentric enhancement of the distal ICA and/or MCA [19]. Together these findings indicate that high-resolution MRI that includes the acquisition of 3D-CISS images could provide supportive information for the accurate diagnosis of MMD, especially in the early angiographic stage.

Management of MMD

Surgical revascularization prevents ischemic attacks by improving the CBF in patients with MMD [44]. The benefits of revascularization surgery for treating MMD have been well established in patients presenting with ischemic symptoms [97–99]. The concept of revascularization surgery for MMD includes both microsurgical reconstruction using an extracranial-intracranial bypass and consolidation for future vasculogenesis by indirect pial synangiosis [100]. Both concepts involve attempting to convert the vascular supply for the brain from the internal carotid system to the external carotid system [100], which is consistent with the physiological nature of MMD according to the angiographic staging of Suzuki and Takaku [1]. Antiplatelet administration can be considered for patients with ischemic symptoms, but there is only weak scientific evidence supporting this approach [44]. Antiplatelet agents are not recommended for hemorrhagic-onset or asymptomatic patients.

Surgical Indications and Procedures for MMD

Surgical Indications

It has been established that direct revascularization surgery such as anastomosis of the superficial temporal artery (STA) and MCA is an effective procedure for MMD patients with ischemic symptoms, being associated with long-term favorable outcomes [97–99]. Revascularization surgery is recommended for MMD patients presenting with cerebral ischemic symptoms (Recommendation grade B) [42]. Direct revascularization and/or combined direct/indirect procedures are recommended for adult MMD patients, while direct, indirect, or combined surgeries are applied to pediatric MMD patients [42]. Revascularization could be considered for hemorrhagic-onset patients, but adequate scientific evidence has been lacking (Recommendation grade C1) [42]. Nevertheless, recent evidence obtained in the Japan Adult Moyamoya trial supports the use of direct revascularization surgery for reducing the risk for rebleeding in adult MMD patients presenting with intracranial hemorrhage [101]. Therefore, the surgical indications for MMD in general are considered to be expanding also to hemorrhagic-onset patients, as was previously indicated for ischemic-onset patients. Finally, revascularization surgery is not applied to asymptomatic patients with MMD because their natural history has not been determined [42].

Surgical Procedures

(1) Indirect Pial Synangiosis

Indirect methods of revascularization are based principally on the idea that neovascularization can be induced from the extracranial arteries to the cortical arteries by placing vascular-rich tissues on the pial brain surface. Various indirect revascularization procedures have been described, including encephalo-myo-synangiosis (EMS), encephalo-galeo-synangiosis, encephalo-duro-arteriosynangiosis (EDAS), and omentum transplantation [102–105]. The EDAS procedure developed by Matsushima et al. [104] involves transplanting a scalp artery with a strip of galea to a linear dural opening made through an osteoplastic craniotomy. There are many variations of indirect revascularization based on this technique. More-complex and extensive indirect procedures that span a larger area of the cortex have also been reported [106]. Indirect revascularization is technically easy and can be performed even by a surgeon with limited experience in microsuturing cerebral vessels. The success of this strategy depends mainly on the natural neovascularization capability of the patient's brain.

(2) Direct Revascularization

Direct bypass involves using a microvascular technique to directly construct the collateral blood flow from extracranial arteries to intracranial cortical vessels. STA-MCA anastomosis, either single- or double-barreled, has been widely used as a standard technique for MMD [107, 108]. Direct bypass surgery results in a rapid increase in the regional CBF in the operated hemisphere. In light of the intrinsic fragility of the vas-

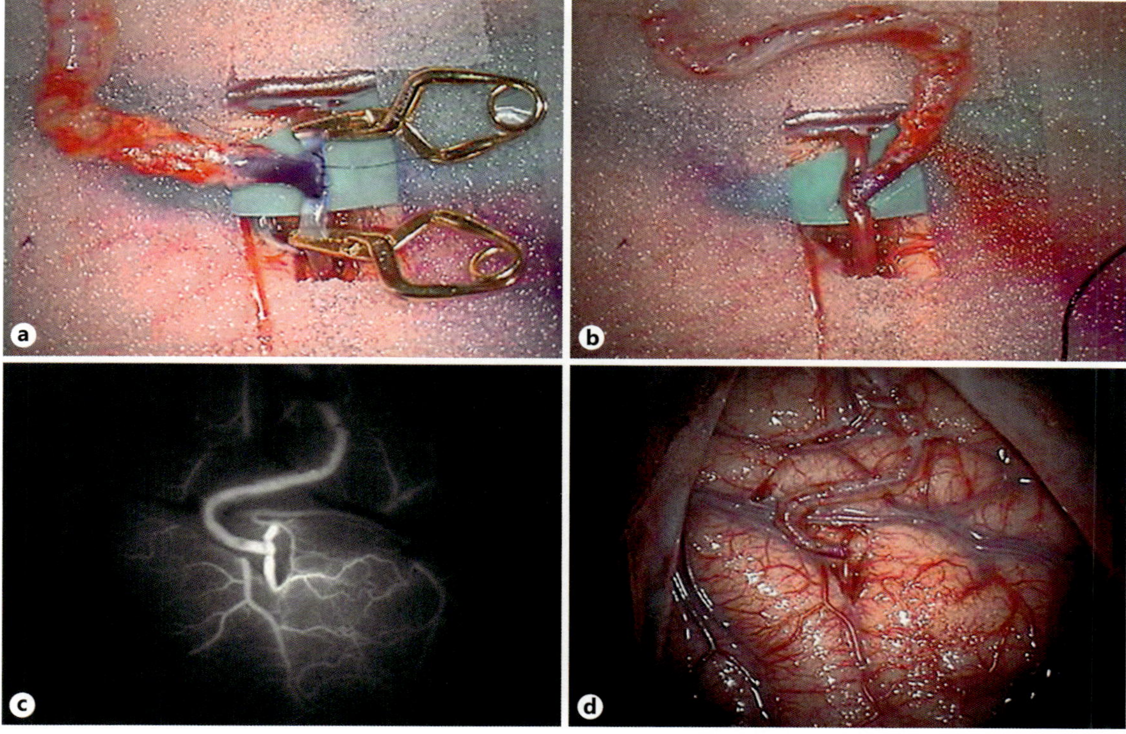

Fig. 3. Intraoperative findings of a right STA-MCA anastomosis in a 27-year-old man presenting with transient ischemic attacks. During (**a**) and after (**b**) the anastomosis procedure. Indocyanine-green videoangiography confirmed the presence of a patent STA-MCA bypass (**c**). Final view (**d**).

cular walls in MMD, such as due to thinness of the medial layer and compromised internal elasticity of the lamina [42], surgeons should ensure that they manipulate the recipient artery gently during the procedure. We have employed direct/indirect combined procedures, such as single STA-MCA anastomosis with EMS, which produced favorable results [109].

The standard procedures of STA-MCA anastomosis for MMD are shown in figure 3, indicating that the procedure is safe and secure with a temporary occlusion time of the recipient artery of 20–30 min. Postoperative single-photon-emission computed tomography (SPECT) usually demonstrates immediate improvement of the CBF in the affected hemisphere that has been operated on (fig. 4).

Perioperative Pathology and Surgical Complications

It is essential to avoid hypercapnia and hypocapnia during surgery in order to reduce the risk of ischemic complications [42]. Surgical complications of MMD include cerebral ischemia and hyperperfusion syndrome [110]. Several pathological mechanisms have been proposed for cerebral ischemia that can occur during the acute stage after surgery. Hayashi et al. proposed a 'watershed shift' phenomenon as an intrinsic type of hemodynamic ischemia occurring in the cortex adjacent to the site of the direct bypass for pediatric MMD [111]. The retrograde blood supply from the STA-MCA bypass may conflict with the anterograde blood flow

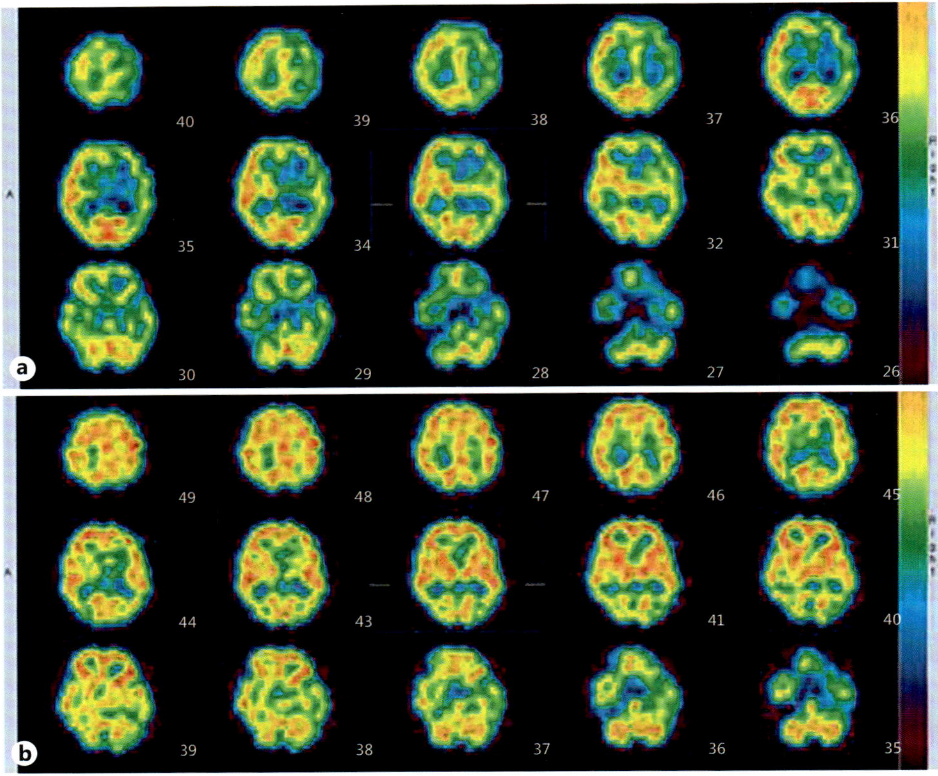

Fig. 4. 123I-IMP-SPECT before (**a**) and after (**b**) a left STA-MCA bypass with EMS in a 65-year-old woman presenting with transient ischemic attacks, demonstrating the improvement in the CBF at 1 day after performing bypass surgery.

from the proximal MCA, and thus result in a temporary decrease in the CBF at the cortex supplied by the adjacent branch of MCA. This watershed shift could result in a cerebral infarction during the perioperative period, especially among pediatric MMD patients [111]. Besides hemodynamic ischemia due to such a watershed shift, thromboembolism from the anastomosed site [112] and mechanical compression by a swollen temporal muscle flap used in EMS could also cause cerebral ischemia during the acute stage [113]. Sufficient hydration, prompt maintenance of the hemoglobin concentration, and antiplatelet administration are essential, especially to avoid the watershed shift and thromboembolic complications during and after surgery [110]. Revision of an indirect bypass such as in EMS should be considered when compression by a swollen temporal muscle pedicle causes an apparent decrease in the CBF [113].

Cerebral hyperperfusion syndrome is one of the most-serious complications of direct revascularization surgery for MMD, especially in adult patients [114–116]. It is well documented that hyperperfusion syndrome after STA-MCA anastomosis is much more common among MMD patients than in patients with atherosclerotic occlusive cerebrovascular diseases [117]. Focal cerebral hyperperfusion can cause a temporary focal neurological deficit in a blood-pressure-dependent manner [110]. The symptoms due to hyperperfusion usually occur between 2 and 6 days after sur-

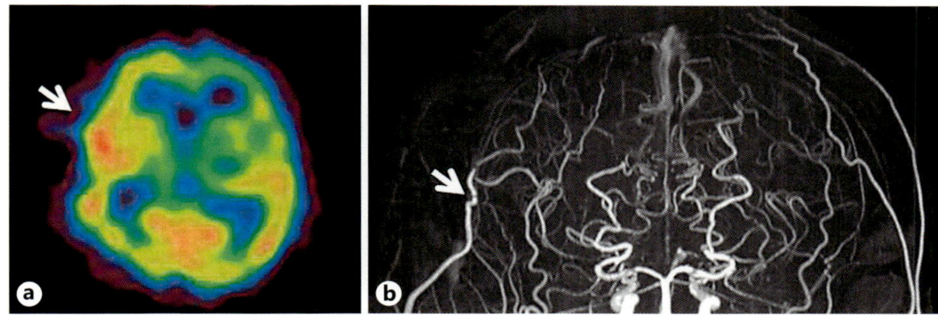

Fig. 5. A 28-year-old man with moyamoya disease underwent STA-MCA bypass surgery. 123I-IMP-SPECT performed 7 days after the surgery demonstrated focal hyperperfusion (arrow in left image) that corresponds to the area of STA-MCA bypass (arrow in right image).

gery. Typical hyperperfusion findings are shown in figure 5. The prognosis of a focal neurological deficit is favorable in most cases, but it should be stressed that focal hyperperfusion can also lead to delayed ICH and/or SAH [118]. The following risk factors for hyperperfusion syndrome in MMD have been reported: adult onset [116, 118], increased preoperative cerebral blood volume [116], hemorrhagic onset [118], surgery on the left hemisphere [119], and smaller diameter of the recipient artery [119]. Controlling the systolic blood pressure to between 110 and 130 mm Hg and the use of minocycline hydrochloride are reported to reduce the risk of hyperperfusion syndrome [119].

Prognosis

Since most stroke episodes are related to hemodynamic insufficiency, ischemic strokes caused by MMD are rarely catastrophic. The mortality rates during the acute stage have been reported to be 2.4 and 16.4% in ischemic and hemorrhagic stroke types, respectively [120]. Although there have been few long-term follow-up studies of patients with MMD, reportedly 75–80% of patients follow a benign course without a significant compromise in their daily activities [121]. However, maladaptation to social or school life is sometimes problematic [122].

Patients who are young at symptom onset (age 3–4 years) appear to have a worse prognosis; they tend to exhibit progressive mental deterioration [123] and frequent infarction [95]. Although the treatment strategy in this age group has not been well established, early surgery has been recommended for this reason [95]. The clinical course of patients with late symptom onset appears to be relatively benign. However, Kuroda et al. [4] followed adult MMD patients (age >20 years) for a mean duration of 73.6 months, and found that disease progression occurred in 15 of 63 patients (23.8%) and in 15 of 86 nonoperated hemispheres (17.4%). The vascular progression occurred in both the anterior and posterior circulations. Eight of the 15 patients with disease progression developed clinical symptoms related to either ischemic or hemorrhagic strokes. Being female was a factor related to the progression. Another study [124] followed 40 asymptomatic MMD patients for a mean duration of 43.7 months, during which 7 experienced ischemic or hemorrhagic strokes, with the annual risk of stroke being 3.2%. Disease progression was closely related to the occurrence of symptoms in this population as well.

These results suggest that the outcome of MMD in adult patients may not be as benign as previously thought, and that patients with MMD should be carefully followed even if they are asymptomatic, although the exact natural history of asymptomatic patients remains to be determined. The AMORE (Asymptomatic Moyamoya Registry) study that is currently underway in Japan is a multicenter observational study aiming to clarify the natural history of asymptomatic MMD [125].

References

1 Suzuki J, Takaku A: Cerebrovascular 'moyamoya' disease. Disease showing abnormal net-like vessels in base of brain. Arch Neurol 1969;20:288–299.
2 Hayashi K, Horie N, Izumo T, Nagata I: A nationwide survey on unilateral moyamoya disease in japan. Clin Neurol Neurosurg 2014;124:1–5.
3 Kelly ME, Bell-Stephens TE, Marks MP, Do HM, Steinberg GK: Progression of unilateral moyamoya disease: a clinical series. Cerebrovasc Dis 2006;22:109–115.
4 Kuroda S, Ishikawa T, Houkin K, Nanba R, Hokari M, Iwasaki Y: Incidence and clinical features of disease progression in adult moyamoya disease. Stroke 2005; 36:2148–2153.
5 Natori Y, Ikezaki K, Matsushima T, Fukui M: 'Angiographic moyamoya' its definition, classification, and therapy. Clin Neurol Neurosurg 1997; 99(suppl 2):S168–S172.
6 Choi HY, Lee JE, Jung YH, Cho HJ, Kim DJ, Heo JH: Progression of isolated middle cerebral artery stenosis into moyamoya disease. Neurology 2007;68:954.
7 Wakai K, Tamakoshi A, Ikezaki K, Fukui M, Kawamura T, Aoki R, Kojima M, Lin Y, Ohno Y: Epidemiological features of moyamoya disease in Japan: findings from a nationwide survey. Clin Neurol Neurosurg 1997;99(suppl 2):S1–S5.
8 Im SH, Cho CB, Joo WI, Chough CK, Park HK, Lee KJ, Rha HK: Prevalence and epidemiological features of moyamoya disease in korea. J Cerebrovasc Endovasc Neurosurg 2012;14:75–78.
9 Ahn IM, Park DH, Hann HJ, Kim KH, Kim HJ, Ahn HS: Incidence, prevalence, and survival of moyamoya disease in Korea: a nationwide, population-based study. Stroke 2014;45:1090–1095.
10 Chen PC, Yang SH, Chien KL, Tsai IJ, Kuo MF: Epidemiology of moyamoya disease in Taiwan: a nationwide population-based study. Stroke 2014;45:1258–1263.
11 Miao W, Zhao PL, Zhang YS, Liu HY, Chang Y, Ma J, Huang QJ, Lou ZX: Epidemiological and clinical features of moyamoya disease in Nanjing, China. Clin Neurol Neurosurg 2010;112:199–203.
12 Duan L, Bao XY, Yang WZ, Shi WC, Li DS, Zhang ZS, Zong R, Han C, Zhao F, Feng J: Moyamoya disease in China: its clinical features and outcomes. Stroke 2012;43:56–60.
13 Uchino K, Johnston SC, Becker KJ, Tirschwell DL: Moyamoya disease in washington state and California. Neurology 2005;65:956–958.
14 Kainth D, Chaudhry SA, Kainth H, Suri FK, Qureshi AI: Epidemiological and clinical features of moyamoya disease in the USA. Neuroepidemiology 2013;40: 282–287.
15 Kuroda S, Houkin K: Moyamoya disease: Current concepts and future perspectives. Lancet Neurol 2008;7:1056–1066.
16 Takagi Y, Kikuta K, Nozaki K, Fujimoto M, Hayashi J, Imamura H, Hashimoto N: Expression of hypoxia-inducing factor-1 alpha and endoglin in intimal hyperplasia of the middle cerebral artery of patients with moyamoya disease. Neurosurgery 2007;60:338–345; discussion 345.
17 Kaku Y, Morioka M, Ohmori Y, Kawano T, Kai Y, Fukuoka H, Hirai T, Yamashita Y, Kuratsu J: Outer-diameter narrowing of the internal carotid and middle cerebral arteries in moyamoya disease detected on 3d constructive interference in steady-state mr image: is arterial constrictive remodeling a major pathogenesis? Acta Neurochir (Wien) 2012;154: 2151–2157.
18 Yuan M, Liu ZQ, Wang ZQ, Li B, Xu LJ, Xiao XL: High-resolution mr imaging of the arterial wall in moyamoya disease. Neurosci Lett 2015;584:77–82.
19 Ryoo S, Cha J, Kim SJ, Choi JW, Ki CS, Kim KH, Jeon P, Kim JS, Hong SC, Bang OY: High-resolution magnetic resonance wall imaging findings of moyamoya disease. Stroke 2014;45:2457–2460.
20 Takagi Y, Kikuta K, Nozaki K, Hashimoto N: Histological features of middle cerebral arteries from patients treated for moyamoya disease. Neurol Med Chir (Tokyo) 2007;47:1–4.
21 Oka K, Yamashita M, Sadoshima S, Tanaka K: Cerebral haemorrhage in moyamoya disease at autopsy. Virchows Arch A Pathol Anat Histol 1981;392: 247–261.
22 Fukui M, Kono S, Sueishi K, Ikezaki K: Moyamoya disease. Neuropathology 2000;20(suppl):S61–S64.
23 Chmelova J, Kolar Z, Prochazka V, Curik R, Dvorackova J, Sirucek P, Kraft O, Hrbac T: Moyamoya disease is associated with endothelial activity detected by anti-nestin antibody. Biomed Pap Med Fac Univ Palacky Olomouc Czech Repub 2010;154:159–162.
24 Guo DC, Papke CL, Tran-Fadulu V, Regalado ES, Avidan N, Johnson RJ, Kim DH, Pannu H, Willing MC, Sparks E, Pyeritz RE, Singh MN, Dalman RL, Grotta JC, Marian AJ, Boerwinkle EA, Frazier LQ, LeMaire SA, Coselli JS, Estrera AL, Safi HJ, Veeraraghavan S, Muzny DM, Wheeler DA, Willerson JT, Yu RK, Shete SS, Scherer SE, Raman CS, Buja LM, Milewicz DM: Mutations in smooth muscle alpha-actin (acta2) cause coronary artery disease, stroke, and moyamoya disease, along with thoracic aortic disease. Am J Hum Genet 2009; 84:617–627.
25 Czabanka M, Pena-Tapia P, Schubert GA, Woitzik J, Vajkoczy P, Schmiedek P: Characterization of cortical microvascularization in adult moyamoya disease. Stroke 2008;39:1703–1709.

26 Kim SJ, Son TO, Kim KH, Jeon P, Hyun SH, Lee KH, Yeon JY, Kim JS, Hong SC, Shin HJ, Bang OY: Neovascularization precedes occlusion in moyamoya disease: angiographic findings in 172 pediatric patients. Eur Neurol 2014;72:299–305.
27 Ikeda H, Sasaki T, Yoshimoto T, Fukui M, Arinami T: Mapping of a familial moyamoya disease gene to chromosome 3p24.2-p26. Am J Hum Genet 1999;64: 533–537.
28 Inoue TK, Ikezaki K, Sasazuki T, Matsushima T, Fukui M: Linkage analysis of moyamoya disease on chromosome 6. J Child Neurol 2000;15:179–182.
29 Yamauchi T, Tada M, Houkin K, Tanaka T, Nakamura Y, Kuroda S, Abe H, Inoue T, Ikezaki K, Matsushima T, Fukui M: Linkage of familial moyamoya disease (spontaneous occlusion of the circle of willis) to chromosome 17q25. Stroke 2000;31:930–935.
30 Sakurai K, Horiuchi Y, Ikeda H, Ikezaki K, Yoshimoto T, Fukui M, Arinami T: A novel susceptibility locus for moyamoya disease on chromosome 8q23. J Hum Genet 2004;49:278–281.
31 Kamada F, Aoki Y, Narisawa A, Abe Y, Komatsuzaki S, Kikuchi A, Kanno J, Niihori T, Ono M, Ishii N, Owada Y, Fujimura M, Mashimo Y, Suzuki Y, Hata A, Tsuchiya S, Tominaga T, Matsubara Y, Kure S: A genome-wide association study identifies rnf213 as the first moyamoya disease gene. Journal of Human Genetics 2011;56:34–40.
32 Miyatake S, Miyake N, Touho H, Nishimura-Tadaki A, Kondo Y, Okada I, Tsurusaki Y, Doi H, Sakai H, Saitsu H, Shimojima K, Yamamoto T, Higurashi M, Kawahara N, Kawauchi H, Nagasaka K, Okamoto N, Mori T, Koyano S, Kuroiwa Y, Taguri M, Morita S, Matsubara Y, Kure S, Matsumoto N: Homozygous c.14576g>a variant of rnf213 predicts early-onset and severe form of moyamoya disease. Neurology 2012;78:803–810.
33 Kim EH, Yum MS, Ra YS, Park JB, Ahn JS, Kim GH, Goo HW, Ko TS, Yoo HW: Importance of rnf213 polymorphism on clinical features and long-term outcome in moyamoya disease. J Neurosurg 2016; 124:1221–1227.
34 Sonobe S, Fujimura M, Niizuma K, Nishijima Y, Ito A, Shimizu H, Kikuchi A, Arai-Ichinoi N, Kure S, Tominaga T: Temporal profile of the vascular anatomy evaluated by 9.4-t magnetic resonance angiography and histopathological analysis in mice lacking rnf213: a susceptibility gene for moyamoya disease. Brain Res 2014;1552:64–71.
35 Kanoke A, Fujimura M, Niizuma K, Ito A, Sakata H, Sato-Maeda M, Morita-Fujimura Y, Kure S, Tominaga T: Temporal profile of the vascular anatomy evaluated by 9.4-tesla magnetic resonance angiography and histological analysis in mice with the r4859k mutation of rnf213, the susceptibility gene for moyamoya disease. Brain Res 2015;1624: 497–505.
36 Ito A, Fujimura M, Niizuma K, Kanoke A, Sakata H, Morita-Fujimura Y, Kikuchi A, Kure S, Tominaga T: Enhanced post-ischemic angiogenesis in mice lacking RNF213; a susceptibility gene for moyamoya disease. Brain Res 2015; 1594:310–320.
37 Fujimura M, Sonobe S, Nishijima Y, Niizuma K, Sakata H, Kure S, Tominaga T: Genetics and biomarkers of moyamoya disease: significance of RNF213 as a susceptibility gene. J Stroke 2014;16: 65–72.
38 Koizumi A, Kobayashi H, Liu W, Fujii Y, Senevirathna ST, Nanayakkara S, Okuda H, Hitomi T, Harada KH, Takenaka K, Watanabe T, Shimbo S: P.R4810k, a polymorphism of RNF213, the susceptibility gene for moyamoya disease, is associated with blood pressure. Environ Health Prev Med 2013;18:121–129.
39 Liu W, Morito D, Takashima S, Mineharu Y, Kobayashi H, Hitomi T, Hashikata H, Matsuura N, Yamazaki S, Toyoda A, Kikuta K, Takagi Y, Harada KH, Fujiyama A, Herzig R, Krischek B, Zou L, Kim JE, Kitakaze M, Miyamoto S, Nagata K, Hashimoto N, Koizumi A: Identification of rnf213 as a susceptibility gene for moyamoya disease and its possible role in vascular development. PLoS One 2011;6:e22542.
40 Wu Z, Jiang H, Zhang L, Xu X, Zhang X, Kang Z, Song D, Zhang J, Guan M, Gu Y: Molecular analysis of RNF213 gene for moyamoya disease in the Chinese Han population. PLoS One 2012;7:e48179.
41 Cecchi AC, Guo D, Ren Z, Flynn K, Santos-Cortez RL, Leal SM, Wang GT, Regalado ES, Steinberg GK, Shendure J, Bamshad MJ, University of Washington Center for Mendelian G, Grotta JC, Nickerson DA, Pannu H, Milewicz DM: RNF213 rare variants in an ethnically diverse population with moyamoya disease. Stroke 2014;45:3200–3207.
42 Research Committee on the P, Treatment of Spontaneous Occlusion of the Circle of W, Health Labour Sciences Research Grant for Research on Measures for Infractable D: Guidelines for diagnosis and treatment of moyamoya disease (spontaneous occlusion of the circle of willis). Neurol Med Chir 2012; 52:245–266.
43 Kim SJ, Heo KG, Shin HY, Bang OY, Kim GM, Chung CS, Kim KH, Jeon P, Kim JS, Hong SC, Lee KH: Association of thyroid autoantibodies with moyamoya-type cerebrovascular disease: a prospective study. Stroke 2010;41:173–176.
44 Bower RS, Mallory GW, Nwojo M, Kudva YC, Flemming KD, Meyer FB: Moyamoya disease in a primarily white, midwestern us population: increased prevalence of autoimmune disease. Stroke 2013;44: 1997–1999.
45 Lamas E, Diez Lobato R, Cabello A, Abad JM: Multiple intracranial arterial occlusions (moyamoya disease) in patients with neurofibromatosis. One case report with autopsy. Acta Neurochir 1978;45:133–145.
46 Tomsick TA, Lukin RR, Chambers AA, Benton C: Neurofibromatosis and intracranial arterial occlusive disease. Neuroradiology 1976;11:229–234.
47 Cramer SC, Robertson RL, Dooling EC, Scott RM: Moyamoya and down syndrome. Clinical and radiological features. Stroke 1996;27:2131–2135.
48 Ganesan V, Kirkham FJ: Noonan syndrome and moyamoya. Pediatr Neurol 1997;16:256–258.
49 Kim YO, Baek HJ, Woo YJ, Choi YY, Chung TW: Moyamoya syndrome in a child with trisomy 12p syndrome. Pediatr Neurol 2006;35:442–445.
50 Kornblihtt LI, Cocorullo S, Miranda C, Lylyk P, Heller PG, Molinas FC: Moyamoya syndrome in an adolescent with essential thrombocythemia: successful intracranial carotid stent placement. Stroke 2005;36:E71–E73.

51 Holz A, Woldenberg R, Miller D, Kalina P, Black K, Lane E: Moyamoya disease in a patient with hereditary spherocytosis. Pediatri Radiol 1998;28:95–97.
52 Salih MAM, Andeejani AMI, Gader AMA, Kolawole T, Palkar V: Moyamoya syndrome-associated with protein-c deficiency. Medical Science Research 1995;23:573–575.
53 Charuvanij A, Laothamatas J, Torcharus K, Sirivimonmas S: Moyamoya disease and protein s deficiency: a case report. Pediatr Neurol 1997;17:171–173.
54 Wang R, Xu Y, Lv R, Chen J: Systemic lupus erythematosus associated with moyamoya syndrome: a case report and literature review. Lupus 2013;22:629–633.
55 Shuja-Ud-Din MA, Ahamed SA, Baidas G, Naeem M: Moyamoya syndrome with primary antiphospholipid syndrome. Medical principles and practice: international journal of the Kuwait University, Health Science Centre 2006;15:238–241.
56 Richards KA, Paller AS: Livedo reticularis in a child with moyamoya disease. Pediatr Dermatol 2003;20:124–127.
57 Czartoski T, Hallam D, Lacy JM, Chun MR, Becker K: Postinfectious vasculopathy with evolution to moyamoya syndrome. J Neurol Neurosurg Psychiatry 2005;76:256–259.
58 Mathew NT, Abraham J, Chandy J: Cerebral angiographic features in tuberculous meningitis. Neurology 1970;20: 1015–1023.
59 Hsiung GY, Sotero de Menezes M: Moyamoya syndrome in a patient with congenital human immunodeficiency virus infection. J Child Neurol 1999;14:268–270.
60 Liu XM, Ruan XZ, Cai Z, Yu BR, He SP, Gong YH: Moyamoya disease caused by leptospiral cerebral arteritis. Chinese Medical Journal 1980;93:599–604.
61 Kim JS, No YJ: Moyamoya-like vascular abnormality in pulmonary sarcoidosis. Cerebrovasc Dis 2006;22:71–73.
62 Joo SP, Kim TS, Lee JH, Lee JK, Kim JH, Kim SH, Kim MK, Cho KH: Moyamoya disease associated with behcet's disease. J Clin Neurosci 2006;13:364–367.
63 Kushima K, Satoh Y, Ban Y, Taniyama M, Ito K, Sugita K: Graves' thyrotoxicosis and moyamoya disease. Can J Neurol Sci 1991;18:140–142.
64 Cerrato P, Grasso M, Lentini A, Destefanis E, Bosco G, Caprioli M, Bradac GB, Bergui M: Atherosclerotic adult moyamoya disease in a patient with hyperhomocysteinaemia. Neurol Sci 2007;28: 45–47.
65 Kestle JR, Hoffman HJ, Mock AR: Moyamoya phenomenon after radiation for optic glioma. J Neurosurg 1993;79:32–35.
66 Halley SE, White WB, Ramsby GR, Voytovich AE: Renovascular hypertension in moyamoya syndrome. Therapeutic response to percutaneous transluminal angioplasty. Am J Hypertens 1988;1: 348–352.
67 Levine SR, Fagan SC, Pessin MS, Silbergleit R, Floberg J, Selwa JF, Vogel CM, Welch KM: Accelerated intracranial occlusive disease, oral contraceptives, and cigarette use. Neurology 1991;41: 1893–1901.
68 Kumar AH, Caplice NM: Clinical potential of adult vascular progenitor cells. Arterioscler Thromb Vasc Biol 2010;30: 1080–1087.
69 Yoshihara T, Taguchi A, Matsuyama T, Shimizu Y, Kikuchi-Taura A, Soma T, Stern DM, Yoshikawa H, Kasahara Y, Moriwaki H, Nagatsuka K, Naritomi H: Increase in circulating cd34-positive cells in patients with angiographic evidence of moyamoya-like vessels. J Cereb Blood Flow Metab 2008;28:1086–1089.
70 Rafat N, Beck G, Pena-Tapia PG, Schmiedek P, Vajkoczy P: Increased levels of circulating endothelial progenitor cells in patients with moyamoya disease. Stroke 2009;40:432–438.
71 Kim JH, Jung JH, Phi JH, Kang HS, Kim JE, Chae JH, Kim SJ, Kim YH, Kim YY, Cho BK, Wang KC, Kim SK: Decreased level and defective function of circulating endothelial progenitor cells in children with moyamoya disease. J Neurosci Res 2010;88:510–518.
72 Jung KH, Chu K, Lee ST, Park HK, Kim DH, Kim JH, Bahn JJ, Song EC, Kim M, Lee SK, Roh JK: Circulating endothelial progenitor cells as a pathogenetic marker of moyamoya disease. J Cereb Blood Flow Metab 2008;28:1795–1803.
73 Lee SC, Jeon JS, Kim JE, Chung YS, Ahn JH, Cho WS, Son YJ, Bang JS, Kang HS, Oh CW: Contralateral progression and its risk factor in surgically treated unilateral adult moyamoya disease with a review of pertinent literature. Acta Neurochir (Wien) 2014;156:103–111.
74 Lee JY, Moon YJ, Lee HO, Park AK, Choi SA, Wang KC, Han JW, Joung JG, Kang HS, Kim JE, Phi JH, Park WY, Kim SK: Deregulation of retinaldehyde dehydrogenase 2 leads to defective angiogenic function of endothelial colony-forming cells in pediatric moyamoya disease. Arterioscler Thromb Vasc Biol 2015;35: 1670–1677.
75 Kang HS, Kim JH, Phi JH, Kim YY, Kim JE, Wang KC, Cho BK, Kim SK: Plasma matrix metalloproteinases, cytokines and angiogenic factors in moyamoya disease. J Neurol Neurosurg Psychiatry 2010;81:673–678.
76 Park YS, Jeon YJ, Kim HS, Chae KY, Oh SH, Han IB, Kim HS, Kim WC, Kim OJ, Kim TG, Choi JU, Kim DS, Kim NK: The role of vegf and kdr polymorphisms in moyamoya disease and collateral revascularization. PLoS One 2012;7:e47158.
77 Wang X, Zhang Z, Liu W, Xiong Y, Sun W, Huang X, Jiang Y, Ni G, Zhou L, Wu L, Zhu W, Li H, Liu X, Xu G: Impacts and interactions of pdgfrb, mmp-3, timp-2, and RNF213 polymorphisms on the risk of moyamoya disease in Han Chinese human subjects. Gene 2013; 526:437–442.
78 Young AM, Karri SK, Ogilvy CS, Zhao N: Is there a role for treating inflammation in moyamoya disease?: a review of histopathology, genetics, and signaling cascades. Front Neurol 2013;4:105.
79 Kim SK, Cho BK, Phi JH, Lee JY, Chae JH, Kim KJ, Hwang YS, Kim IO, Lee DS, Lee J, Wang KC: Pediatric moyamoya disease: an analysis of 410 consecutive cases. Ann Neurol 2010;68:92–101.
80 Horn P, Bueltmann E, Buch CV, Schmiedek P: Arterio-embolic ischemic stroke in children with moyamoya disease. Childs Nerv Syst 2005;21:104–107.
81 Kim JM, Lee SH, Roh JK: Changing ischaemic lesion patterns in adult moyamoya disease. J Neurol Neurosurg Psychiatry 2009;80:36–40.
82 Hishikawa T, Tokunaga K, Sugiu K, Date I: Assessment of the difference in posterior circulation involvement between pediatric and adult patients with moyamoya disease. J Neurosurg 2013; 119:961–965.
83 Cho HJ, Jung YH, Kim YD, Nam HS, Kim DS, Heo JH: The different infarct patterns between adulthood-onset and childhood-onset moyamoya disease. J Neurol Neurosurg Psychiatry 2011;82: 38–40.

84 Suzuki J, Kodama N: Moyamoya disease – a review. Stroke 1983;14:104–109.

85 Nah HW, Kwon SU, Kang DW, Ahn JS, Kwun BD, Kim JS: Moyamoya disease-related versus primary intracerebral hemorrhage: [corrected] location and outcomes are different. Stroke 2012;43:1947–1950.

86 Kikuta K, Takagi Y, Nozaki K, Sawamoto N, Fukuyama H, Hashimoto N: The presence of multiple microbleeds as a predictor of subsequent cerebral hemorrhage in patients with moyamoya disease. Neurosurgery 2008;62:104–111; discussion 111–112.

87 Mori N, Miki Y, Kikuta K, Fushimi Y, Okada T, Urayama S, Sawamoto N, Fukuyama H, Hashimoto N, Togashi K: Microbleeds in moyamoya disease: susceptibility-weighted imaging versus t2*-weighted imaging at 3 tesla. Invest Radiol 2008;43:574–579.

88 Sun W, Yuan C, Liu W, Li Y, Huang Z, Zhu W, Li M, Xu G, Liu X: Asymptomatic cerebral microbleeds in adult patients with moyamoya disease: a prospective cohort study with 2 years of follow-up. Cerebrovasc Dis 2013;35:469–475.

89 Ikezaki K, Matsushima T, Kuwabara Y, Suzuki SO, Nomura T, Fukui M: Cerebral circulation and oxygen metabolism in childhood moyamoya disease: a perioperative positron emission tomography study. J Neurosurg 1994;81:843–850.

90 Hogan AM, Kirkham FJ, Isaacs EB, Wade AM, Vargha-Khadem F: Intellectual decline in children with moyamoya and sickle cell anaemia. Dev Med Child Neurol 2005;47:824–829.

91 Imaizumi C, Imaizumi T, Osawa M, Fukuyama Y, Takeshita M: Serial intelligence test scores in pediatric moyamoya disease. Neuropediatrics 1999;30:294–299.

92 Seol HJ, Wang KC, Kim SK, Hwang YS, Kim KJ, Cho BK: Headache in pediatric moyamoya disease: review of 204 consecutive cases. J Neurosurg 2005;103:439–442.

93 Park-Matsumoto YC, Tazawa T, Shimizu J: Migraine with aura-like headache associated with moyamoya disease. Acta Neurol Scand 1999;100:119–121.

94 Baik JS, Lee MS: Movement disorders associated with moyamoya disease: a report of 4 new cases and a review of literatures. Mov Disord 2010;25:1482–1486.

95 Olesen J, Friberg L, Olsen TS, Andersen AR, Lassen NA, Hansen PE, Karle A: Ischaemia-induced (symptomatic) migraine attacks may be more frequent than migraine-induced ischaemic insults. Brain 1993;116:187–202.

96 Yamada I, Suzuki S, Matsushima Y: Moyamoya disease: Comparison of assessment with mr angiography and mr imaging versus conventional angiography. Radiology 1995;196:211–218.

97 Houkin K, Kuroda S, Nakayama N: Cerebral revascularization for moyamoya disease in children. Neurosurg Clin N Am 2001;12:575–584, ix.

98 Irikura K, Miyasaka Y, Kurata A, Tanaka R, Yamada M, Kan S, Fujii K: The effect of encephalo-myo-synangiosis on abnormal collateral vessels in childhood moyamoya disease. Neurol Res 2000;22:341–346.

99 Ishikawa T, Houkin K, Kamiyama H, Abe H: Effects of surgical revascularization on outcome of patients with pediatric moyamoya disease. Stroke 1997;28:1170–1173.

100 Fujimura M, Tominaga T: Current status of revascularization surgery for moyamoya disease: Special consideration for its 'internal carotid-external carotid (ic-ec) conversion' as the physiological reorganization system. Tohoku J Exp Med 2015;236:45–53.

101 Miyamoto S, Yoshimoto T, Hashimoto N, Okada Y, Tsuji I, Tominaga T, Nakagawara J, Takahashi JC, Investigators JAMT: Effects of extracranial-intracranial bypass for patients with hemorrhagic moyamoya disease: results of the Japan adult moyamoya trial. Stroke 2014;45:1415–1421.

102 Karasawa J, Kikuchi H, Furuse S, Sakaki T, Yoshida Y: A surgical treatment of 'moyamoya' disease 'encephalo-myo synangiosis'. Neurol Med Chir 1977;17:29–37.

103 Takeuchi S, Abe H, Ozawa T, R T: Surgical treatment for moyamoya disease. Surgical effect of encephalo-galeo-synangiosis on moyamoya disease. Surgery for Cerebral Stroke 2000;28:98–103.

104 Matsushima Y, Fukai N, Tanaka K, Tsuruoka S, Inaba Y, Aoyagi M, Ohno K: A new surgical treatment of moyamoya disease in children: a preliminary report. Surg Neurol 1981;15:313–320.

105 Karasawa J, Kikuchi H, Kawamura J, Sakai T: Intracranial transplantation of the omentum for cerebrovascular moyamoya disease: a two-year follow-up study. Surg Neurol 1980;14:444–449.

106 Park JH, Yang SY, Chung YN, Kim JE, Kim SK, Han DH, Cho BK: Modified encephaloduroarteriosynangiosis with bifrontal encephalogaleoperiosteal synangiosis for the treatment of pediatric moyamoya disease. Technical note. J Neurosurg 2007;106:237–242.

107 Miyamoto S, Kikuchi H, Karasawa J, Nagata I, Yamazoe N, Akiyama Y: Pitfalls in the surgical treatment of moyamoya disease. Operative techniques for refractory cases. J Neurosurg 1988;68:537–543.

108 Karasawa J, Kikuchi H, Furuse S, Kawamura J, Sakaki T: Treatment of moyamoya disease with sta-mca anastomosis. J Neurosurg 1978;49:679–688.

109 Fujimura M, Tominaga T: Lessons learned from moyamoya disease: outcome of direct/indirect revascularization surgery for 150 affected hemispheres. Neurol Med Chir 2012;52:327–332.

110 Fujimura M, Tominaga T: Significance of cerebral blood flow analysis in the acute stage after revascularization surgery for moyamoya disease. Neurol Med Chir 2015;55:775–781.

111 Hayashi T, Shirane R, Fujimura M, Tominaga T: Postoperative neurological deterioration in pediatric moyamoya disease: watershed shift and hyperperfusion. J Neurosurg Pediatrics 2010;6:73–81.

112 Fujimura M, Kaneta T, Tominaga T: Efficacy of superficial temporal artery-middle cerebral artery anastomosis with routine postoperative cerebral blood flow measurement during the acute stage in childhood moyamoya disease. Childs Nerv Syst 2008;24:827–832.

113 Fujimura M, Kaneta T, Shimizu H, Tominaga T: Cerebral ischemia owing to compression of the brain by swollen temporal muscle used for encephalo-myo-synangiosis in moyamoya disease. Neurosurg Rev 2009;32:245–249; discussion 249.

114 Fujimura M, Kaneta T, Mugikura S, Shimizu H, Tominaga T: Temporary neurologic deterioration due to cerebral hyperperfusion after superficial temporal artery-middle cerebral artery anastomosis in patients with adult-onset moyamoya disease. Surg Neurol 2007;67:273–282.
115 Kim JE, Oh CW, Kwon OK, Park SQ, Kim SE, Kim YK: Transient hyperperfusion after superficial temporal artery/middle cerebral artery bypass surgery as a possible cause of postoperative transient neurological deterioration. Cerebrovasc Dis 2008; 25:580–586.
116 Uchino H, Kuroda S, Hirata K, Shiga T, Houkin K, Tamaki N: Predictors and clinical features of postoperative hyperperfusion after surgical revascularization for moyamoya disease: a serial single photon emission ct/positron emission tomography study. Stroke 2012;43:2610–2616.
117 Fujimura M, Shimizu H, Inoue T, Mugikura S, Saito A, Tominaga T: Significance of focal cerebral hyperperfusion as a cause of transient neurologic deterioration after extracranial-intracranial bypass for moyamoya disease: comparative study with non-moyamoya patients using n-isopropyl-p-[(123) i]iodoamphetamine single-photon emission computed tomography. Neurosurgery 2011;68:957–964; discussion 964–955.
118 Fujimura M, Mugikura S, Kaneta T, Shimizu H, Tominaga T: Incidence and risk factors for symptomatic cerebral hyperperfusion after superficial temporal artery-middle cerebral artery anastomosis in patients with moyamoya disease. Surg Neurol 2009;71:442–447.
119 Fujimura M, Niizuma K, Inoue T, Sato K, Endo H, Shimizu H, Tominaga T: Minocycline prevents focal neurological deterioration due to cerebral hyperperfusion after extracranial-intracranial bypass for moyamoya disease. Neurosurgery 2014;74:163–170; discussion 170.
120 Yonekawa Y, Taub E: Moyamoya disease: status 1998. Neurologist 1999;5: 13–23.
121 Yonekawa Y, Kahn N: Moyamoya disease. Adv Neurol 2003;92:113–118.
122 Imaizumi T, Hayashi K, Saito K, Osawa M, Fukuyama Y: Long-term outcomes of pediatric moyamoya disease monitored to adulthood. Pediatr Neurol 1998;18:321–325.
123 Moritake K, Handa H, Yonekawa Y, Taki W, Okuno T: [follow-up study on the relationship between age at onset of illness and outcome in patients with moyamoya disease]. No Shinkei Geka 1986;14:957–963.
124 Kuroda S, Hashimoto N, Yoshimoto T, Iwasaki Y, Research Committee on Moyamoya Disease in J: Radiological findings, clinical course, and outcome in asymptomatic moyamoya disease: results of multicenter survey in Japan. Stroke 2007;38:1430–1435.
125 Kuroda S, Group AS: Asymptomatic moyamoya disease: literature review and ongoing amore study. Neurol Med Chir 2015;55:194–198.

Jong S. Kim, MD, PhD
Department of Neurology, Asan Medical Center, University of Ulsan
Asanbyeongwon-gil 86, Songpa-gu
Seoul 138-736 (Korea)
E-Mail jongskim@amc.seoul.kr

Author Index

Subject Index

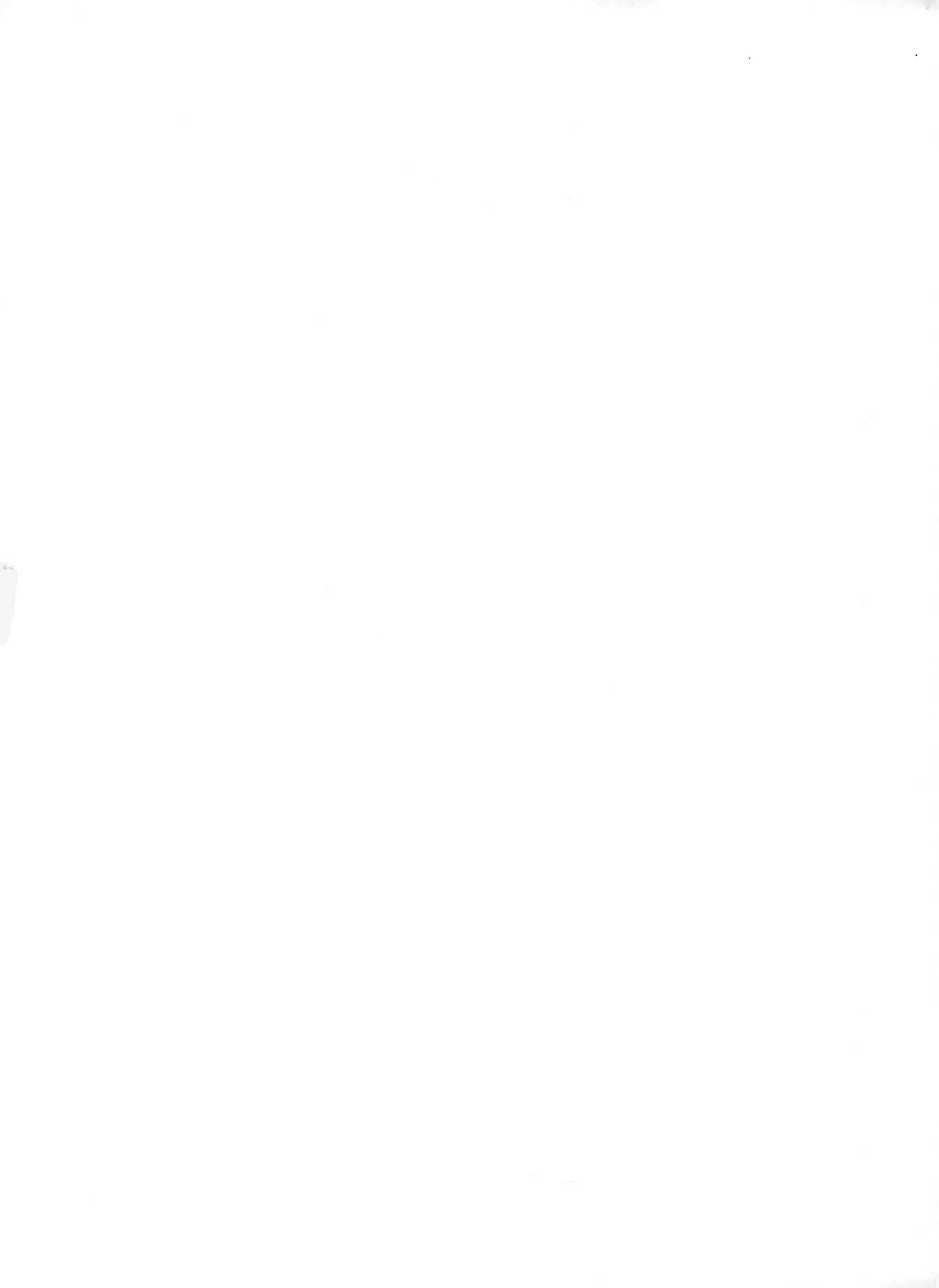